AF326830

Atlas of
COMMON
SUBLUXATIONS
of the
HUMAN
SPINE
and
PELVIS

A NOTE TO THE READER

The micrographs that appear in the Atlas can be viewed in color on the CRC Web page. To access this material go to http:\\www.crcpress.com/ and then to the prompt for "Updates and Downloads". Follow the prompts to the area reserved from the Atlas. The color photographs can be viewed on the Web page or downloaded to your files

Atlas of
COMMON SUBLUXATIONS of the HUMAN SPINE and PELVIS

William J. Ruch, D.C.

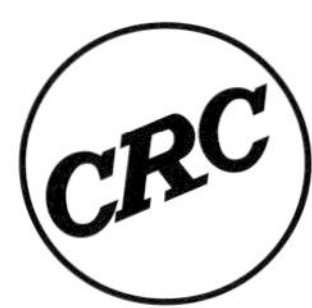

CRC Press

Boca Raton   New York   London   Tokyo

Publisher/Life Sciences:	Robert B. Stern
Project Editor:	Carrie L. Unger
Editorial Assistant:	Carol Messing
Marketing Manager:	Susie Carlisle
Direct Marketing Manager:	Becky McEldowney
Cover design:	Denise Craig
PrePress:	Gary Bennett
Manufacturing:	Sheri Schwartz

Library of Congress Cataloging-in-Publication Data

Ruch, William J.
    Atlas of common subluxations of the human spine and pelvis / William J. Ruch
      p. cm.
    Includes bibliographical references and index.
    ISBN 0-8493-3117-X
    1. Spine—Abnormalities—Atlases.   2. Spine—Wounds and injuries—Atlases.   I. Title.
    [DNLM: 1. Spine—pathology—atlases.   2. Spinal Injuries—physiopathology—atlases   3. Dislocation—physiopathology—
atlases   WE 17 R899a   1997]
    RZ265.S64R83 1996
    617.5′6—dc20
    DNLM/DLC
    for Library of Congress   96-46124
                                                    CIP

DEDICATION

This book is dedicated to the memory of Norman N. Goldstein, Ph.D. His gift was guidance, inspiration, and encouragement even in his final days.

Biographical Information

*William J. Ruch, D.C. has been in private practice at North Oakland
Chiropractic Clinic in Oakland, California for nine years.
Dr. Ruch graduated from the University of San Francisco with a B.S. in Biology
in 1975 and received his D.C. from Life Chiropractic College West in 1986.
Dr. Ruch is a member of the International Chiropractic Association, the
American Back Society and an instructor for Chiropractic Biophysics Inc.
Dr. Ruch spent seven years developing spinal and pelvic dissection procedures
and has studied, photographed and X-rayed more than two hundred and fifty
human cadavers in the course of his research. His extensive photographic
library of these studies form the core material for this book. He taught
dissection of the human spine at Life Chiropractic College West for 6 1/2 years
during which time he amassed the extensive knowledge of spinal and pelvic
pathophysiology upon which the text heavily relies. He has authored nine
articles on clinical anatomy in the Journal of Clinical Chiropractic, and has had
several of his cadaver specimen and X-ray photographs published in the book
Clinical Chiropractic by G. Plaugher , Williams and Wilkins, 1993.*

Colophon:

Designed by William Ruch and Paul Marcus.

Typography and layout by Paul Marcus\ General Eclectics, Berkeley, California.

Photo Masking by Paul Marcus, Shereen Harris, and Olivia Destandau

Original illustrations by Susan Davis

Indexed by Shereen Harris

This book was designed and produced on Apple Macintosh® computers.
Layout was done with QuarkXPRESS®; original text editing was done in Microsoft Word®.
Dr. Ruch's original slides were scanned to Kodak Photo CD®s and were cropped, rotated, scaled, and
masked using Adobe® Photoshop®, which was also used to create the original illustrations. Incidental
art was created in Adobe® Illustrator® and Macromedia FreeHand®. Color plates were separated with
PixelCraft ColorAccess® software. Proof copies were made on an Apple LaserWriter® Pro 630 and a
Hewlett-Packard 550C® inkjet printer. Indexing was done from electronic proofs made in Adobe
Acrobat® format.
Review copies were printed and collated on a Xerox DocuTech® high-speed imager from PostScript™
files saved to disk.

Body copy set in Sabon and **Bold** 10pt on 12pt leading.

Captions set in Helvetica 9 pt on 11 pt.

Titles and headers set in **ITC Serif Gothic Bold** and **Black**.

Hardware/Software references are for information only and imply no warranty nor endorsement of those products.
All names are trademarks of their respective companies.

An Atlas Of Common Subluxations
Of The Human Spine And Pelvis

IN THE ANTERIOR TO POSTERIOR VIEW
WITH MID-SAGITTAL SECTIONS OF SPECIMENS AND X-RAYS

TABLE OF CONTENTS

Preface vii

Acknowledgment viii

Introduction ix

Biographical Information xi

Colophon (Production Notes) xi

CHAPTER ONE
Normal Human Spine: Structure and Dynamics

The Three Spinal Tissues 2

    The Vertebral Column 2

    The Thecal Sac 3

    The Spinal Cord 7

Motion of the Vertebral Column 10

CHAPTER TWO
Pathophysiology of the Human Spine

Spinal Subluxation and the Central Nervous System 11

CHAPTER THREE
Subluxations of the Cervical Spine

Discussion 23

Expanded Table of Contents of the Atlas of Subluxations of the Cervical Spine 27

Section I: Subluxations with Lordotic Cervical Curve (9) 30

Section II: Subluxation with Loss of Lordotic Curve (Straight or Military Neck) (3) 46

Section III: Subluxation with Reversed or Kyphotic Curve (12) 52

    Upper Cervical Subluxations 52

    Mid-Cervical Subluxations 58

    Lower Cervical Subluxations 62

CHAPTER FOUR

Subluxations of the Thoracic Spine

Discussion 77

Expanded Table of Contents of the Atlas of Subluxations of the Thoracic Spine 83

Section I: Subluxations with a Normal Thoracic Curve 86

Section II: Subluxation with a Reversal of the Upper Curve 88

Section III: Subluxation with a Reversal of the Lower Curve 94

Section IV: Subluxations with Antrolesthesis of the Upper and Lower Thoracic Vertebrae . 100

Section V: Hyperkyphosis of the Thoracic Curve 106

Additional MRIs and X-rays 112

CHAPTER FIVE

Subluxations of the Lumbar Spine

Discussion 117

Expanded Table of Contents of the Atlas of Lumbar Subluxations 125

Section I: Subluxations of the Lumbar Spine with a Lordotic Curve 128

Section II: Subluxations of the Lumbar Spine with a Loss of Lordotic Curve. 156

Section III: Subluxations of the Lumbar Spine with a Reversal of the Lordotic Curve 168

Additional X-ray/MRI Comparison. 176

CHAPTER SIX

Subluxations of the Pelvic Girdle

Discussion 179

Visceral Implications of Pelvic Subluxation 180

The Sacrum 181

The Sacroiliac Joints 183

The Pubic Symphysis 185

Pelvic Motion. 187

Pelvic Tilt and Imaging. 188

The Lumbosacral Relationship 189

Physiological Subluxations 191

Flexion/ Extension Rotations 192

Non-Physiological Subluxations 192

Anterior to Posterior Pelvic Shearing. 192

Superior to Inferior Pelvic Shearing. 193

The Geriatric Pelvis 201

Intrasacral Subluxations 202

Glossary. 205

References 219

Index 225

PREFACE

The purpose of this book is to help the Chiropractic/Medical/Legal communities better understand the nature of the subluxation of the spine. The subluxation of vertebrae can have dramatic health consequences and can permanently alter an individual's quality of life. The goal of this book is to positively influence anatomically based therapeutic intervention for spinal subluxations.

This book is the result of my work in the Life-West Chiropractic College Anatomy Laboratory. There I was able to dissect all or part of the spines of 240 individuals. The pictures depicted are the result of the photographic record I made of 130 of these individuals.

As a chiropractic student I received far less instruction on the human spine and spinal cord in contrast to many classes on the heart and kidney. When I lecture to practicing physicians, I find they know more about the internal workings of the kidney than about the motion of the spinal cord in the canal with normal postural changes. Treatment of the spine should be based on the most comprehensive understanding possible. Knowledge of the anatomical and dynamic facts of the human spine and pelvis is limited in the teaching institutions of this country, both chiropractic and medical. One world renowned medical school has the cadavers remain supine for the entire human dissection course. When asked about instruction of the anatomy of the prone back and spine, the instructor said "they can look in a book if they are interested." He went on to add that, "we are so pressed for time that the students are given the choice between dissecting and being tested on either the arm or the leg, not both, because the anatomy is similar." Most medical personnel throw pills at almost all musculoskeletal problems, because the teachers can't teach what they don't know. In chiropractic college I was told we couldn't look at the intervertebral discs because "we don't have time."

I went into the lab on my own time to learn what I needed to know. In one of the first specimens I sectioned, I found the spinal cord tethered against the whole anterior canal wall, obliterating the anterior spinal artery. Only months from graduating, I realized I was seriously undereducated for my profession. I was saddened and, to say the least, frightened.

My laboratory studies illustrated that vertebral column deformities can alter the shape of spinal cord tissue and it's vascular structures. My work as a doctor has shown me that these conditions impair circulation and generate neurological loss of function. I have been fortunate to be able to combine the two experiences.

The need for this knowledge to be distributed to practicing doctors is essential. I see primitive treatment being done by chiropractors, physicians, and surgeons alike because of lack of understanding of the anatomy and dynamics of the human spine. My hope is that this book will help to remedy this deficiency.

ACKNOWLEDGMENT

I would like to thank Life Chiropractic College-West for allowing this project to take place; without the laboratory and cadavers this study could not have occurred. The Life Chiropractic College-West Library has been very helpful with my never ending requests. I would also thank the many students, now doctors, who gave their valuable time in the anatomy laboratory to help this project. Especially helpful were Drs. Gordon Partridge, Jim Zallaha, Peter Fisk, Alvin Dolley, Steve Milligan, and Danielle and Martien Crozier. There were many more than I can name now but I hope they all get valuable use of this book and know that their work and efforts bore fruit. I deeply appreciate the doctors who reviewed the text, wrote valuable comments and supportive letters. They are Drs. Walter Freeman, Chuck Masarsky, Glen Harrison, Don Harrison, and Gerald Clum. I also want to thank attorneys John Starbuck, Paul Silver, and Jack Silver for their review comments, which were extremely helpful in clarifying the text. I would also like to thank Dr. Linda Fraley for taking me back to school, Gary Lewis of X-Ray Systems, Inc. of San Jose, Ca. for donating the x-ray equipment to the anatomy laboratory, Dr. Jane Robinson for surveying and organizing all the material, Mitchell Boyce for getting my whole computer system up and running and making it "dummy proof," Jacqueline Ellis for teaching me how to "double click" and all the rest, Deirdre McCarthy for showing me through Photoshop, Donna Robbins for all the typing, editing, and support, Brian Lewis for his help with the terminology, Susan Davis for her work on the illustrations, and Olivia Destandau for help with the graphics. Without any one of you this book could not have been finished. Invaluable work on the final phases of this book were the typesetting, picture editing, and indexing by Paul Marcus and Shereen Harris of General Eclectics. There were many people, over the years, who were encouraging and supportive. I have been so fortunate they are too numerous to name. I thank you all.

William J. Ruch, D. C.
Oakland, California
August, 1996

INTRODUCTION

Subluxation of the vertebrae consists of injury to the ligaments, discs, cartilage, joint capsules, tendons, and other supporting tissues. Its occurrence initiates inflammation, muscle spasms, pain, and immobility. Subluxation of the vertebrae is the etiology of spinal osteoarthritis and can influence the shape of the spinal cord and brainstem and alter nervous system blood supply. This book illustrates the future degenerative consequences of subluxation. Deterioration of the vertebral column following loss of normal alignment can impair circulation of blood and cerebral spinal fluid in the spinal cord leading to pain and loss of neurological control. Today's trauma can be a serious health factor twenty years from now.

This book is organized into six chapters. The first two chapters detail the principles and anatomical and physiological facts used in the next four chapters. The atlases of Chapters 3, 4, and 5 are primarily paired pictures of a specimen with the X-rays I took of that specimen. Most of the dissections of the spines involved sagittal sectioning of the cervical spine and the thoracic spine. The remaining lumbar-pelvic section was dissected to show the combined muscular and nervous tissues that cross the whole region. The sections were cut in a mid-sagittal plane (as close as we could get) and X-rayed from the lateral view. A-P X-rays were also taken before sectioning but are not part of this presentation. There are characteristic patterns of subluxations and I have tried to classify these and document the more common types of changes that occur in all the structures of the spine. The pictures are arranged in the order of progressive severity of dislocation and degeneration. There are many ways in which the spine can subluxate (deviate) from normal. The normal spine has an architecture that can be described in the X-Y-Z planes (the Cartesian coordinate system). This book focuses on deviation in the Z plane (anterior to posterior direction) but there are some Y plane problems pointed out (inferior to superior direction). The sixth chapter, on the pelvis, deals with innominate rotation around the X axis (flexion/extension subluxations) and shearing dislocations in the Z and Y planes.

The book also contains advanced imaging (CT Scan and MRI) of sections of the spine and pelvis, some with their associated X-rays. These X-rays, CT Scans, and MRIs are of my patients, and I am grateful for their kind cooperation in allowing these images to be used for educational purposes.

I believe there are a number of professions that can benefit from this book besides chiropractic. Medical personnel need to know the biomechanics of the spine in emergency rooms, as well as orthopedic and neurosurgeons in operating rooms. Legal personnel evaluating injured claimants can have graphic material that shows the extent of soft tissue damage, as well as future degenerative conditions that can be expected post traumatically. Insurance personnel and nursing supervisors can get a more accurate picture of the future health care needs of their policy holders.

The chiropractic profession needs to have a better understanding of the dynamic principles and anatomic structures of the human spine and pelvis to better serve their patients. I hope this book can contribute to our abilities to understand the pathology of subluxations and to correct them.

CHAPTER ONE

Normal Human Spine:

Structure and Dynamics

This chapter will discuss the normal spinal column as a complex and dynamic structure. The normal physiology and anatomy must be studied before one can understand the pathological affects of sub-luxation complexes. Emphasis will be placed on the physiology of the motion of the central nervous system and its supporting tissues within the normal spinal column.

The shape of the spinal column and canal, posture, and the pressures on the spinal cord are intimately related. Poor posture is not merely a reflection of personality or character. It can be a reflection of altered spinal curves and misplaced body masses. Examples are displacement of the head in relation to the rib cage and displacement of the rib cage in relation to the pelvis. The displacements deform the spinal column and result in joint dysfunction. What is not commonly understood is the resulting disruption of the spinal cord, which brings with it impaired sensor and receptor function.

The spinal column has three systems of integrated tissues. Under normal conditions, each system moves differently and has distinct dynamic qualities from the others (**See Figure 1-1**). When healthy and normal, the three systems move synchronously and in harmony. Several of the causes which change the spinal column from the normal state are car accidents, compulsory education, and deforming our bodies to modern life.

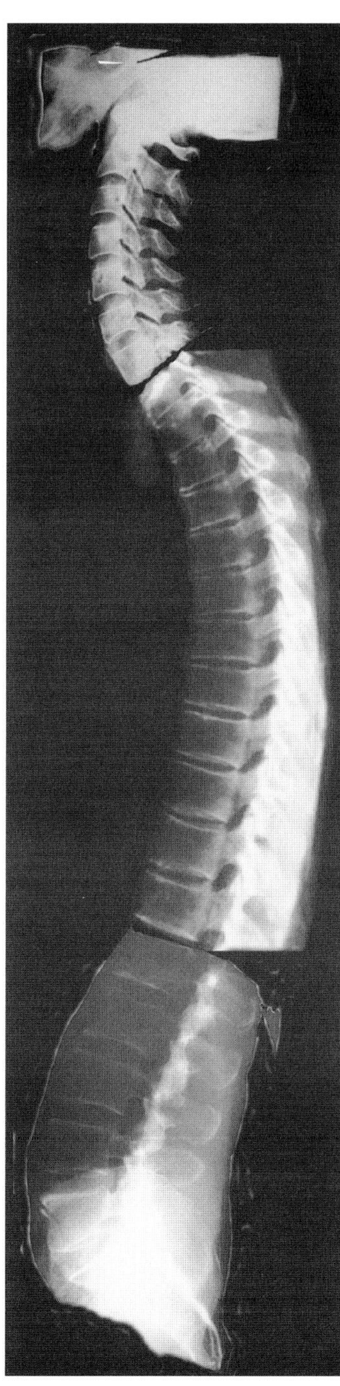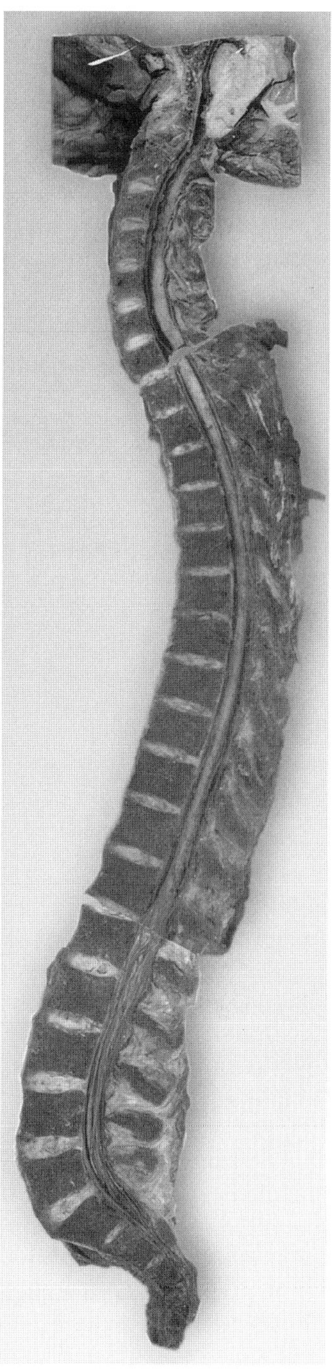

Figure 1-1
NEAR NORMAL SPINE
The normal spinal column has lordotic curves in the cervical and lumbar regions and kyphotic curves in the thoracic and sacral regions. The pons, brainstem, and spinal cord are all a continuous structure. There is space in the spinal canal between the spinal cord and the front of the canal in the neutral postion. There is slight disc degeneration in the anterior of every disc. Disc height is normal with some very slight anterior disc bulging.

THE THREE SPINAL TISSUES

The three spinal tissues are

- the vertebral column itself with the vertebrae, discs, ligaments, facets, capsules, cartilage, and muscles.
- the thecal sac, consisting of the dura mater-arachnoid mater tube or envelope of the central nervous system.
- the brain stem, spinal cord and nerve roots ("pons-cord tissue tract," as Dr. Alf Breig calls the lower central nervous tissue). This is from the clivus of the occiput to the spinal canal and to the sacrum and coccyx. It is continuous tissue from the pons to the conus medularis and caudae equinae.

Each system (**See Figure 1-2**) has a different way of moving based on its structure. Structure and function go together, and each has completely different tissues and handles motion in a unique way. We will discuss the structure and motion of each system in conjunction with the absolute or global motion of the normal spinal column.

The Vertebral Column

The first system is the vertebral column. One aspect of the vertebral column not well appreciated is the "3 point weight bearing" system of most of the vertebrae (**See Figure 1-3**). The occipital-atlas is a 2-point-joint system, as is essentially the atlanto-axial joint. The C2-C3 joints become a 3-point weight bearing system and thus it remains down to the L5-sacral joints. Studies indicate that the normal vertebral body/disc unit bears about 36% of the body weight and each of the two facets bear about 32%. Altered weight bearing changes this relationship and causes altered bone remodeling. We know that gravitational force is involved with normal physiology (space travel causes osteoporosis). Therefore altered gravitational forces (altered weight bearing) create altered bone. Subluxations change the weight bearing of the involved joints. Altered posture and reduced viability are reflections of the subluxations.

The vertebral column is a much investigated system. Studies attempt to describe vertebral column motion with various terms, but all will agree that the motion between each vertebrae accumulates to give overall or absolute motion. This motion involves compression of the cartilaginous interfaces between the vertebrae at all the joint structures. Normal motion acts as a pump to promote the physiological forcing of fluid exchange, nutrient supply, and waste elimination. When motion is prevented, pathology results (**See Page 10**).

Segmental motion combines to give global or "absolute motion," like bending forward. The motion of the vertebra varies with the section of the vertebral column. Because the cartilaginous

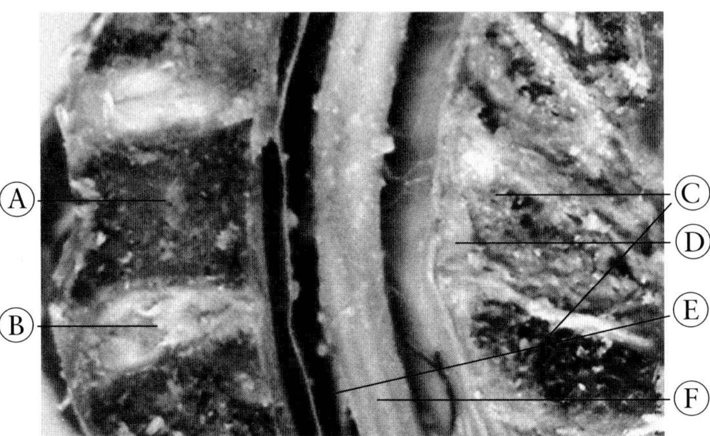

Figure 1-2

THE THREE SYSTEMS OF THE HUMAN SPINE:

1 -THE VERTEBRAL COLUMN
- (A) Vertebral body
- (B) Disc
- (C) Spinous process
- (D) Ligamentum flavum

2-THE MENINGES OR THECAL SAC
- (E) Thecal wall

3-PONS-CORD TISSUE TRACT
- (F) Spinal cord

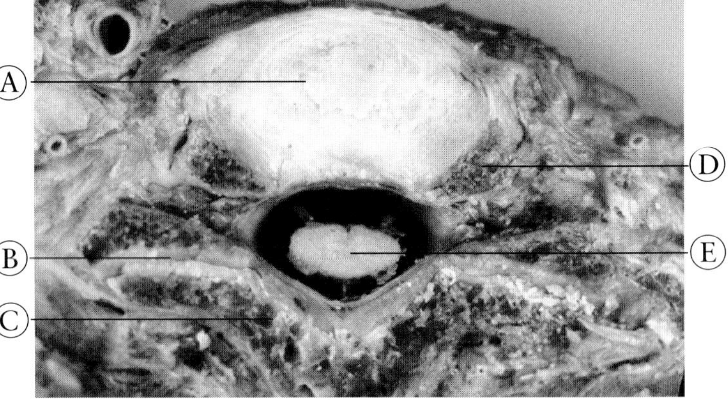

Figure 1-3

THREE POINT WEIGHT BEARING

Three point weight bearing in the cervical spine, the posterior articulations or facets provide weight bearing support as well as the body and disc.

- (A) Disc
- (B) Posterior articulation or facets
- (C) Lamina
- (D) Uncinate process
- (E) Spinal cord

facets are in different planes of orientation, and the discs are of different sizes and shapes, the cervical vertebrae move differently than the thoracic vertebrae, which in turn move differently than the lumbar vertebrae. The motion between each pair of vertebrae, (segmental motion) such as C4 and C5, T4 and T5, or L4 and L5, is unique, each contributing to flexion, extension and twisting of the whole spine (global or absolute motion).

The Thecal Sac

The second system, the thecal sac, is connected to the top, bottom, and right and left sides of the spinal canal, changing shape during motion (**See Figure 1-6**). The changes of the spinal canal in normal motion are transmitted to the thecal sac as deforming forces. A common example is when pulling on a balloon (motion) one expects it to change shape (deform).

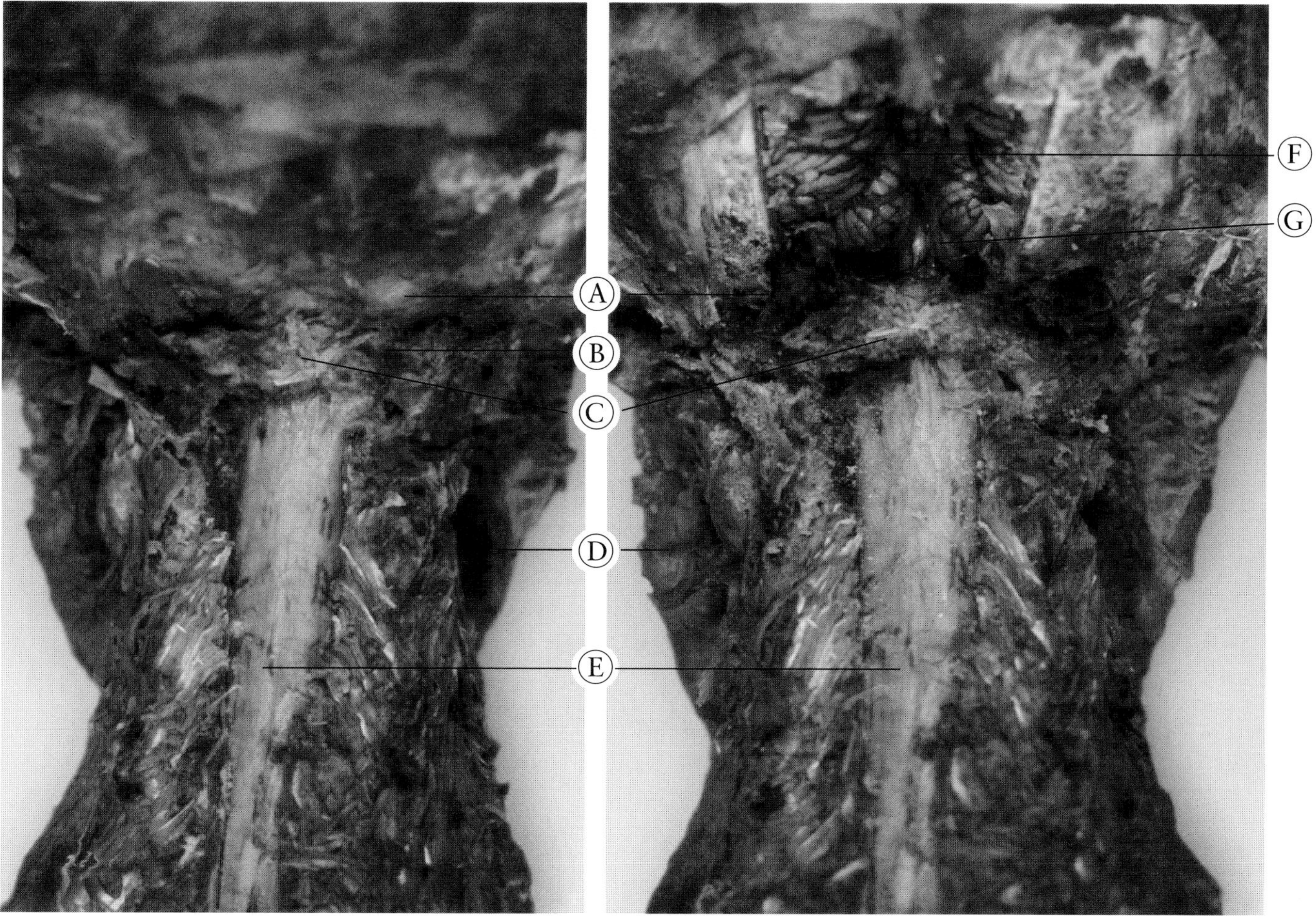

a. b. Figure 1-4

NORMAL ANATOMICAL RELATIONSHIPS OF THE SKULL AND VERTEBRAL COLUMN

Photo (a). Laminectomized specimen with skin removed from back of skull, to show relationships of structures. (Posterior view.)
  (A) Base of Skull (Occiput)
  (B) Vertebral artery
  (C) Atlas
  (D) Mandible
  (E) Thecal Sac

Photo (b). Same specimen with occiput partially removed to show the cerebellum.
  (F) Cerebellum
  (G) Inferior Cerebellar Artery

The term "thecal" or "theca" is used to describe the combined dura/arachnoid mater and other supportive structures. The dura mater is the tough enclosing membrane of the sac. The arachnoid mater is the inner lining of the sac. The "subdural space," between the dura and arachnoid mater, is a potential space (**See Figure** 1-8).

This space doesn't really exist in a normal spinal column. That is why the term "theca" is used to describe this seemingly single structure with the dura mater on one side and the arachnoid mater on the other. Pathological conditions can separate these structures, but normally they act or function as a single structure.

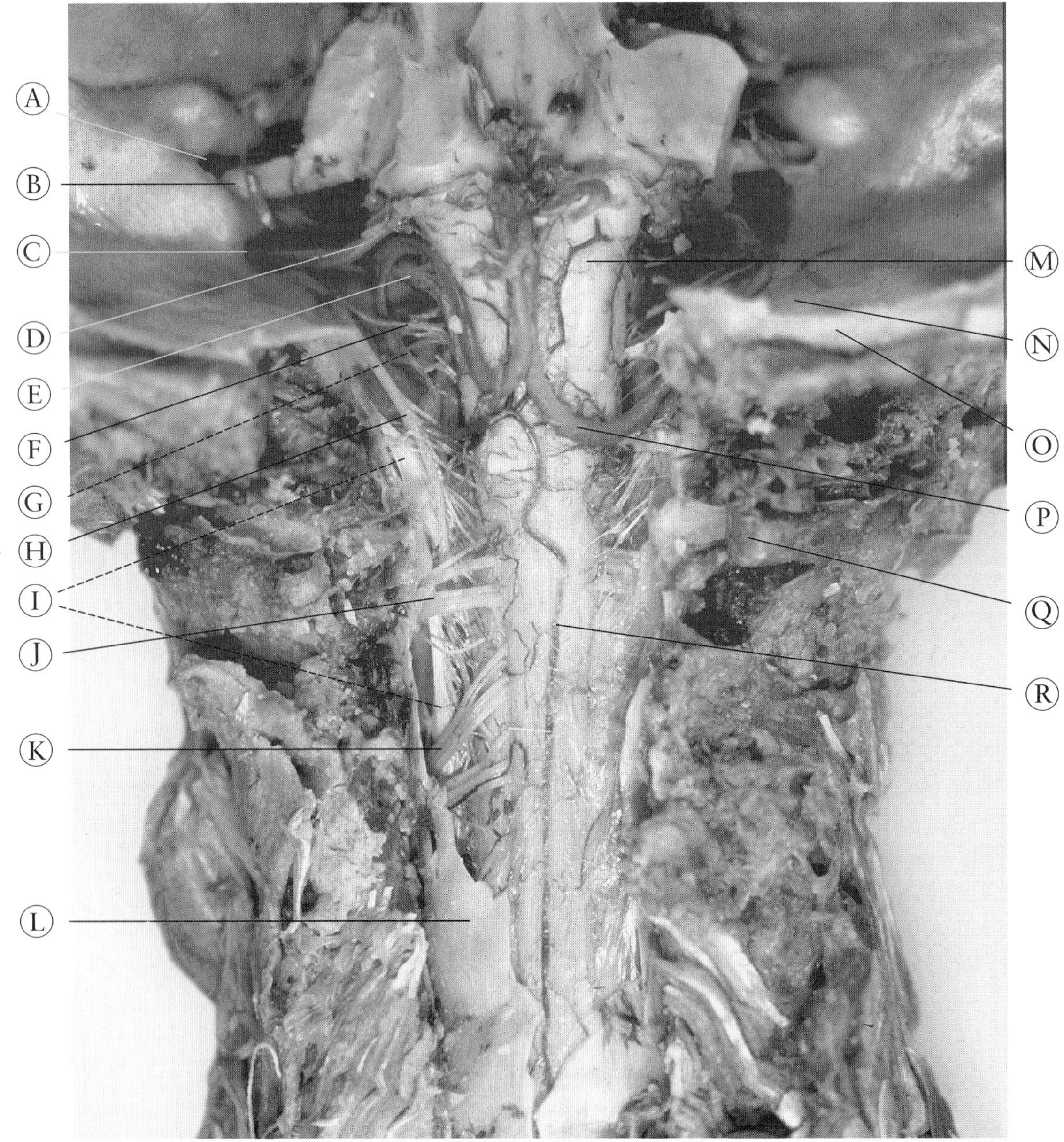

c.

Figure 1-5*

NORMAL ANATOMICAL RELATIONSHIPS, continued

Photo (c). Same specimen with occiput opened and cerebellum removed, with the skull in the neutral position relative to the neck.

(A) Internal Auditory Meatus	(G) C1 nerve rootlets	(M) Brainstem
(B) Acoustic Nerve(VIII)	(H) Spinal Accessory Nerve (XI)	(N) Cerebellar Fossa
(C) Jugular Foramen	(I) Dentate Ligament	(O) Occiput (cut edge)
(D) Glossopharyngeal Nerve(IX)	(J) C2 Nerve rootlets	(P) Inferior Cerebellar Artery
(E) Vagus Nerve(X)	(K) C3 Nerve rootlets	(Q) Arch of Atlas
(F) Hypoglossal Nerve (XII)	(L) Thecal sac (dural side)	(R) Dorsal Spinal Artery

*Color representation of the above figure appears after numbered page 80.

"Meninges" is a collective term used to describe all the supporting tissue of the central nervous system. This includes the thecal sac (theca), the pia mater, the dentate ligaments (AKA denticulate), arachnoid trabeculae, a web of fibers in the subarachnoid space attaching to the arachnoid mater, and pia mater that holds the cerebral spinal fluid (CSF) as a cushion for the spinal cord. The median septum is a single sheet of tissue in the posterior canal between the cord and the theca. The meninges provide support and confer shape to the cord tissue.

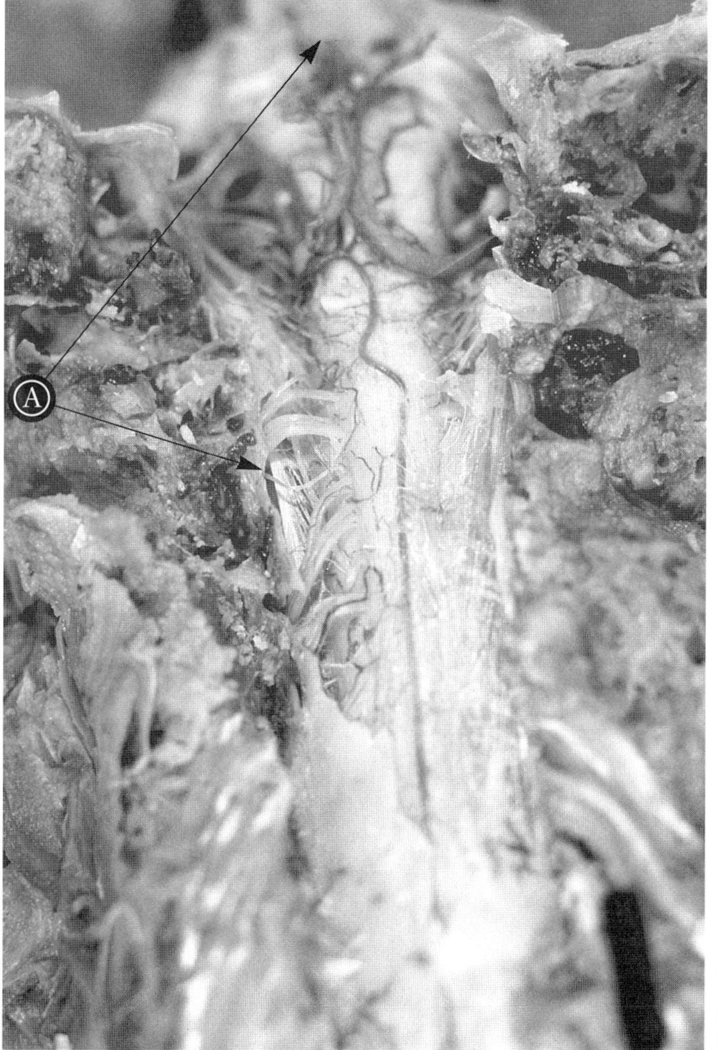

a.

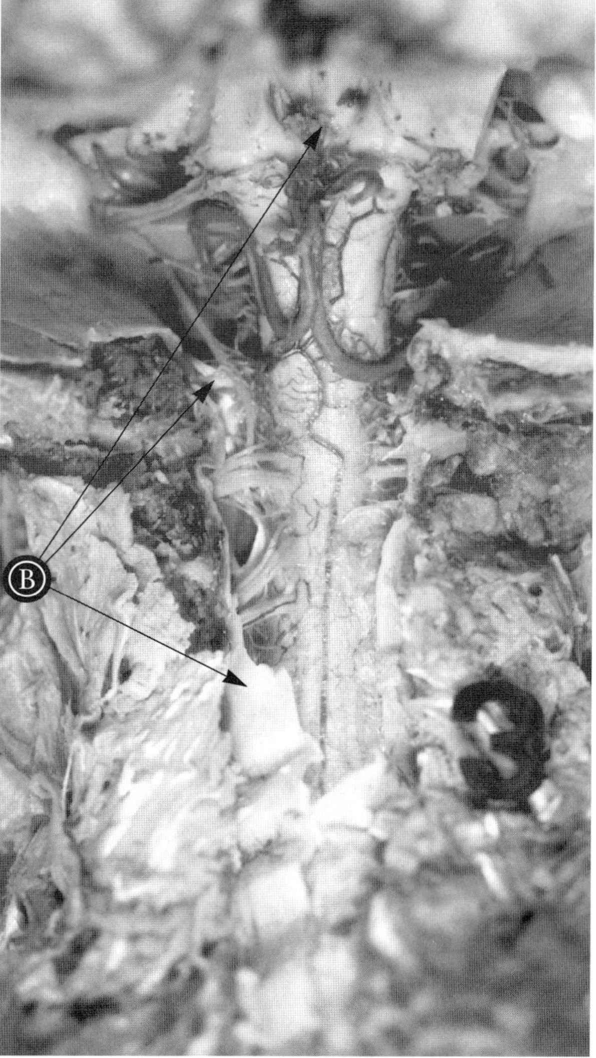

b.

Figure 1-6*

EFFECTS OF HEAD FLEXION AND EXTENSION ON THE CENTRAL NERVOUS SYSTEM

(a). Flexion(head tipped forward) increases the distance between the occiput and the coccyx, therefore lengthening the neural canal and the stretching the cord and brainstem.
  (A) Note stretching of the dentate ligament and the movement of the brainstem down toward the occiput. Note positions of Dentate Ligament, Brainstem, Base of Occiput, Arch of Atlas (refer to **Figure** 1-5 for keys to anatomical structures)

(b). Extension (head tipped backward) decreases the distance between the occiput and the coccyx, shortening and relaxing the cord and brainstem.
  (B) Note the relaxed left dentate ligament, the folded, relaxed dura mater (thecal sac), and the distance of the brainstem from the occiput. Note positions of Dentate Ligament, Brainstem, Base of Occiput, Arch of Atlas, Thecal sac.

*Color representation of the above figure appears after numbered page 80.

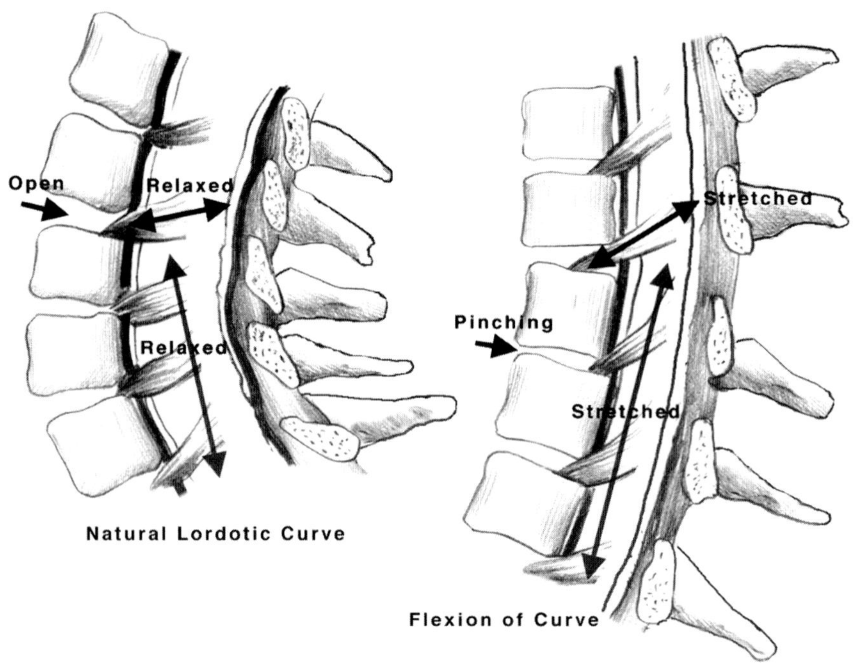

Figure 1-7

Extension of a lordotic curve in comparison to flexion. The closeness of the lamina and spinous processes in extension shortens the posterior aspect of the canal. Compare the flexion position with the large space between each lamina and spinous process. The spinal cord and thecal sac go from being on the inside of a concavity to the outside of a convexity.

There are some significant effects of absolute motion on the spinal cord. Vertebral column flexion (forward) increases the length of the spinal canal and spinal cord. The net distance from the foramen magnum to the coccyx increases with each individual. The amount of change can be 2-3 inches from extreme extension (shortened position) to extreme flexion (lengthened position). **See Figure 1-6.** This is accomplished in the vertebral column by lamina and facet separation and posterior disc height increase. **See Figure 1-7.** Also, in lateral flexion, the concave side is shortened and the convex side is lengthened. For instance, in right lateral flexion, the right side of the spinal canal is shorter in length than the left side of the canal. Absolute motion changes the shape of the spinal canal.

The thecal sac is made of the same tissue from top to bottom and has normal tube dynamics. It deforms as a tube in flexion and extension. Its net length will vary inversely with the diameter. The longer the tube gets, the narrower it becomes, while the shorter the tube gets, the wider it becomes. The volume remains relatively the same throughout the various positions the vertebral column can assume. Loss of the normal spinal architecture can change this relationship with mechanical and hydrualic pressures that result in pathology.

The thecal sac in the normal spinal column should be attached to the foramen magnum and upper cervical spine and coccyx. In between, it should be free of attachment to the vertebrae. This is not strictly true because the nerve root sheath of every nerve root is an extension of the thecal sac which attaches to the intervertebral foramen (IVF) and distal tissue. **See Figure 1-8.** These other attachments create slightly different dynamics than independent tubular structures.

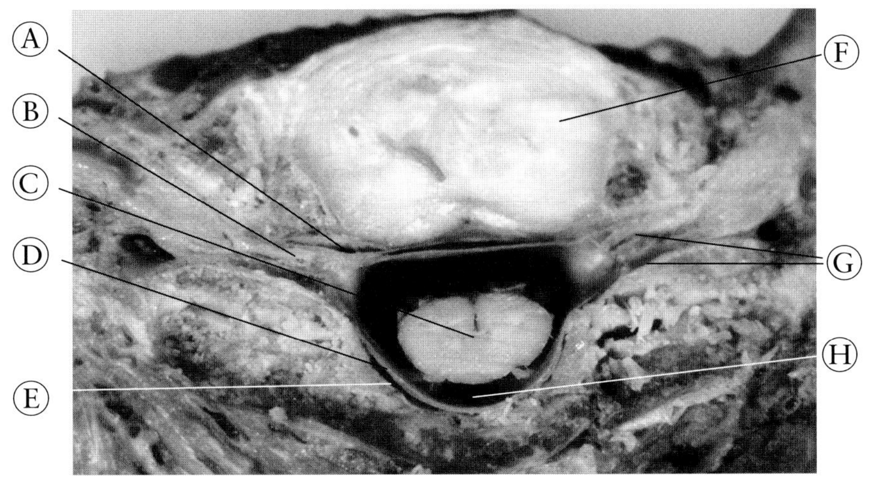

Figure 1-8
NORMAL ANATOMICAL RELATIONSHIPS - AXIAL VIEW
Axial section through the C7-T1 disc. See how the epineural sheath around the nerve root in the I.V.F. is an extension of the thecal sac. This shape and position of spinal cord is normal.

(A) Nerve root sheath
(B) Nerve root
(C) Spinal cord
(D) Thecal sac
(E) Epidural space
(F) Disc
(G) Intervertebral foramen (I.V.F.)
(H) Subarachnoid space

THE SPINAL CORD

The third system, the "pons-cord" tissue tract, includes the entire spinal cord from the conus medularis to the brain stem and the pons. It also includes the nerve rootlets that gather to form the nerve roots. This is all continuous tissue. The spinal cord and much of the nervous tissue of the central nervous system is actually an amorphous, gelatin-like substance. The spinal cord is attached to the thecal sac via the pia mater, spinal nerve rootlets, dentate ligaments arachnoid mater, and the filum terminale.

As the thecal sac changes in shape with normal position change of the individual, the pons-cord tissue tract also changes in shape and position. In forward flexion, the cord moves anteriorly in the canal and increases in overall length. This motion can change the relationship between the nerve roots and the foraminae. The anterior to posterior diameter of the cord decreases and the right-to-left diameter increases. The dentate ligaments, being only on the right and left side of the cord, cause a different action in lateral flexion and rotation. As the person bends and/or rotates to one side, the dentate ligament on the concave or shortened side relaxes while the dentate ligament of the convex side is stretched. This pulls the cord to the convex or longer side of the canal away from the pinching and compressing side of the spine. This change in the shape of the cord changes the shape of the tiny arteries and acts as a pump. This normal pumping action pushes the red blood cells and nutrients through the cord tissue, creating the blood flow that occurs in the lower central nervous system.

As stated earlier, when the spinal column is healthy, the three systems move in harmony. Segmental vertebral column motion is unique, differing with the section under observation. Deforming forces of the vertebral column during normal motion are transmitted through the thecal sac as a uniform motion. Despite the uneven, unique inter-segmental motion of the vertebrae, the motion of the thecal sac, under normal conditions, transmits a uniform force to the spinal cord. This is a very important point. Standing with just cranial flexion will stretch the meninges and cord all the way to the caudae equinae. The spinal cord needs and requires uniform distribution of this motion along its entire length for normal function. This leads to a distribution of forces to the whole "pons-cord tissue tract," thus helping to reduce the occurrence of deforming forces severely affecting one part of the cord and causing nervous tissue injury. The nervous tissue also needs this motion and changing shape to deliver adequate nutrients, because the motion acts as a pump for the whole CNS.

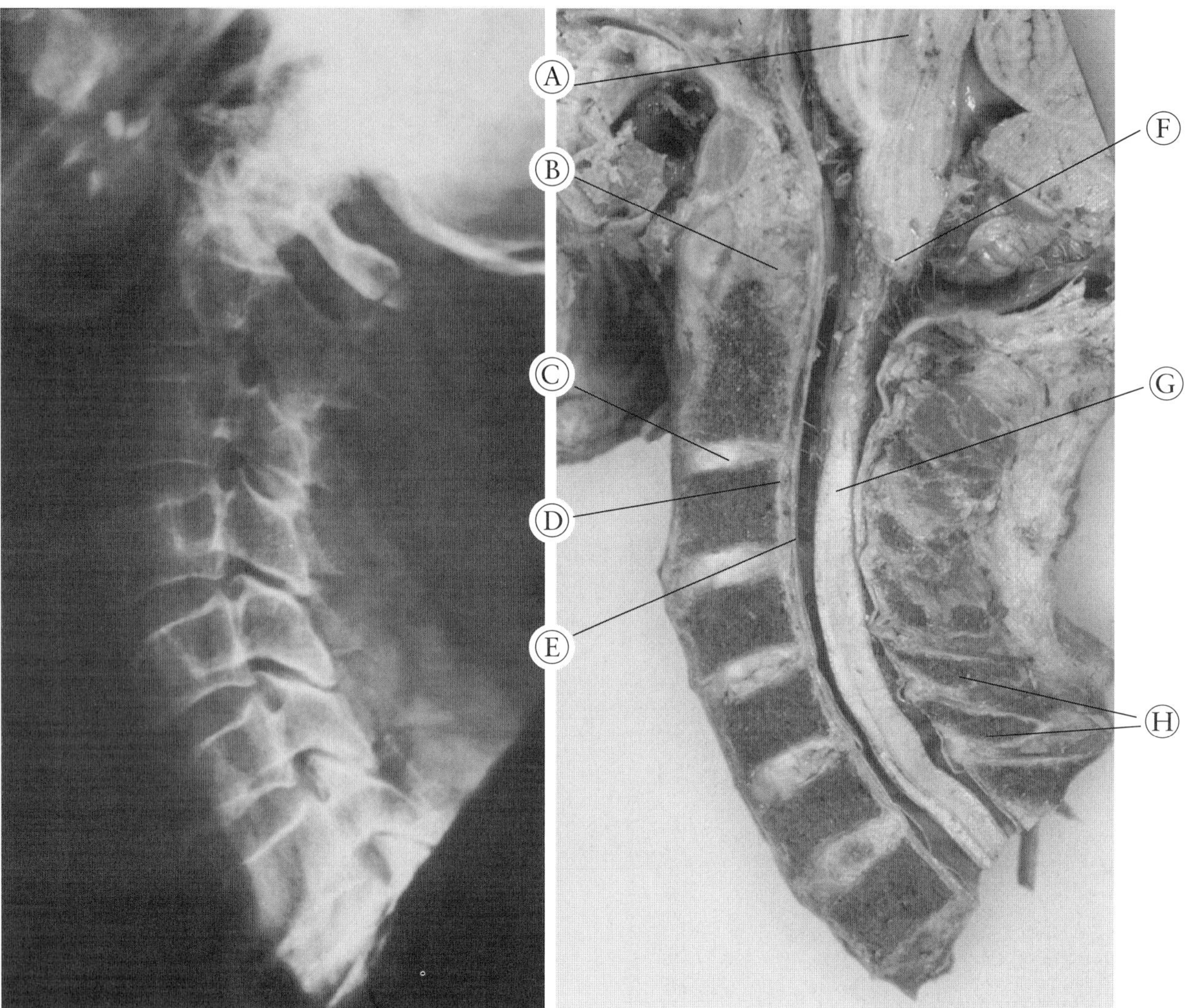

Figure 1-9

NORMAL SPINAL CORD - CANAL RELATIONSHIP

In this individual, the spinal cord does not completely fill the vertebral canal. Minor -posterior disc bulging (as at C5-C6 and C6-C7) has occurred without directly impinging on the cord, so this individual may have experienced only minor symptoms or none at all. Note the healthy cervical curve.

(A)	Pons	(E)	Thecal sac
(B)	Dens of C2	(F)	Brainstem
(C)	Disc of C2-C3	(G)	Spinal cord
(D)	Posterior longitudinal ligament	(H)	Spinous processes

There are individual differences or variations in the diameter of the spinal cord and in the diameter of the vertebral canal. **See Figures 1-9 and 1-10.** One severe difference is called congenital canal stenosis. Some of the clinical implications are that the anatomical variation can manifest itself as different symptoms with the same diagnosis or trauma. Two people sitting next to each other in a car when it is rear-ended can have completely different responses to the injury. They can have different symptoms, complaints, and recovery times. This is the basis for using "syndromes" to describe the range of effects of types of injuries. Some of the symptoms will be present in certain people and not in others even in the same accident.

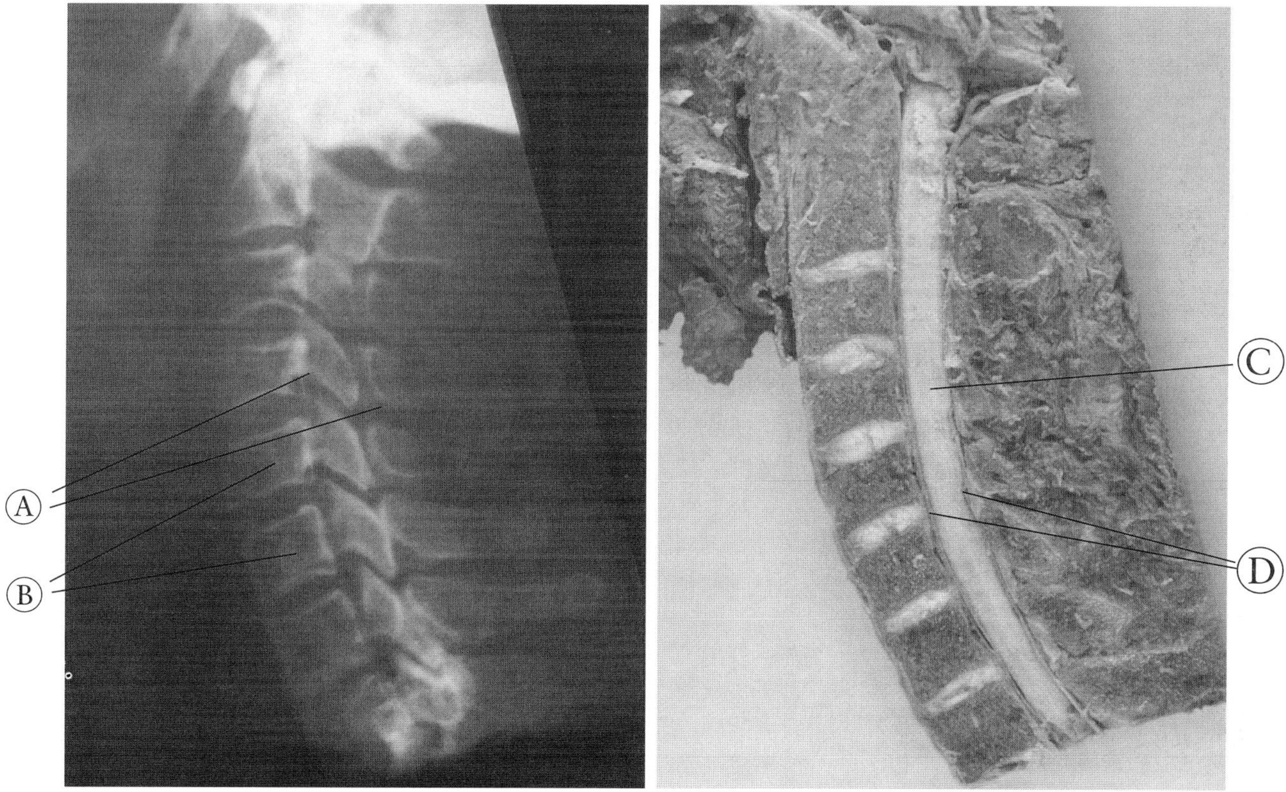

Figure 1-10
Cervical spinal canal narrowing or stenosis.
The relationship between the size of the canal and spinal cord can vary between individuals. In this specimen the spinal cord occupies the entire canal. Any changes in the shape in the wall of the canal can have significant neurological consequences.
  (A) Narrow spinal canal
  (B) Slight antrolisthesis of C6 relative to C5
  (C) Spinal cord
  (D) Slightly narrowed spinal cord

Motion of the Vertebral Column

The discs of the vertebral column are for allowing flexibility of the spinal column so the head and eyes can interact with the environment. This flexibility is essential to vascular flow in the capillaries of the spinal cord. The bending, twisting, and turning an individual does is important for the nutrient and oxygen delivery to the axons and neurons of the central nervous system. This motion is also essential to the health of the discs and ligaments of the vertebral column. They also require motion for nutrient and oxygen exchange. Studies show forced immobility initiates degenerative changes of the joint tissues. The fibrocytes that maintain the tissue are starved with stasis. So the discs deliver motion to the spinal column, not shock absorbing function. The flexibility they exhibit is necessary for their health as well as that of the nervous tissue.

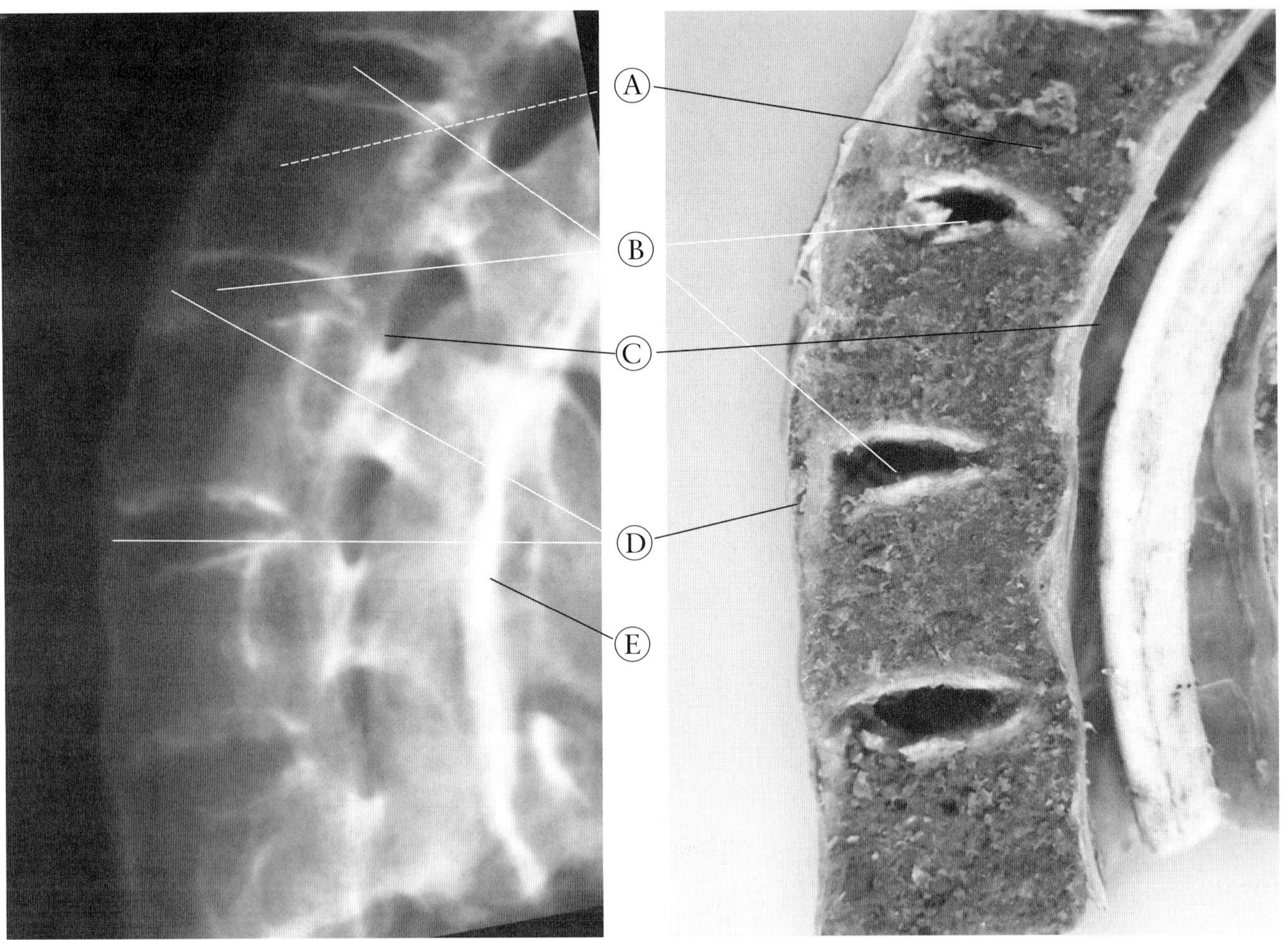

a.

b.

Figures 1-11 A & B
LOSS OF MOTION RESULTS IN LOSS OF JOINT TISSUE

An X-ray and specimen of a cervical spine with fusion of all the ligaments and resulting loss of the discs and other joint tissues

  (A) Vertebral bodies
  (B) Disc spaces
  (C) Calcified posterior longitudinal ligament
  (D) Calcified anterior longitudinal ligament
  (E) Facets or zygopophyseal joints are fused

CHAPTER TWO

Pathophysiology Of The Human Spine

Spinal Subluxation and the Central Nervous System

Subluxation is a term used to describe the loss of normal joint integrity. It is less than a luxation or a complete loss of integrity and less than a dissociation of two adjacent bones joined by an articulation. In the case of the human spine, a subluxation involves two adjoining vertebrae, the disc, and two pairs of facets or gliding joints. This loss of normal integrity results in the disruption of the connecting soft tissues, spasmodic contractions consisting of "guarding responses" to joint distress by the surrounding musculature. Joint spaces often become reduced, and range of motion becomes limited, often accompanied by pain and inflammation.

In the mid-sagittal plane of the human spine, the most common patterns of subluxation are a complete retrolisthesis (**See Figure 2-1**), a

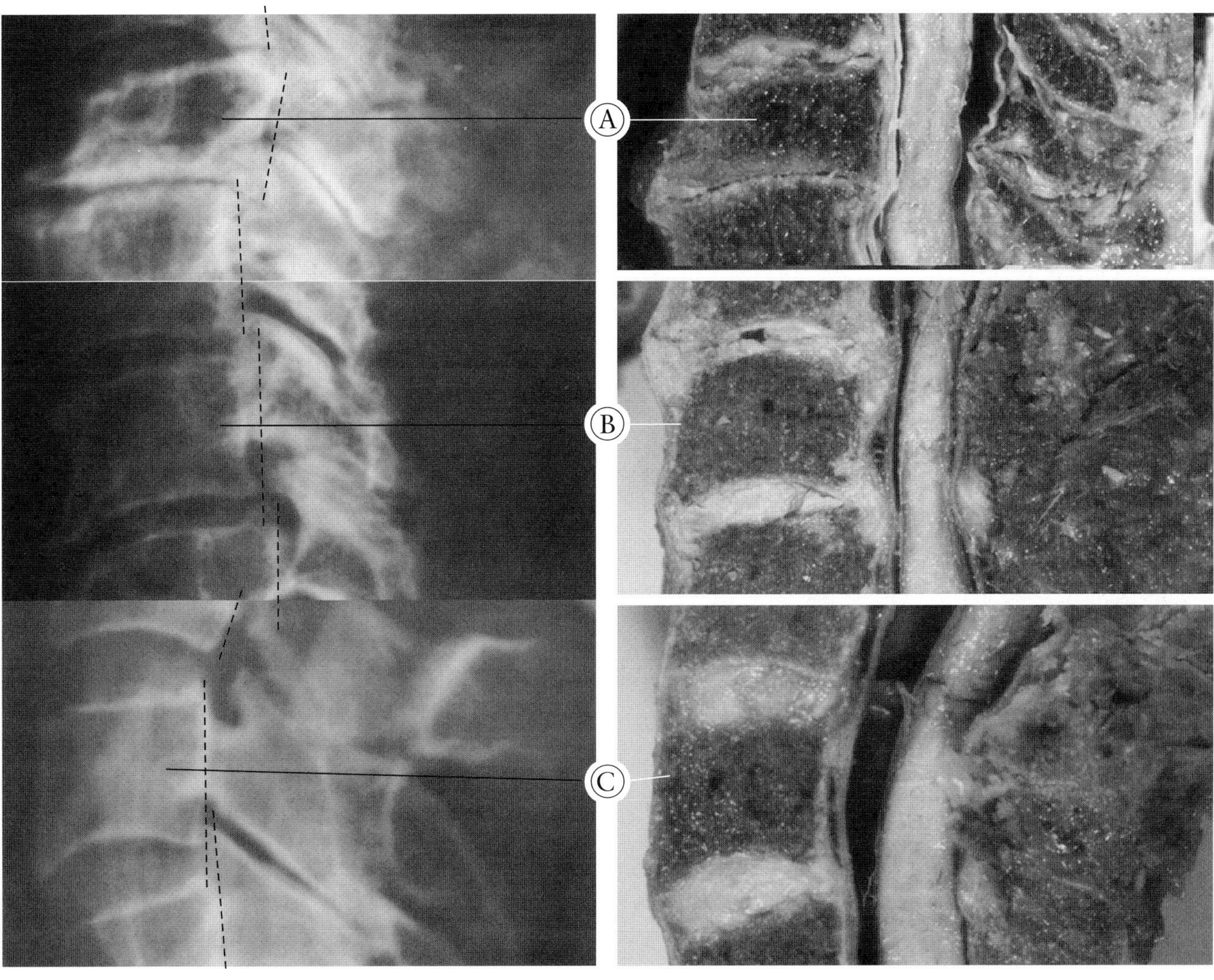

Figure 2-1
TYPES OF COMMON SUBLUXATIONS
Subluxation of vertebrae involve the three joints of two adjacent vertebrae: a disc and two zygopophyseal joints. Note the pathological changes of the zygopophyseal joints as well as the discs.

(A) A complete retrolisthesis: the body of this vertebrae is posterior to both the superior and inferior segments.
(B) Stairstepped retrolisthesis: this vertebrae is posterior to the superior vertebrae but anterior to the inferior.
(C) A complete anterolisthesis: this vertebrae is anterior to both the superior and inferior segments.

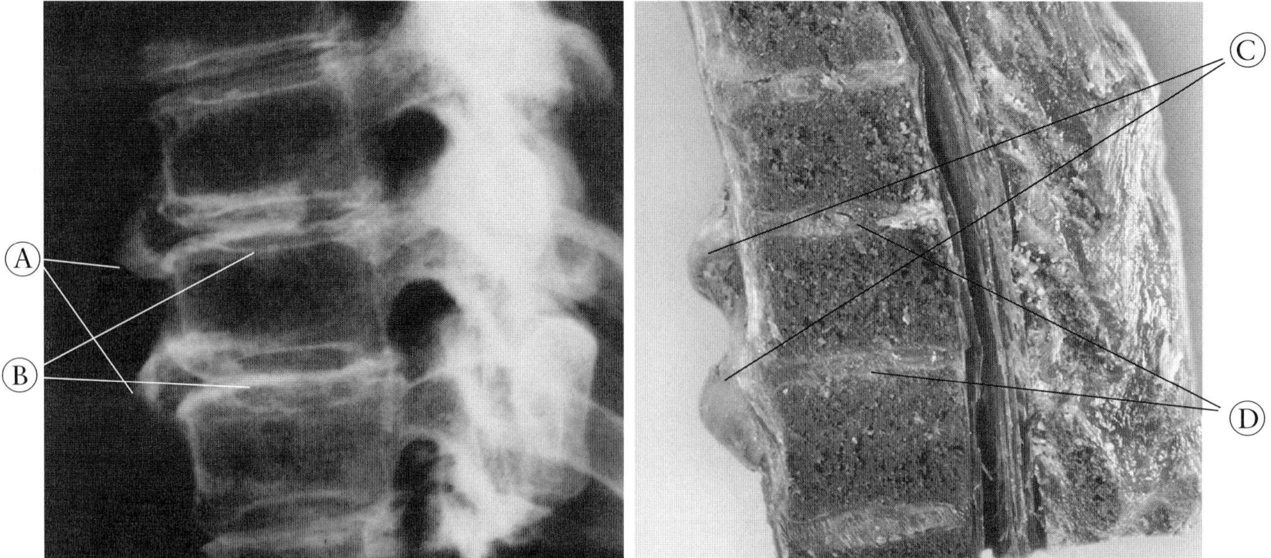

Figure 2-2
This illustrates disc bulging and endplate changes.
The endplate damage indicates trauma that has healed but has left injured soft tissues. The instability and altered mechanics of the injured joints results in chronically degenerative changes. Pictured here is a pair of bulging discs with their X-rays indicating calcification of the A.L.L. and discs.

(A) Osteophytes   (C) Bulging discs
(B) Damaged endplates   (D) Dessicated discs

stairstepped retrolisthesis, and a complete anterolesthesis. These occur in all combinations to form subluxation complexes when more than two vertebrae are involved. This is the etiology of osteoarthritis of the spine, degenerative joint disease, and spondylosis. Loss of normal joint integrity alters weight bearing of the joints, puts abnormal stress on soft tissues and bones, and initiates degenerative processes. In time the vertebral body develops "spurs" or "osteophytes" of various types.

We are used to looking at vertebral bodies from two dimensions, the A-P and lateral X-ray. The end plate changes are three dimensional and are the responses to the loss of normal weight bearing (See Chapter 1). The subluxation of a vertebrae can do one of two things to a joint: hyperload the joint or unload the joint. Both conditions will cause the bone and joint tissue to change. Normal motion is interrupted, causing deterioration of all avascular structures, ligaments, cartilage, and other connective tissue. This is also true for the facets or zygopophyseal joints. A retrolisthesis hyperloads at least one disc and puts shearing forces on the anterior longitudinal ligament (A.L.L.), the posterior longitudinal ligament (P.L.L.), the annular rings, nucleus pulposus, cartilage plates, and capsular ligaments. The bulging, twisting, and straining tissue attached to the end plates pull, push, and stretch it. It worsens with time, becoming irreversible (See Figure 2-2). Pictured are two bulging discs in the anterior-lateral direction with calcification of part of the A.L.L. and end plate.

The complete retrolisthesis usually causes more disc degeneration, end plate changes, facet sclerosis, and spinal canal changes. The stairstepped retrolisthesis is more common and associated with disc bulging, spinal curve, and spinal canal changes. The anterolisthesis is not as common and can be associated with either or both of the other types.

The change from normal alignment in the cervical spine can also have vascular consequences. The shape of the vertebral artery can become longer and more narrow than normal from kyphotic deformity of the cervical spine. Mechanical distress can generate a sympathetic "storm" and a regional vasoconstriction causing irritation of the arterial wall of the vertebral artery and its tributaries, the sinuvertebral. In **Figure 2-4**, an axial cut was made at the middle of the body of C2 below the superior articulating facets but above the transverse processes. Viewed from below, it is apparent that C1 is rotated relative to C2 and the inferior articulating facet of C1 on the left is contacting and compromising the vertebral artery. The vertebral arteries are the blood supply to the cervical spinal cord and any impairment can have adverse results. Poor vascular circulation from pressure on the arteries that supply the spinal cord and pressure on the spinal tissue itself is a natural consequence of subluxation of the spine. Pain can be only one of the many results of hypoxia of the spinal cord tissue.

Multiple subluxations of the vertebral column can have a profound effect on the quality of movement, nutrition, and general health of the central nervous system. This effect occurs due to the basic anatomical fact that the shape of the vertebral column creates the shape of the spinal canal which in turn determines the shape of the lower central nervous system (spinal cord, brainstem and nerve roots). Subluxation of the vertebrae changes the shape of the vertebral canal. Usually this change is an increase in length of the canal. The more change, the greater the effect on the central nervous system and the spinal cord.

The amount of change due to subluxation can vary with the individual, the number of vertebrae involved, and how the curves are altered. There seems to be substantial natural variation between the diameter of the canal and diameter

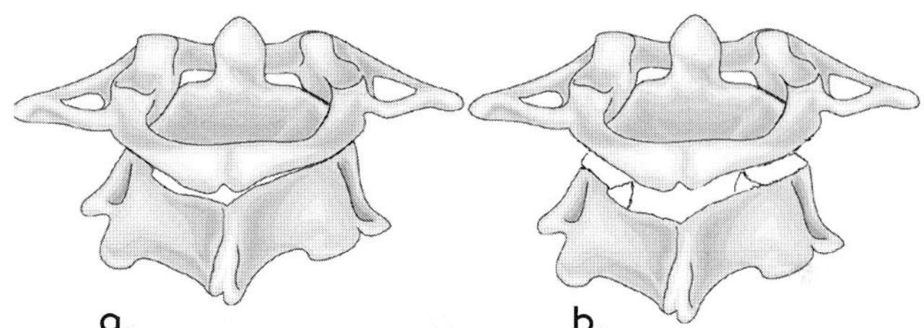

Figure 2-3

(a). Posterior view of C1 and C2.
(b). Plane of cut Figure 2-4 has through C1 and C2.
     Figure 2-4 is top section looking from underneath.

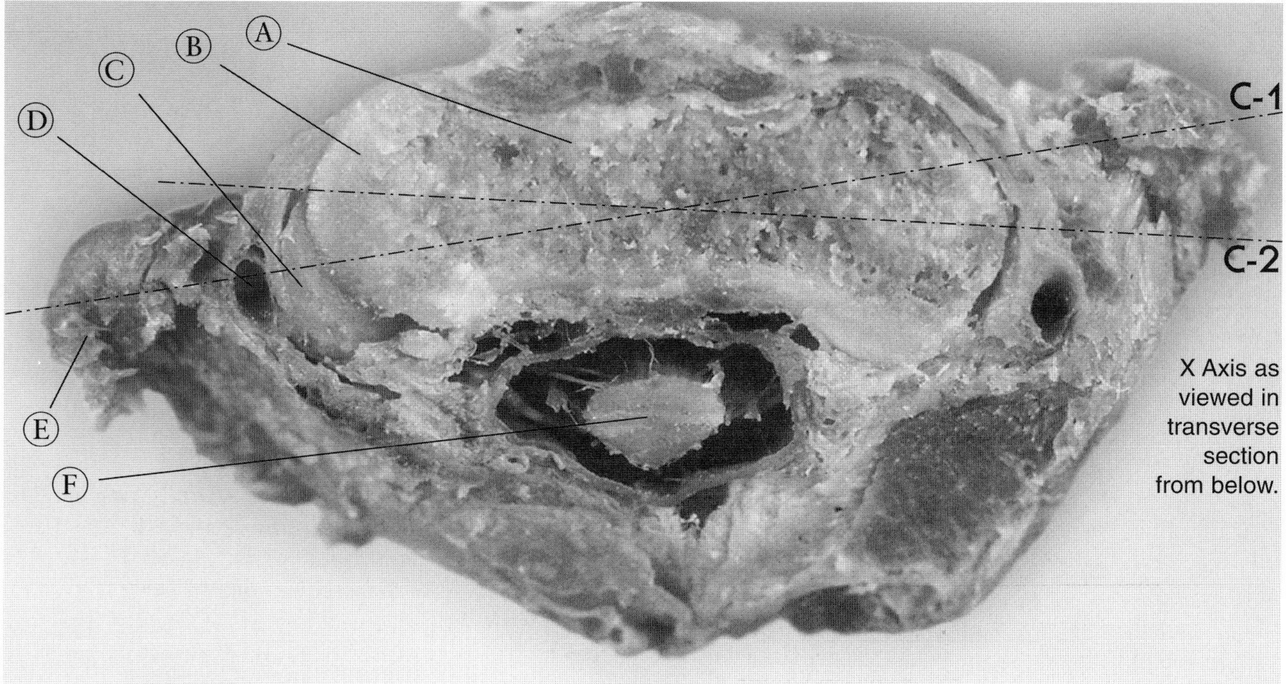

Figure 2-4
SUBLUXATION OF C1-2

Rotation of C1 to C2 with occlusion of the vertebral artery by C1 inferior facet.

(A) Body of C2
(B) Superior articulating facet of C2
(C) Inferior articulating facet of C1
(D) Vertebral artery
(E) Transverse process of C1
(F) Spinal cord

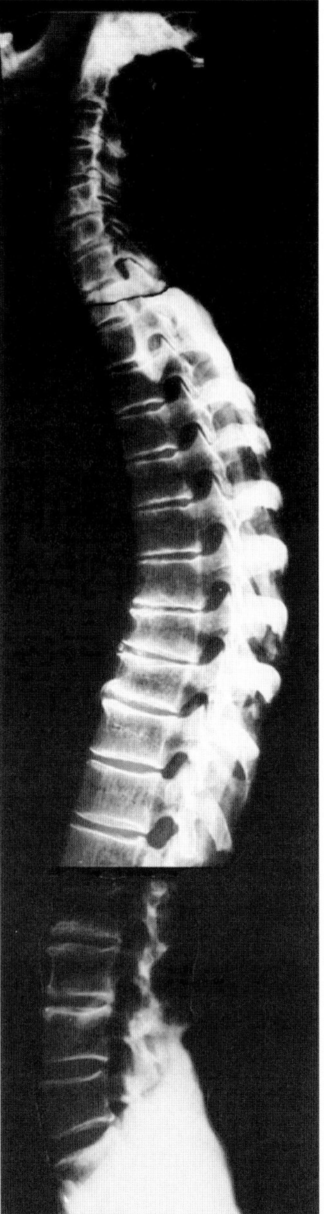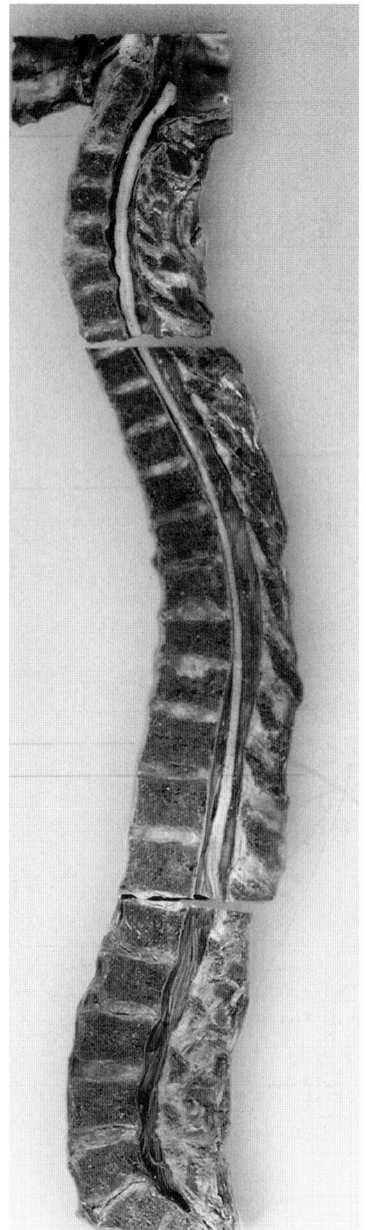

of the spinal cord. The space between the bony canal and the spinal cord can also vary with individuals (**See Chapter 1**). This explains how some people can tolerate more change due to subluxation than others. In some cases this space, or forgiveness of the system, can explain why relatively minor subluxations can cause distress on one person's nervous system, while a second person can tolerate radical changes in the vertebral column with little or no distress. In the case of this second person one might be able to elicit some symptoms on exam but generally in the second case the person seems to enjoy good health.

Figure 2-5
VERTEBRAL COLUMN WITH MULTIPLE
SUBLUXATIONS WITH CURVES MAINTAINED
NOTE: Discs usually don't degenerate unless there are subluxations or they have suffered some architectural disturbance. Healthy discs occur next to pathological ones, so age can't be a factor. There is a reduced cervical curve with posterior and anterior disc bulging and loss of disc height.
1. Note: cord impressions without significant stenosis.
2. Tractioned cord in upper thoracic despite almost "normal" curve; all discs with various levels of degeneration: note posterior wall intradural adhesions entrapping vascular structures.
3. Reduced lumbar curve and loss of disc height and hydration.

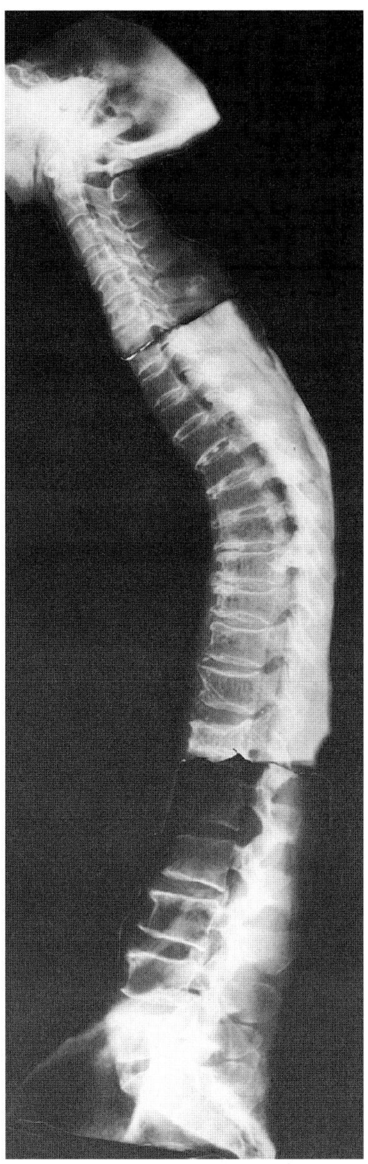

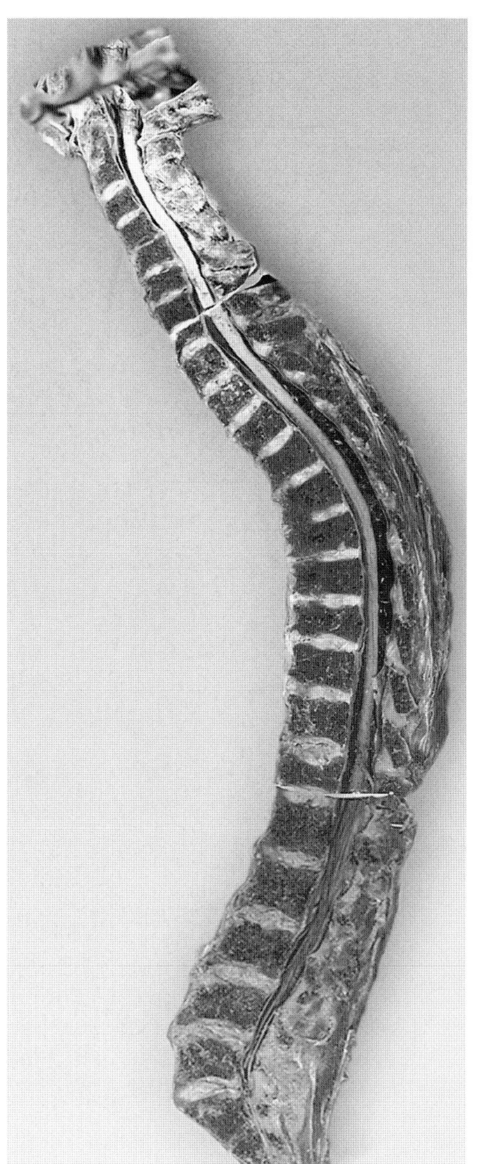

Figure 2-6
VERTEBRAL COLUMN WITH MULTIPLE SUBLUXATIONS AND LOSS OF CURVES

Here we see a reversal of cervical curve with canal stenosis and cord contact at C5-6. The thoracic spine has progressive anterior spurring with hyperkyphosis from altered weight bearing and osteoporosis. Increased thoracic curve changes due to compression fractures T6-T12.
Note: hypertrophy of A.L.L. T5-T12:
Note cord/canal contact T5-T9. Discs have dark brown areas that correspond to calcified appearance on X-ray. Loss of lumbar curve adds to flexion deformity of entire vertebral column and resulting poor posture.

The normal architectural features of lordotic and kyphotic curves is an essential component of the human spine (**See Figures 2-5 and 2-6**). In **Figure 2-5**, there are near normal curves so that the multiple misalignments and bulging discs are not seriously impinging the cord. The increased thoracic curvature and reduced cervical and lumbar curves have tractioned the thoracic section of the spinal cord into the anterior wall of the canal. One can observe the normal posture of this individual. In **Figure 2-6** there is altered curvature of all sections and a resulting "poor posture," and a bent forward or flexion deformity of the spinal column.

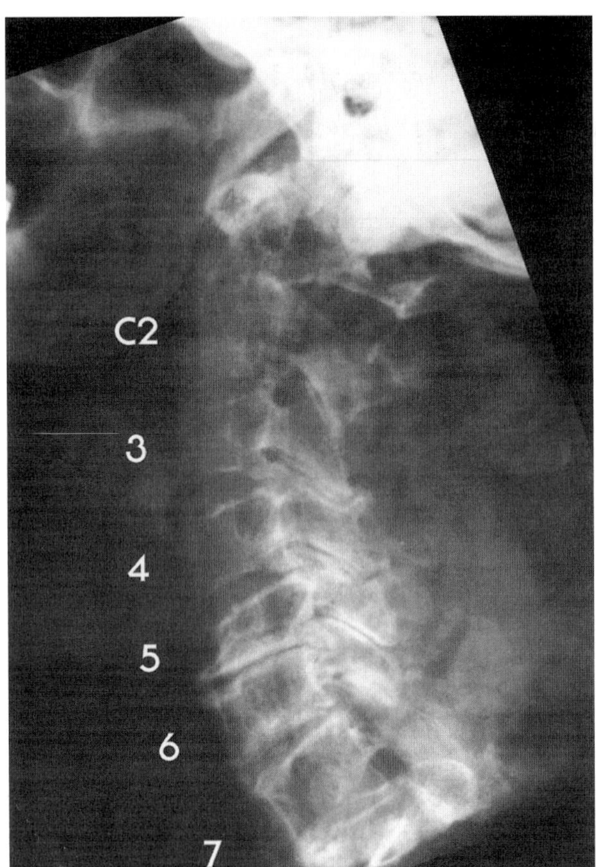

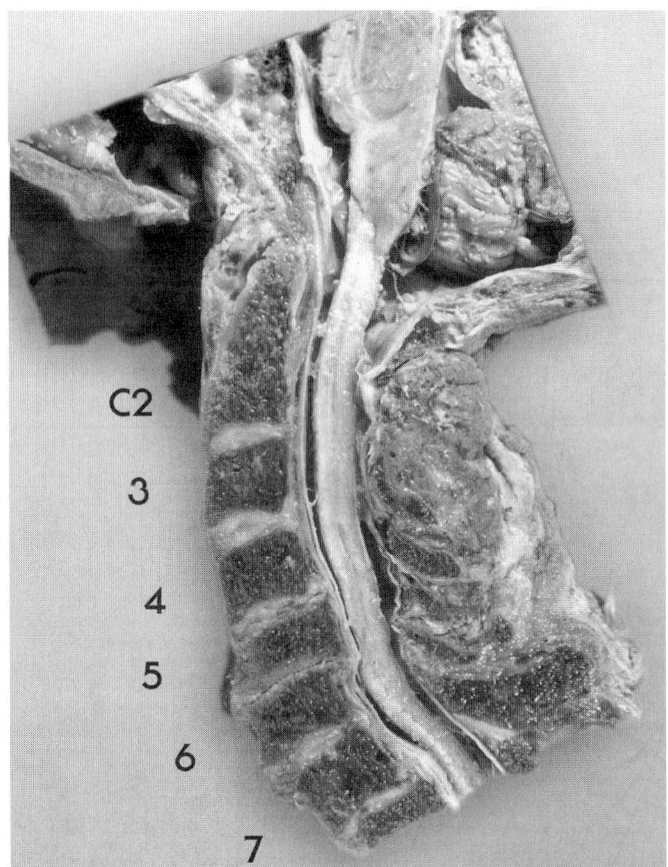

Figure 2-7

MULTIPLE SUBLUXATIONS WITH CURVE REDUCTION AND CORD CONTACT

The lower cervical spine has by far the most injuries and degenerative changes of any section of the spine. Both in the cadavers and in our patients in clinical practice, the C4-C5 and C5-C6 segments show the greatest relative anteroposterior displacement in the entire cervical spine (Hadley, 1964). They are also remote from the head, and therefore are more vulnerable to whiplash than the upper segments.

Note the canal stenosis of the cervical region as a result of the reversal of the lordotic curve and osteophytic changes. This change in the shape of the canal is an increase in its length. The anterior portion of the cervical spinal cord is in contact with the anterior wall of the canal as is the mid thoracic cord from T5 to T9. This condition is viewed in the neutral position. Any postural change into more flexion, as sitting in a chair, increases the traction and vascular compromise of the cord and nerve roots.

Looking at **Figure 2-7**, we see a lateral cervical X-ray and specimen. These figures have the discs, ligaments, and a central nervous system still intact. This is called a mid sagittal section.

What we see is a change in the normal relationship of the vertebrae C3-C4, mostly C4-C5, C-5-C6, and C6-C7. These are very common subluxation patterns. Notice the amount of change in only the subluxated segments. This cannot be completely explained due to age because C1, C2, C3 joint complexes are the same age as C4, C5, C6.

The change in the position of the vertebrae C4, C5, C6 causes an alteration in the shape of the canal that affects the cervical cord enlargement or bulge. The cervical spine is compressed in this region and the canal narrows due to the displacement of the vertebrae posterior to each other. An example is the C5 posterior inferior

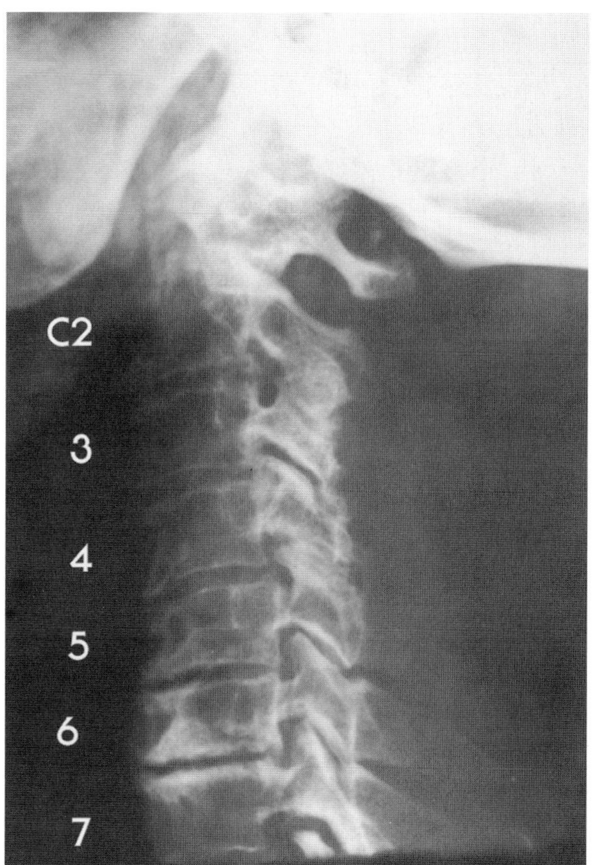

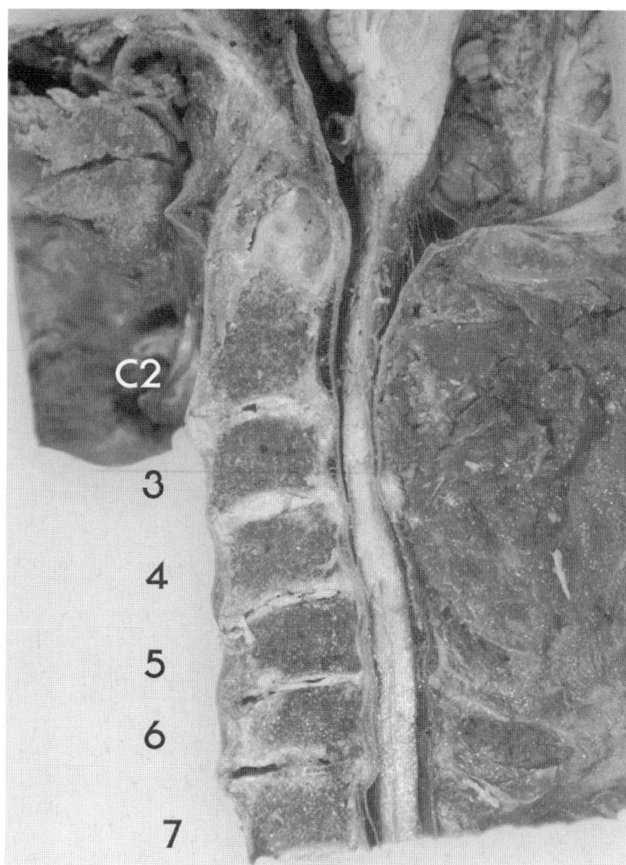

Figure 2-8
MULTIPLE SUBLUXATIONS WITH A REVERSAL OF THE CERVICAL CURVE
Loss of curve starts with C2-3 and a complete retrolisthesis of C5 to C4 and C6 with cord compromise C4-C7. Vertebral body enlargement forms stenosis of the canal and significant anterior spurring of C4-7. C6 retro to C7 with cavitation and near fusion of disc.

body being closer to the superior spinal laminar junction of C6. This is coupled with the fact that the A to P diameter of C5's body has increased by almost 20%, due to altered weight bearing which is a major result of subluxation. Many studies show that bone remodels to stress. When weight bearing or stress is altered, the bone changes its shape to accommodate the weight bearing. The result will be disc degeneration and eventual fusion. This condition can lead to cervical myelopathy with various symptoms of the upper extremities and may also have a serious effect on the rest of the spinal cord function.

Figure 2-8 is another specimen with its associated X-ray showing more advanced degeneration. Multiple subluxations of a long standing nature have a profound effect on the central nervous system and in the shape of the vertebral canal. We see in both specimens a radical change, especially in **Figure 2-8's** X-ray. This is a result of the subluxations that have altered the curvature. These subluxations have created a flexion deformity of the cervical spine.

In **Figure 2-9** are shown a cervical MRI and X-ray of a patient. There are some similarities between **Figure 2-8** and **Figure 2-9**. The history of the patient is when working at a desk, he had parasthesia bilaterally to the fingers, weakness, diminished reflexes, shoulder and neck pain, and some pain in his arms. The MRI of this patient was taken in the recumbent position, not in the position that created the symptoms. He got relief by lying down on his back.

The patient in **Figure 2-10** has a similar problem, getting relief by laying down on her back. Here we have a mid-sagittal view of the entire spine seen in the position in which it was taken. The spinal cord is in the anterior portion of the canal from C3 to T10. The patient gets relief (head, neck, stomach, and back pain) in this position. Her problem is aggravated while seated at her desk with her neck flexed forward. In both cases, signs of spinal cord distress are seen

while in a position that relieves symptoms. In both these cases, cervical flexion increased symptoms. Because of the loss of the normal curve that is already in this multiple subluxated cervical spine, a longer than normal canal is created, with flexion stretching the spinal cord and pressing it into the bulging discs and osteophytes. The cord is elevated to the anterior portion of the canal even in the recumbent position. This is not normal. The anterior spinal artery can be compressed by the posterior osteophytes and bulging discs. This contact can be reduced when the patient is lying on his or her back and the cervical spine or lumbar spine is in extension (**See Figure 2-11**). The reversal of the cervical curve (or kyphosis) can lengthen the

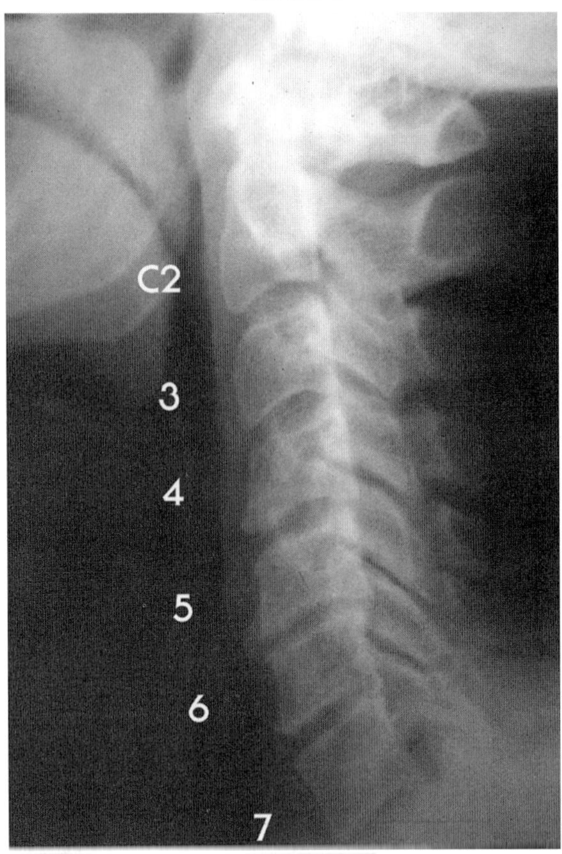

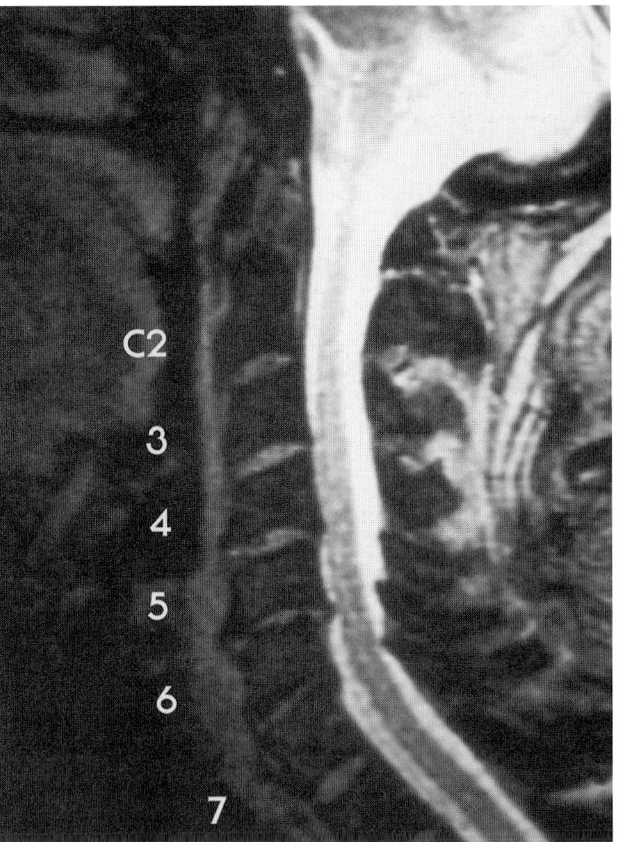

Figure 2-9

CERVICAL X-RAY AND MRI STUDY WITH LOSS OF LORDOSIS

The lateral X-ray of this patient clearly shows the loss of curvature, multiple subluxations, loss of disc height, and posterior osteophytes. This MRI shows loss of curvature ("military neck") resulting from posterior subluxations at C3 retro to C2, C4 retro to C3 and C5 retro to C6.

Note the loss of disc height and posterior spurring. The spinal cord is much smaller in diameter than the vertebral canal, but it is the tethering or stretching of the cord against C3-5 that makes these significant problems. The posterior disc bulging and osteophytes of C3-5 are actually in contact with the spinal cord in the neutral supine position, a position of relief for this patient of bilateral parasthesia in the upper extremities. His symptoms were brought on by sitting at his desk doing paper work.

We have to extrapolate his changing positions to the changing length of the vertebral canal.

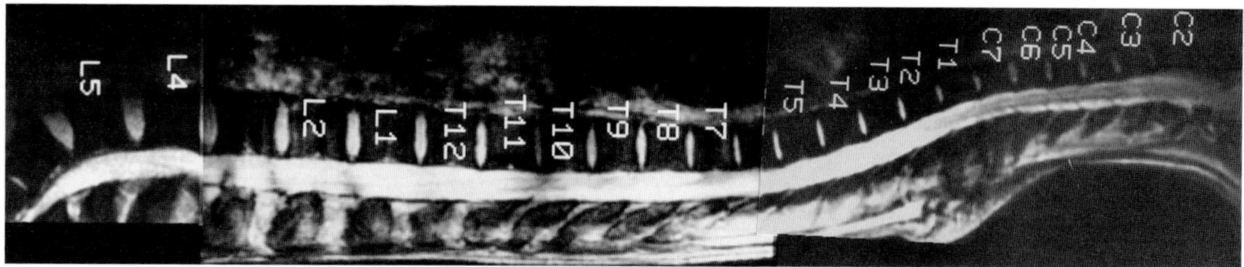

Figure 2-10

MIDSAGITTAL MRI STUDY OF THE ENTIRE VERTEBRAL COLUMN SEEN IN THE POSITION THE STUDY WAS TAKEN

The anteriority of the cord in the canal from C4 to T9 (tethering) shows the overall effect of the reverse curve is tethering of cord and the hypokyphotic curve of the thoracic spine in standing or supine views. Aligned segments with reduced curve. Anterior location of the spinal cord in the canal in the supine view through most of the thoracic spine.

Loss of lordotic curve in the lumbar spine is a flexion deformity or a lengthening of the canal.

Note sacral disc. Central nervous system tension is transferred to caudae equinae all the way to the IVFs. We need to extrapolate postural change from supine to flexed (seated or other) positions.

Note: Anterior cord displacement in the "neutral position." Patient actually gets relief in this position, all flexion irritates her condition.

Figure 2-11
CERVICAL X-RAY AND MRI STUDY SHOWING REVERSAL OF CURVE

Cervical MRI and X-ray of same individual showing reversal of lordotic curve or a cervical kyphosis. Note the straightening of the brainstem to thoracic cord, a complete retrolisthesis of C5, large interspinous distance from C3-7, enlargement of C5 body due to hyper loading and bulging discs. Consider the anatomic and physiologic changes with active, persistent cervical flexion as required by many jobs.

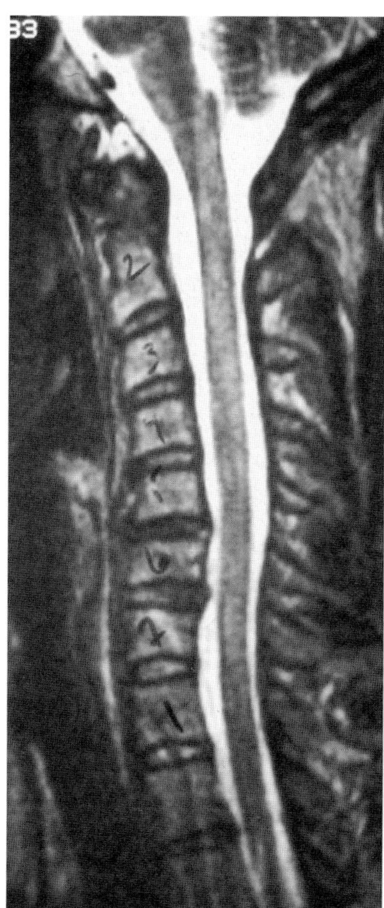

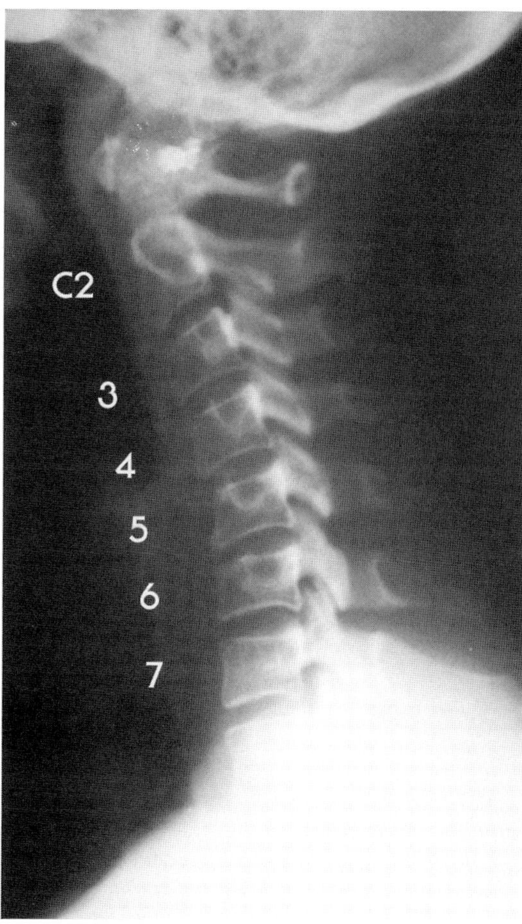

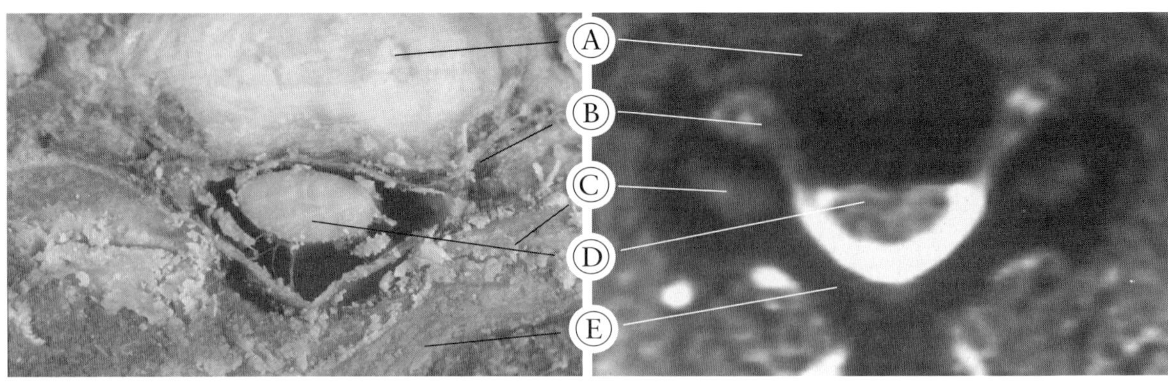

a.

b.

Figure 2-12 A & B
AXIAL VIEWS OF TETHERED CORD

(a). This specimen is being viewed at the C7 level. Note the anterior canal wall contact and flattening of the spinal cord. This individual was in a neutral position when dissection and photo were taken. Can the ventral horn neurons be fully vascularized?

(A) Disc
(B) Nerve root
(C) Facet
(D) Spinal cord
(E) Lamina

(b). This MRI of an axial view at the C5 level clearly shows the spinal cord tethered against the anterior wall of the vertebral canal. At this level, the cord has lost its normal almost round appearance. It is severely flattened and vulnerable to even slight posterior disc bulging and minor osteophytes. Can we assume the anterior spinal artery has any blood flow?

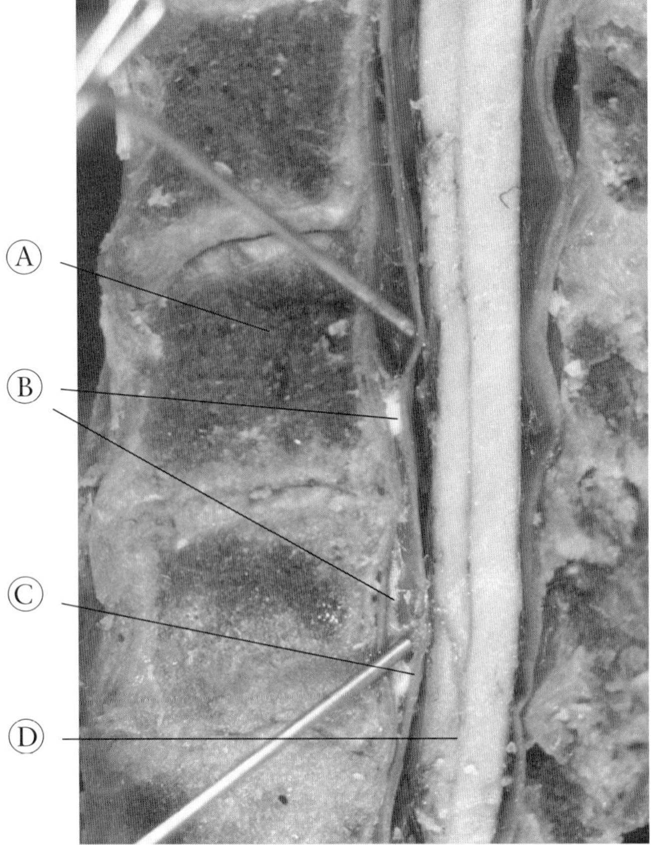

Figure 2-13A
EPIDURAL ADHESIONS/ANTERIOR WALL
Epidural adhesions between the anterior vertebral canal wall and the thecal sac (Dura Mater). These tissues are supposed to be freely moveable relative to each other. The adhesions are the result of chronic inflammation due the subluxations of the vertebra and end stage DJD.

(A) Body of vertebra
(B) Epidural adhesions
(C) Thecal wall
(D) Spinal cord

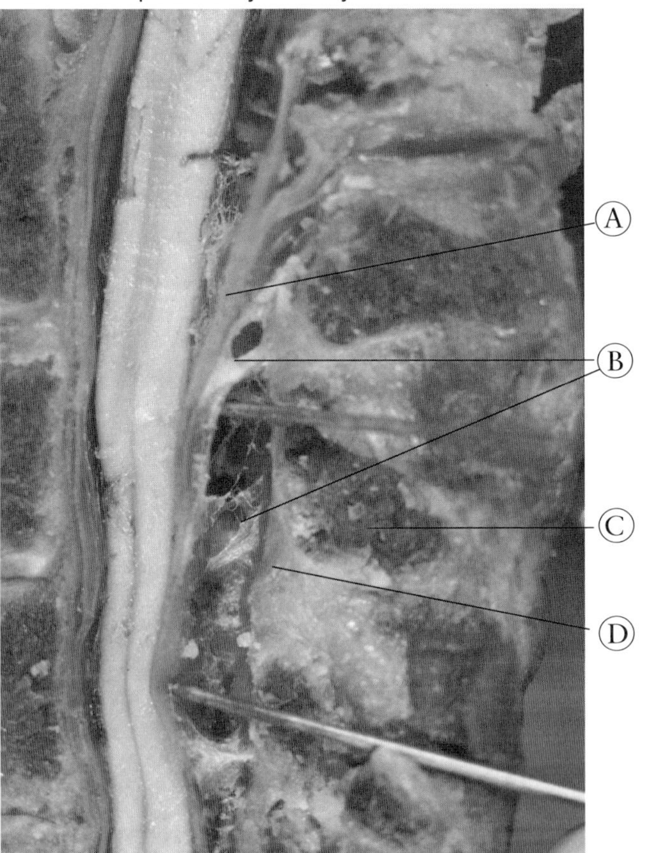

Figure 2-13B
EPIDURAL ADHESIONS/POSTERIOR WALL
Epidural adhesions in the posterior portion of the vertebral canal. These adhesions are the result of chronic inflammatory states in the posterior joints and soft tissues of the vertebral column in the thoracic region and even the thecal sac, pia mater, nerve rootlets, and arteries.

(A) Thecal wall
(B) Epidural adhesions
(C) Spinous process
(D) Ligamentum flavum

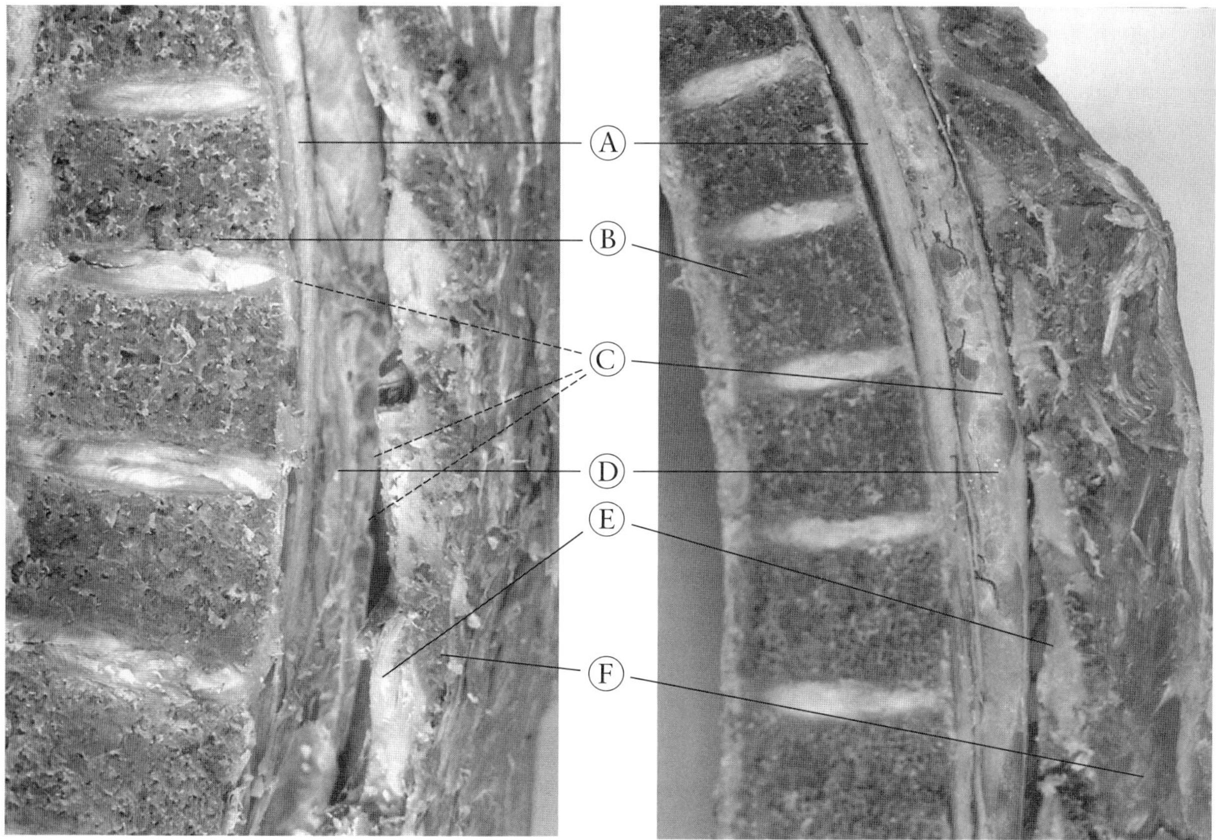

Figure 2-14   Figure 2-15

INTRATHECAL OR SUBARACHNOID ADHESIONS

Both of these specimens show posterior subarachnoid adhesions in the thoracic region of the vertebral column. They each have tethered the spinal cord with large contact areas against the canal wall. Since the posterior canal wall lengthens more, the stretch or irritation is greater in the posterior hemisphere of the thecal sac.

(A) Spinal cord
(B) Vertebral bodies
(C) Thecal wall
(D) Subarachnoid adhesions
(E) Ligamentum flavum,
(F) Spinous processes.

canal in the cervical area and the entire spinal cord. Note the straight appearance of the spinal cord and brain stem, the increased distance between the spinous processes of C3-7, the subluxation complex involving C3-7, bulging discs of the involved segments, and osteoarthritic change of C5, a complete retrolisthesis. The components of the cervical subluxation complexes alter lordotic curves. The resulting effects on the central nervous system cause profound health care changes.

In **Figure 2-12A** we see the displaced spinal cord in a specimen at the C7 level with the ventral surface of the spinal cord in contact with the anterior wall of the spinal canal. This is a deforming of the anterior and lateral tracts of the cord, and can not be considered normal. In **Figure 2-12B** the axial MRI view is at C5 showing the spinal cord flattened against the anterior

wall of the canal. There is a deforming of the vascular as well as neural structures. The animal studies are clear. When the cord is deformed, altered conductivity results. When this happens, there are two main components; duration and intensity. How long a period the condition persists is important because the studies show decreased conductivity with increase in time of deforming force. The intensity is obviously a factor. When the increase in tethering or compression occurs, the conductivity decreases. There was a 70% incidence of all degrees and forms of cord deformation in the random population of 116 cadavers.

Another complication of the deforming effects of subluxation complexes of the vertebral column is inflammation and resulting adhesions. In **Figure 2-13** you see epidural adhesions that have developed because of chronic inflammation.

There are obvious subluxations with end stage disc degeneration. In **Figure 2-13A** the dura mater (the outside of the thecal sac) is adhered to the P.L.L. This condition severely impairs the normal independent motions of the thecal sac and the vertebral column. (**See Chapter 1**). The adhesions can be extensive in the spinal canal. **Figure 2-13B** shows adhesions of the dura mater to the lamina and ligamentum flavum in the posterior wall of the canal. This has to be a further restrictive condition to normal motion and physiology. There are two main factors at work here: the degeneration of the disc and ligament tissue as essentially an inflammatory condition, and the abnormal mechanics of vertebral motion putting unusual stress on the thecal sac and other meningeal structures. This causes an inflammation of the meninges inside the subarachnoid space (**See Figures 2-14 and 2-15**). Here are two specimens with subarachnoid adhesions. In both cases, the thoracic cord is tethered against the anterior wall of the canal. This condition, more than any other, chronically pulls or stretches the posterior elements of

the thecal sac. The persistent irritation causes inflammation and adhesions of the pia mater, arachnoid mater, median septum, and the arachnoid trabeculae. In both cases, the cervical curve is altered by subluxation complexes. The tractioning and irritation of the thoracic cord and meningeal tissues is one major result. Also, there must be impaired CSF flow in this area along with the altered biomechanics of the CNS. See **Figure 2-16** for the MRI appearance in the thoracic spine. Note the imaging density of the adhesions is similar to that of the spinal cord. *In situ* the adhesions are dense and entrap arterioles and nerve rootlets.

As demonstrated, subluxation of the vertebral column has many aspects that interfere with normal health. The vertebral column is a complex structure with many types of tissues, that when healthy, work in harmony. Alteration of the normal architectural features of the vertebral column can have severe health consequences that can advance with increasing duration and intensity.

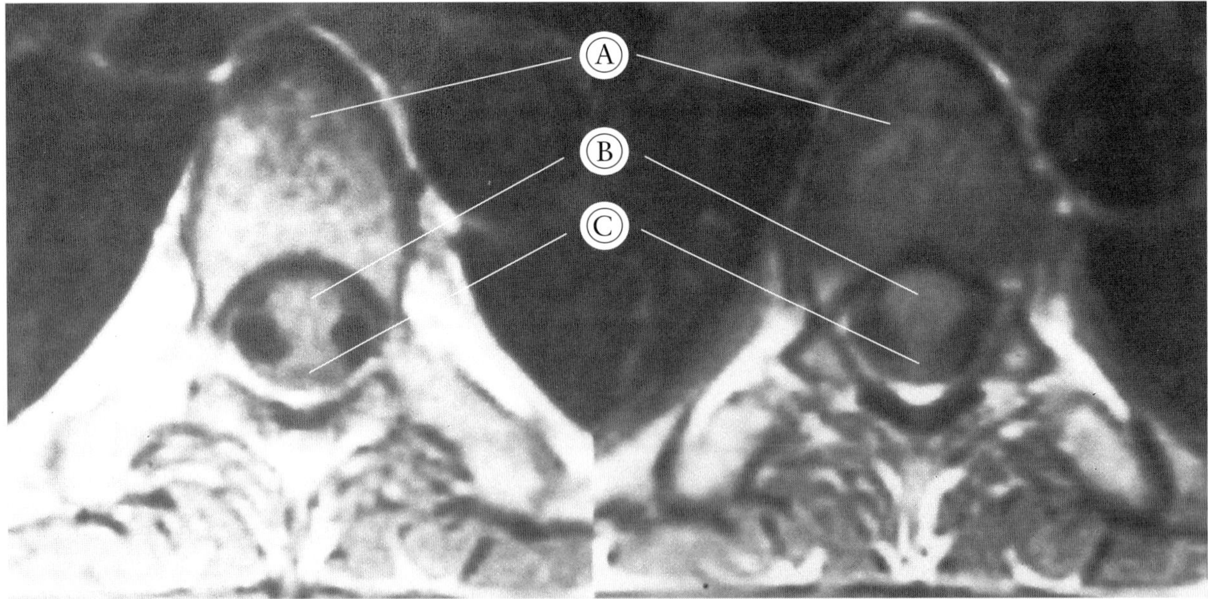

Figure 2-16

THORACIC SPINE: MRI AXIAL VIEWS OF TETHERED SPINAL CORDS
Note subarachnoid adhesions and cord-canal contact in the recumbent position, the spinal cord is in the wrong part of the canal for this position.
   (A) Vertebral body
   (B) Spinal cord
   (C) Subarachnoid or intrathecal adhesions

CHAPTER THREE
Subluxations Of The Cervical Spine

Discussion

The motion and support of the head are main features of the unique joint complexes of the cervical spine. The alteration of the normal architecture aligning the head with the thoracic spine is the primary cause of degenerative change. The blood supply of the cervical spine, face, and lower head are controlled by the integrity of the vertebral column (**See Figure 3-1**). The changes caused by subluxation of the cervical vertebrae can result in headaches as a patient complaint. The cervicogenic origins of most headaches are only partially appreciated by the health care community. Blood flow to vital parts of the central nervous system can alter due to subluxations of the cervical spine. Headaches can also be caused by head to thorax misalignment with the SCM spasm that can develop and compress the external jugular vein. This decreases or stops blood drainage from the face and side of the head. Some headaches are caused by inflammation of the tendinous attachments of the SCM into the mastoid process due to chronic spasm.

When the head is accelerated in a different way from the thorax, the cervical spine will deform. This is commonly refered to as whiplash, but I prefer the term "buckling." Buckling is an engineering term that conveys partial collapse of an architectural structure, an accurate description of the results of the head being suddenly accelerated 20 miles an hour faster and in a different direction than the thorax. The result is anterior to posterior as well as rotational misalignments. With preservation of the normal lordotic curve, the cervical spine undergoes none of the changes of osteoarthritis, even in old age. Most osteoarthritis of the spine is the result of uncorrected subluxations and remolded bones and joints due to the chronically altered weight bearing. Osteoarthritic

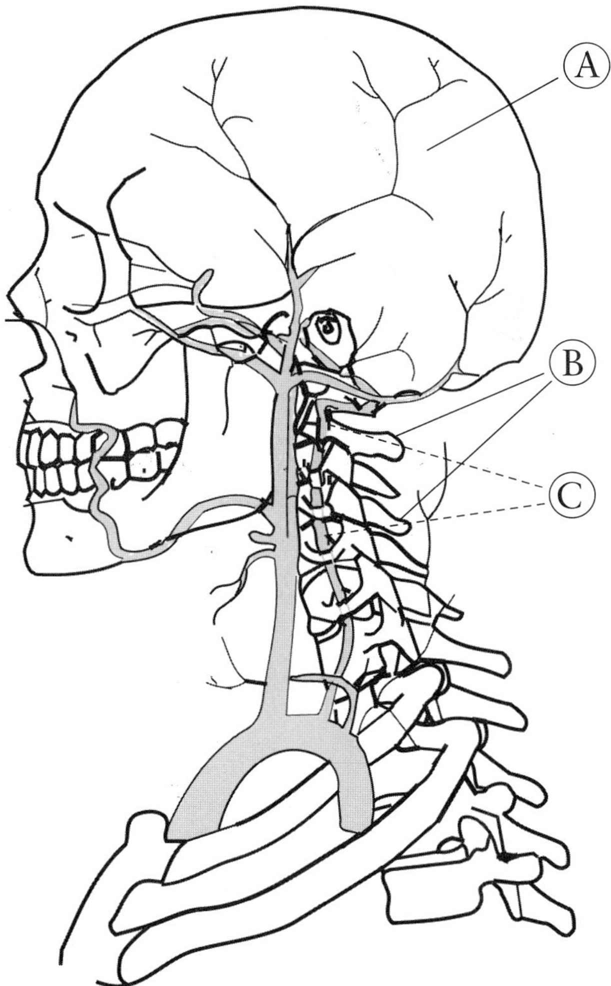

Figure 3-1

The head and cervical spine can misalign and have altered structure. The vertebral artery and other vascular and nervous system structures can suffer a change in function. Note the position of the vertebral artery and its relationship to the cervical spine and the head. These arteries supply the spinal cord, vertebrae, ligaments, and brainstem with blood.

(A) Head
(B) Cervical spine
(C) Vertebral artery

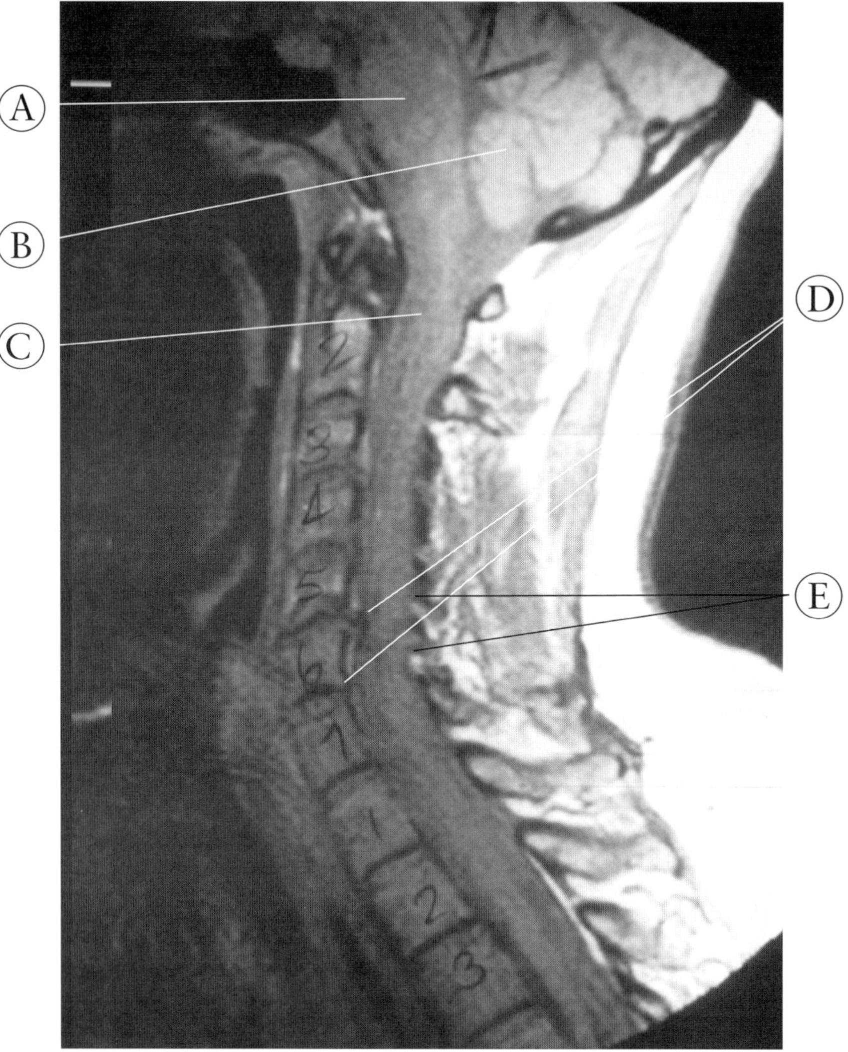

Figure 3-2

This is an MRI of a cervical spine, lower head, and upper thoracic spine. The subluxated sixth vertebra has formed posterior osteophytes. The retrolisthesis of C6, the posterior osteophytes, and the lamina of C-7 have created a canal stenosis.

(A) Brainstem
(B) Cerebellum
(C) Spinal cord
(D) Posterior osteophytes
(E) Lamina

changes include disc degeneration, spinal canal stenosis, intervertebral foramen narrowing, uncinate process hypertrophy, and facetal sclerosis (**See Figure 3-2**). Loss of joint alignment or subluxation of the cervical vertebrae results in changes to all the tissues of the affected segments. This also has unfortunate consequences for areas of the central nervous system (**See Figure 3-3**). The subluxations alter the course of the vertebral arteries and tributaries and therefore alter the blood flow in those vascular structures (**See Chapter 2**). The subluxations can change the shape of the spinal cord, brainstem, and pons (**See Figure 3-4**). Altered shape and blood supply to the central nervous system can change its function. The factors that can lead to altered function include the type of anatomical relationships, the degree of change, and the time or duration of subluxation. Some patients have all factors working against them, while others are more fortunate.

The cervical spine has more capacity to change in length than the other portions of the spine. The posterior cervical canal wall has more flexion-extension range of motion than any other part of the vertebral column. The center of the cervical canal can lengthen 3 cm. from full extension to full flexion. That is nearly half the total change possible for the whole spine. The loss of the lordotic curve can add 1 to 2 cm. or more of length to the whole canal, permanently stretching the spinal cord, brainstem, pons, and nerve roots. With certain flexed postures or positions, an over-stretching of the lower CNS can take place.

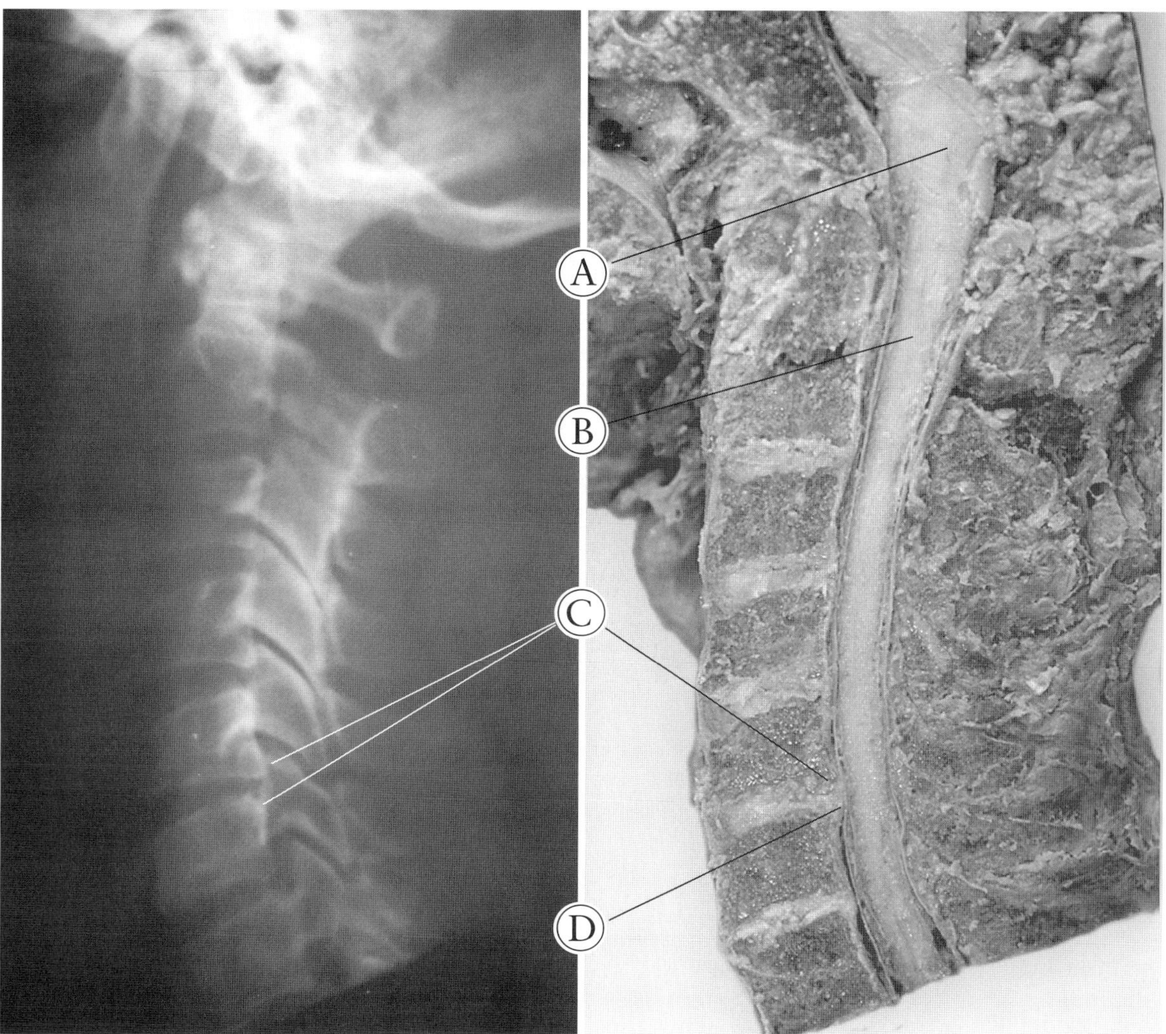

Figure 3-3

This specimen has a reduced canal diameter and a large lower central nervous system. The combination has created a spinal canal stenosis. The brainstem is compressed and there is a hypolordotic or reduced cervical curve. The C5-6 disc bulge is a minor change in the anterior canal wall. C5 and C6 are subluxated and the disc and end plates have remolded and reduced the canal at that point. In this situation a small disc bulge can be clinically significant.

   (A) Brainstem
   (B) Spinal cord
   (C) End plate changes
   (D) C5-6 disc bulge

Head to thorax misalignment can alter the shape of neurological and vascular structures of the neck and their function. This could also happen to the pharynx and larynx which are attached to the anterior longitudinal ligament at the back of the esophagus. **See Figure 3-5.**

The mandible is moved by the muscles of mastication. The inferior muscular groups hold the mandible in place by attachments to the hyoid bone and the sternum and clavicles. Subluxation of the cervical spine can alter that arrangement and normal mandibular motion will be impossible.

The specimens presented are common patterns of subluxation; however, this is not a complete depiction of all types of subluxation.

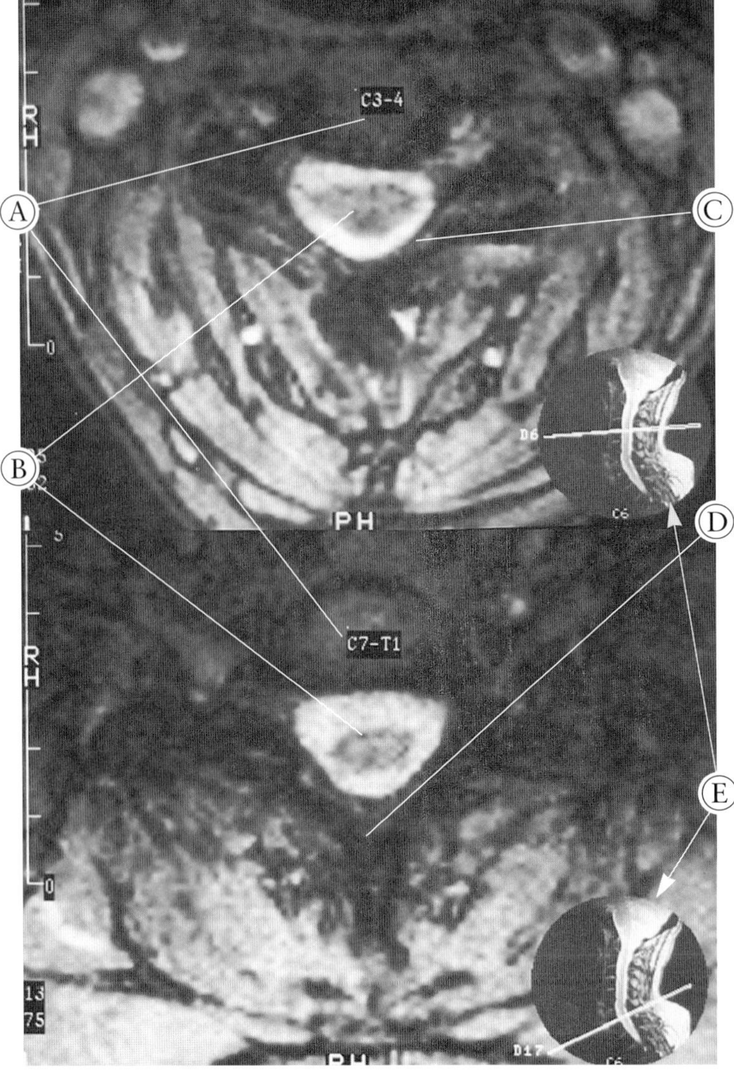

Figure 3-4
Two MRI axial views of the cervical spine. These views show a stretched spinal cord. The upper picture is a view at C3-4. The left to right diameter of the spinal cord is elongated. The dentate ligaments have narrowed and pulled on each side of the spinal cord, making it wider. The lower picture is taken at the C7-T1 level and also shows a widened cord.
- (A) Vertebral body
- (B) Spinal cord
- (C) Lamina
- (D) Spinous process
- (E) Picture key showing the level viewed and angle of scan

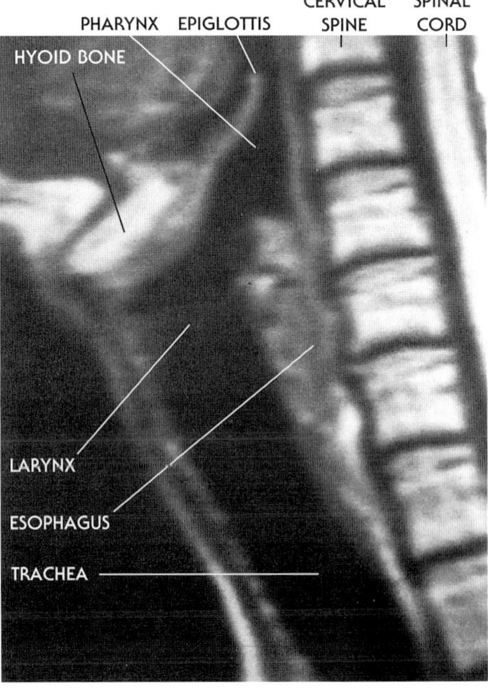

Figure 3-5
Cervical Spine/Soft-Tissue Attachments
The throat: esophagus, hyoid bone, larynx, and other structures attach directly to the anterior of the cervical spine. These structures can be altered in shape and length with head-to-thorax misalignment.

CHAPTER THREE — EXPANDED TABLE OF CONTENTS
Atlas of Subluxations of the Cervical Spine
SECTION I:
Subluxations with lordotic cervical curve (8 pairs)

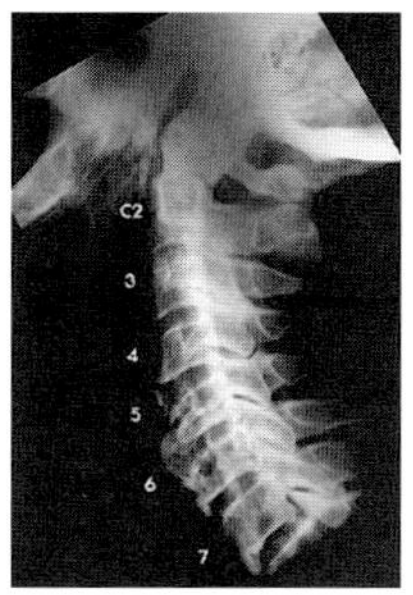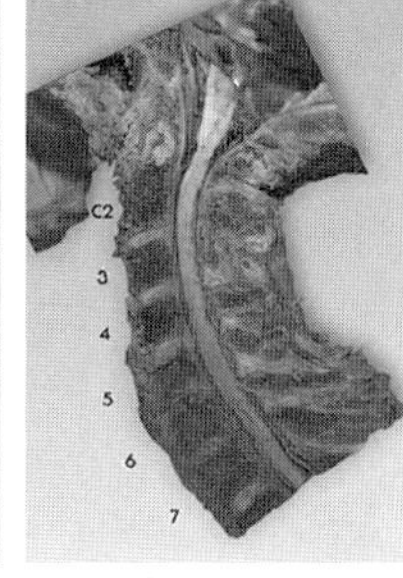

Plates 3-1 A & B
SUBLUXATIONS WITH LORDOTIC
CERVICAL CURVE

Pg. 30-31

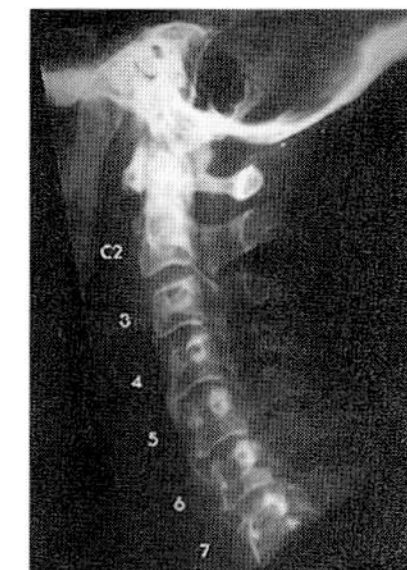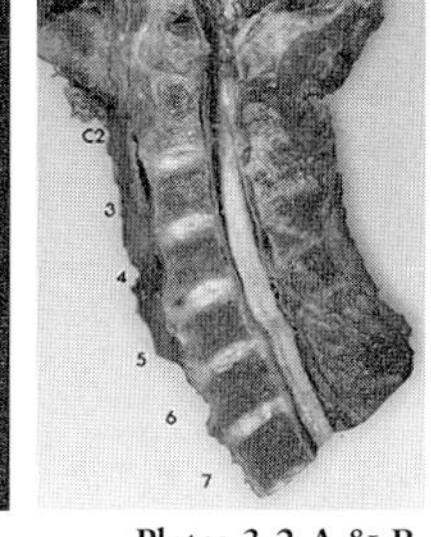

Plates 3-2 A & B
SUBLUXATIONS WITH LORDOTIC
CERVICAL CURVE

Pg. 32-33

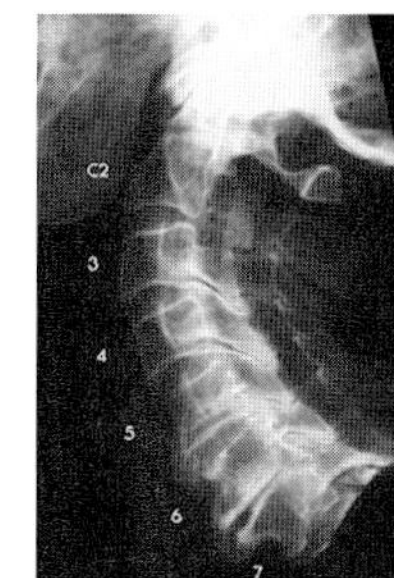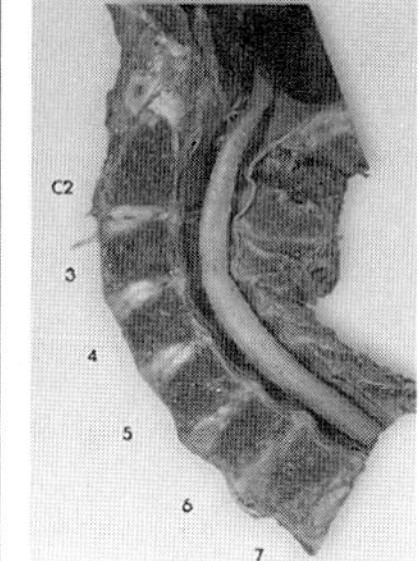

Plates 3-3 A & B
SUBLUXATIONS WITH LORDOTIC
CERVICAL CURVE

Pg. 34-35

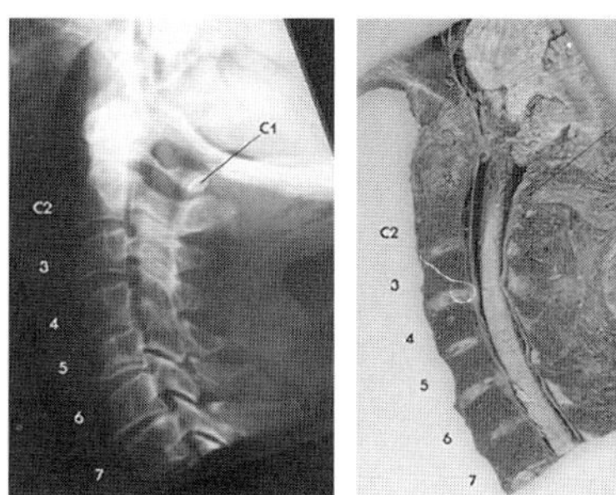

Plates 3-4 A & B
SUBLUXATIONS WITH LORDOTIC
CERVICAL CURVE

Pg. 36-37

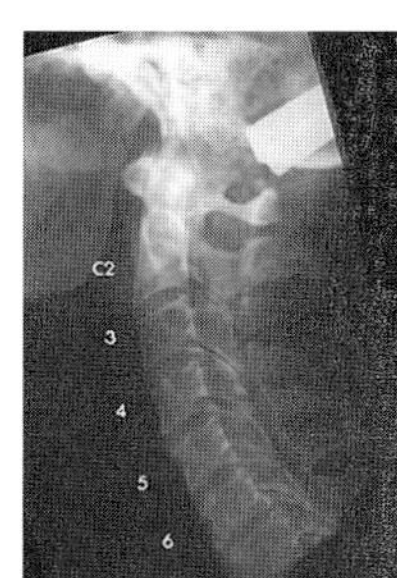

Plates 3-5 A & B
SUBLUXATIONS WITH LORDOTIC
CERVICAL CURVE

Pg. 38-39

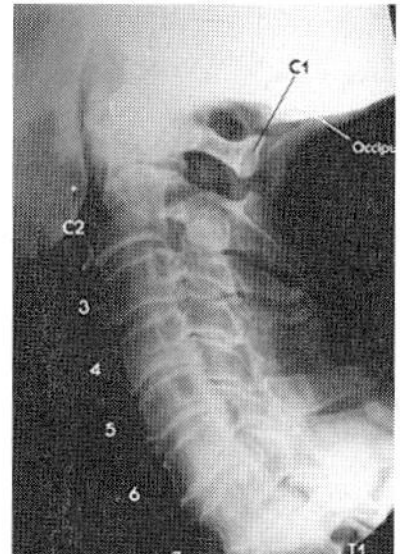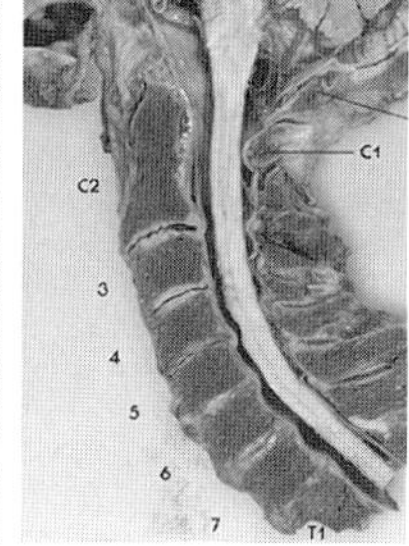

Plates 3-6 A & B
SUBLUXATIONS WITH LORDOTIC
CERVICAL CURVE

Pg. 40-41

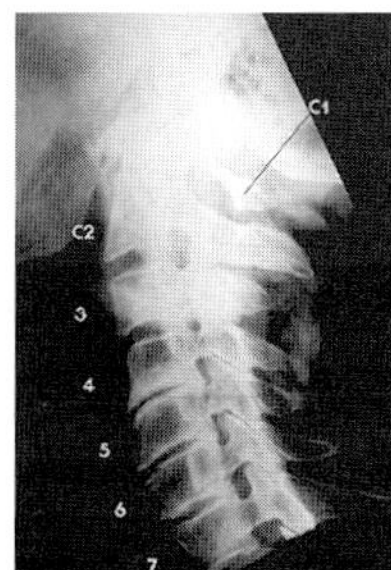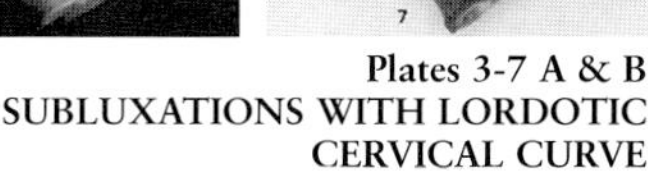

Plates 3-7 A & B
SUBLUXATIONS WITH LORDOTIC
CERVICAL CURVE

Pg. 42-43

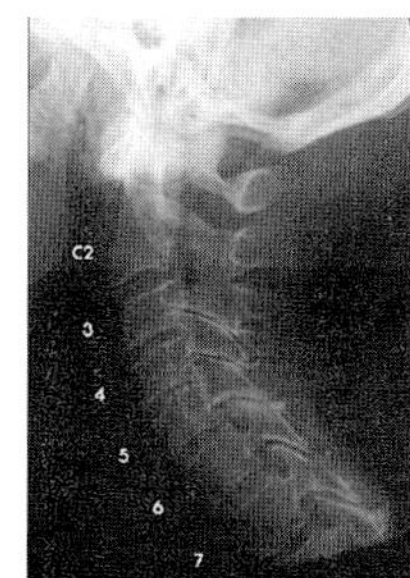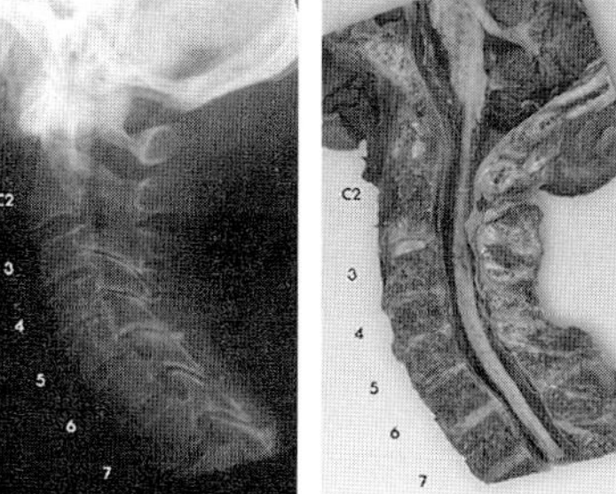

Plates 3-8 A & B
SUBLUXATIONS WITH LORDOTIC
CERVICAL CURVE

Pg. 44-45

CHAPTER THREE — EXPANDED TABLE OF CONTENTS
Atlas of Subluxations of the Cervical Spine
SECTION II:
Subluxations with loss of lordotic curve (straight or military neck) (3 **pairs**)

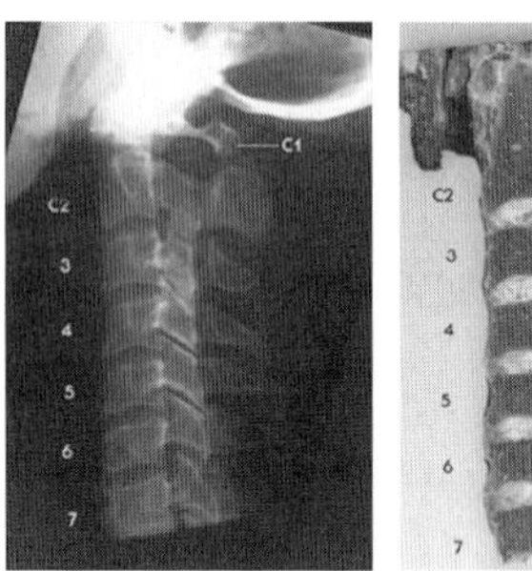

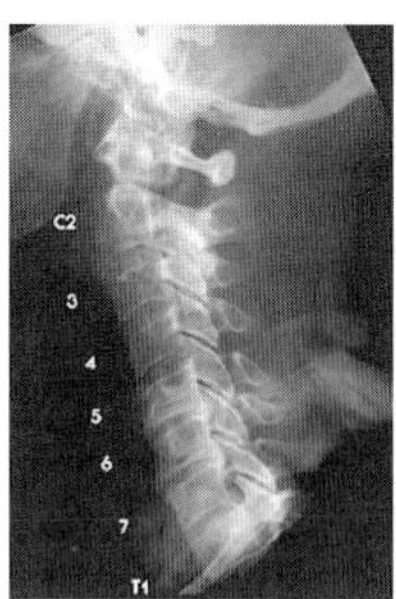

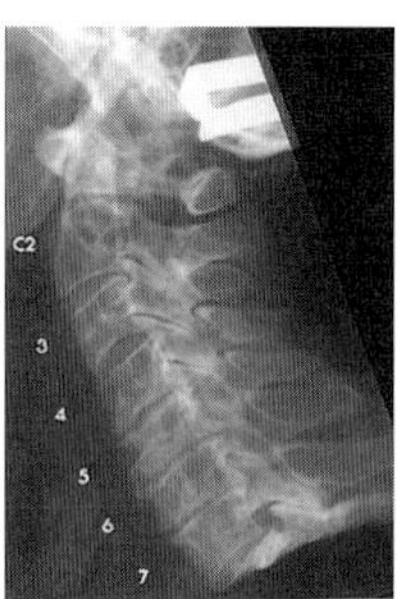

Plates 3-9 A & B
SUBLUXATIONS WITH LOSS OF
LORDOTIC CURVE
(Straight or military neck)
Pg. 46-47

Plates 3-10 A & B
SUBLUXATIONS WITH LOSS OF
LORDOTIC CURVE
(Straight or military neck)
Pg. 48-49

Plates 3-11 A & B
SUBLUXATIONS WITH LOSS OF
LORDOTIC CURVE
(Straight or military neck)
Pg. 50-51

SECTION III:
Subluxations with reversed or kyphotic curve (12 pairs)

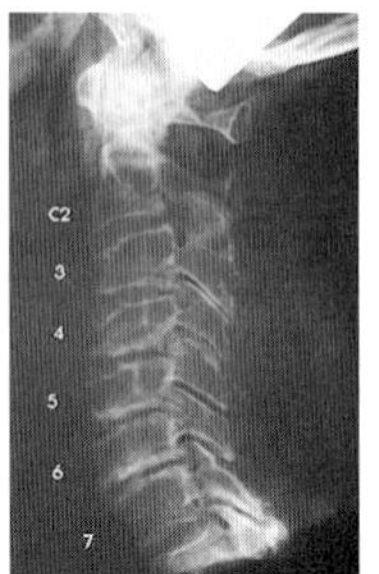

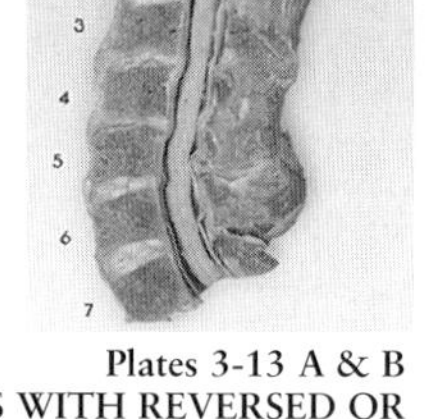

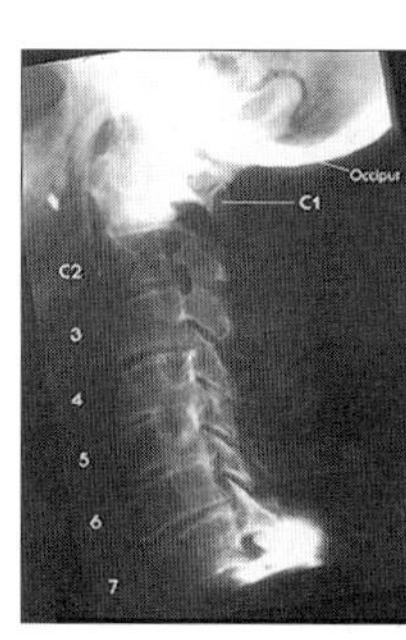

Plates 3-12 A & B
SUBLUXATIONS WITH REVERSED OR
KYPHOTIC CURVE
Upper cervical subluxations
Pg. 52-53

Plates 3-13 A & B
SUBLUXATIONS WITH REVERSED OR
KYPHOTIC CURVE
Upper cervical subluxations
Pg. 54-55

Plates 3-14 A & B
SUBLUXATIONS WITH REVERSED OR
KYPHOTIC CURVE
Upper cervical subluxation
Pg. 56-57

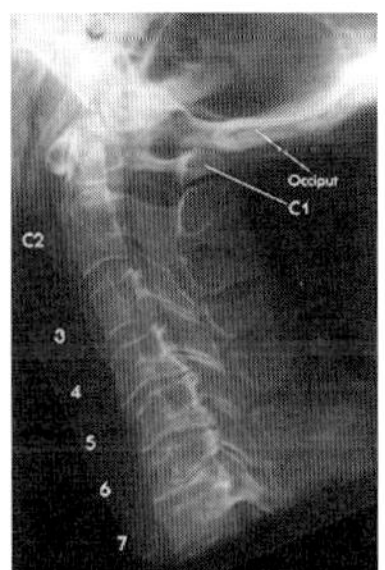

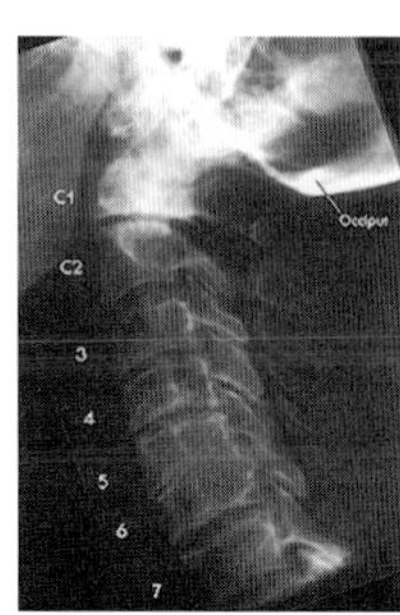

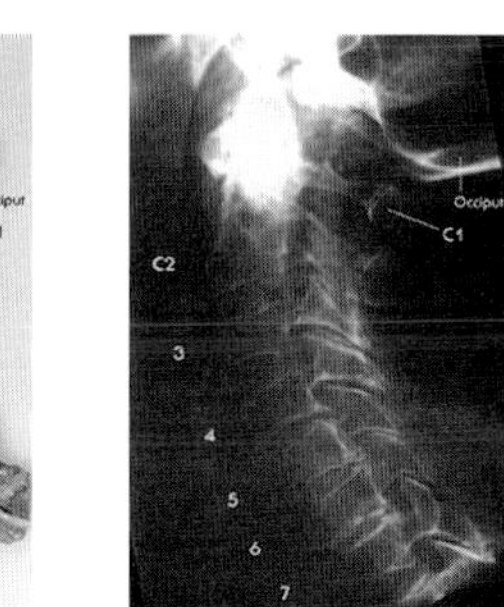

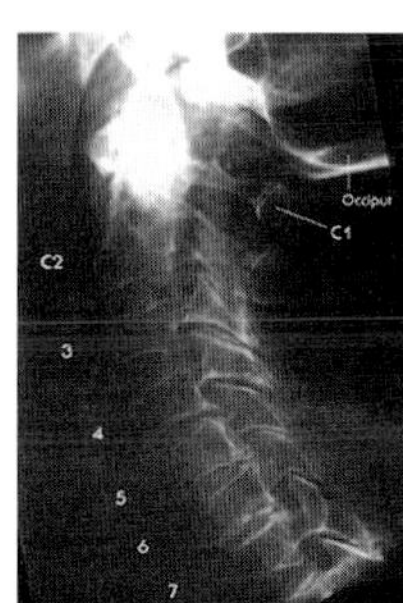

Plates 3-15 A & B
SUBLUXATIONS WITH REVERSED OR
KYPHOTIC CURVE
Mid-cervical subluxations
Pg. 58-59

Plates 3-16 A & B
SUBLUXATIONS WITH REVERSED OR
KYPHOTIC CURVE
Mid-cervical subluxations
Pg. 60-61

Plates 3-17 A & B
SUBLUXATIONS WITH REVERSED OR
KYPHOTIC CURVE
Lower cervical subluxations
Pg. 62-63

CHAPTER THREE — EXPANDED TABLE OF CONTENTS
Atlas of Subluxations of the Cervical Spine

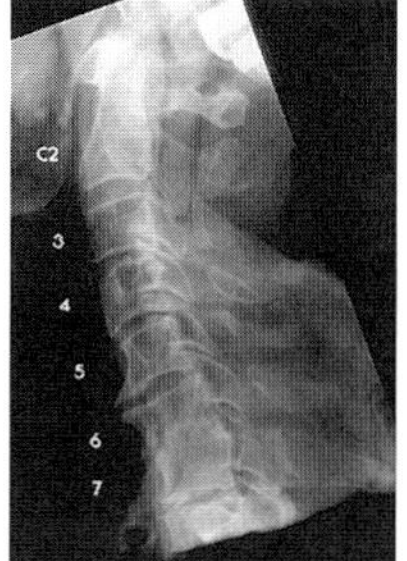 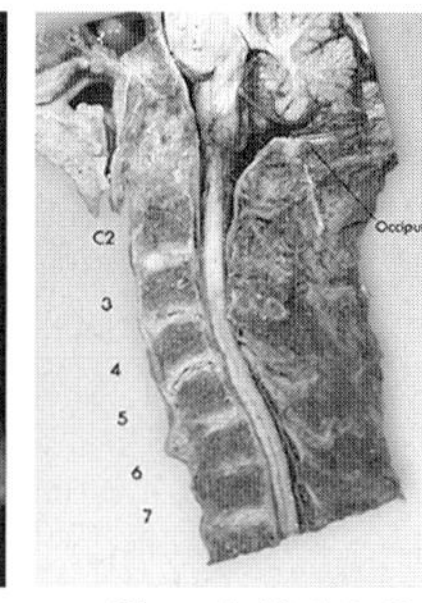

Plates 3-18 A & B
SUBLUXATION WITH REVERSED OR
KYPHOTIC CURVE
Lower cervical subluxations

Pg. 64-65

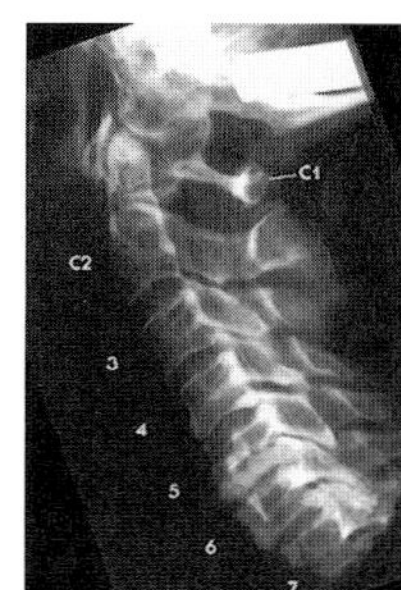 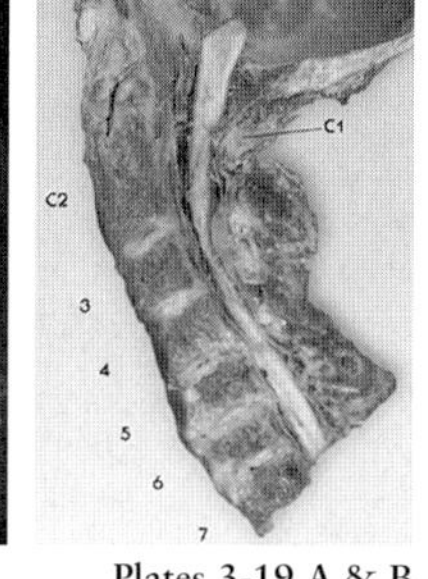

Plates 3-19 A & B
SUBLUXATIONS WITH REVERSED OR
KYPHOTIC CURVE
Lower cervical subluxations

Pg. 66-67

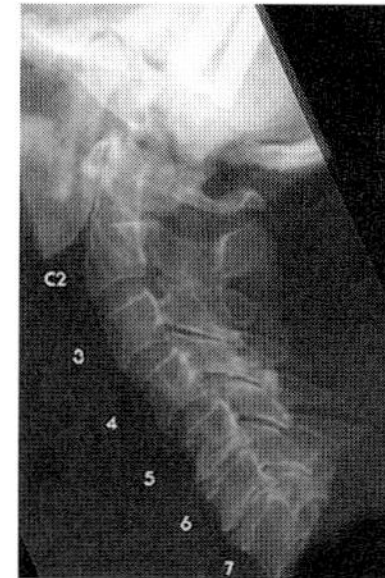 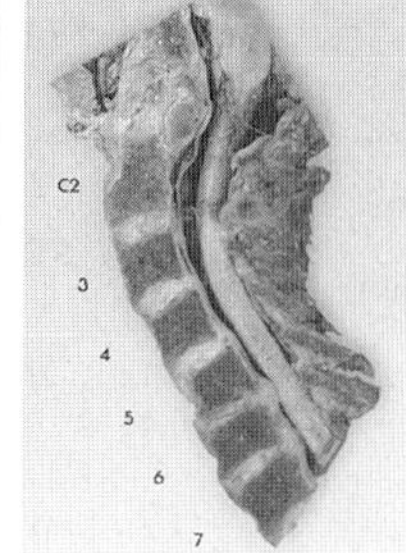

Plates 3-20 A & B
SUBLUXATIONS WITH REVERSAL OR
KYPHOTIC CURVE
Lower cervical subluxations

Pg. 68-69

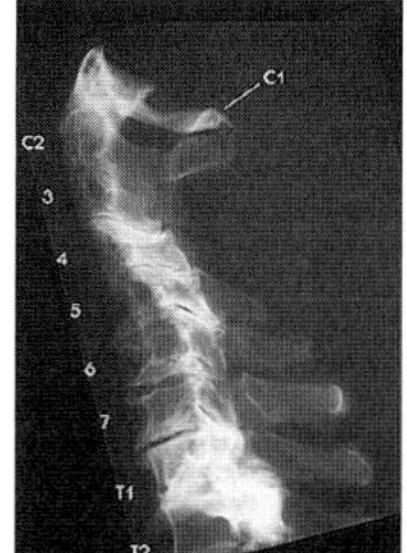 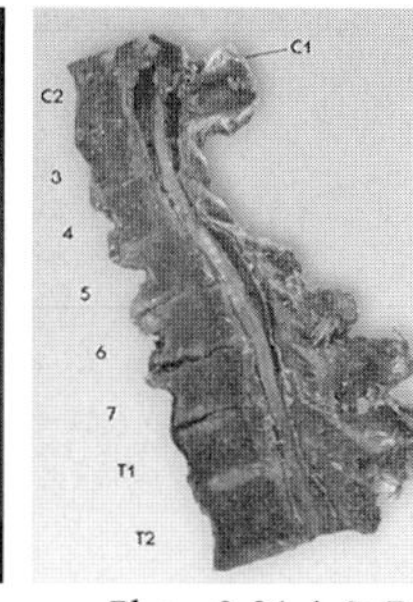

Plates 3-21 A & B
SUBLUXATIONS WITH REVERSED OR
KYPHOTIC CURVE
Mid-cervical subluxations

Pg. 70-71

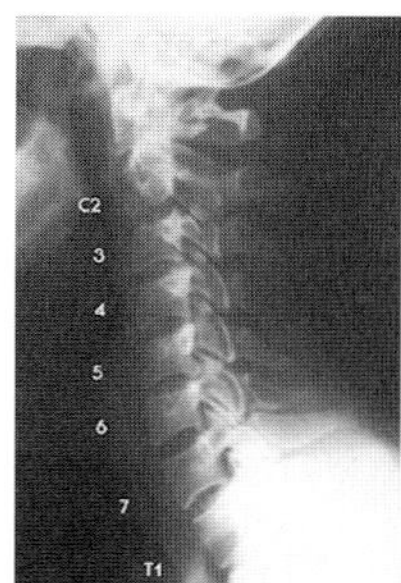

Plates 3-22 A & B
SUBLUXATION WITH REVERSAL OR
KYPHOTIC CURVE
An X-ray and MRI comparison

Pg. 72-73

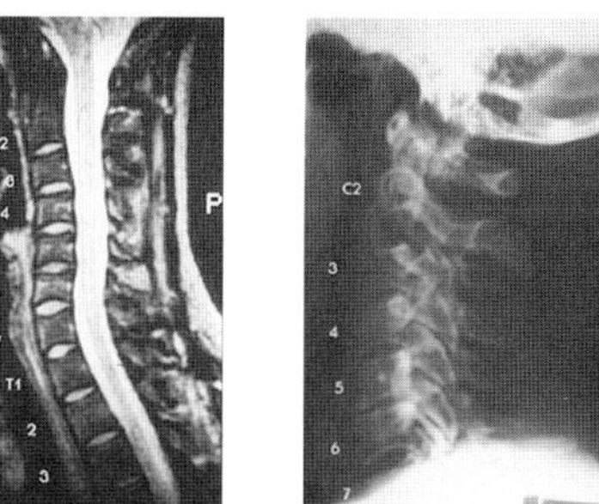 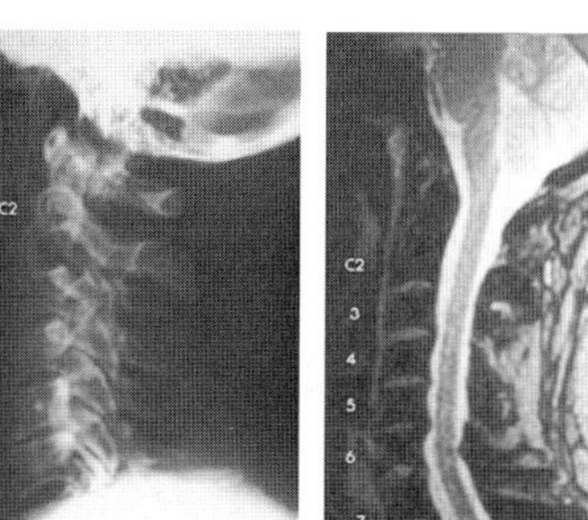

Plates 3-23 A & B
SUBLUXATION WITH REVERSAL OR
KYPHOTIC CURVE
An X-ray and MRI comparison

Pg. 74-75

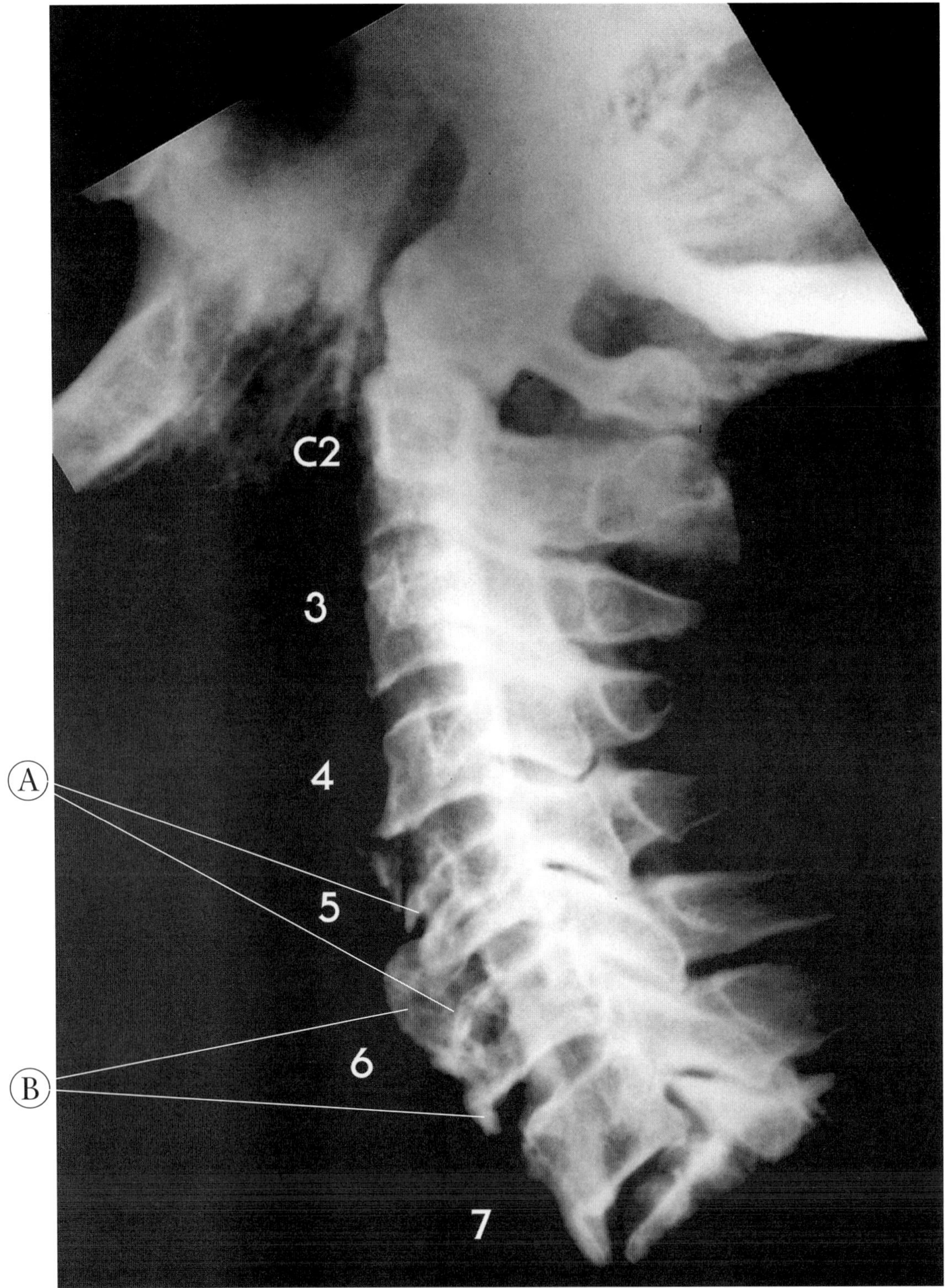

Plates 3-1 A & B

SUBLUXATIONS WITH LORDOTIC CERVICAL CURVE

This is an example of a modest lordotic cervical curve with signs of old trauma. Note the vertebral alignment, congenital stenosis, with virtually no posterior disc bulging. All of the cervical discs are substantial and hydrated despite the signs of old trauma. The discs had plenty of time to degenerate post accident but are healthy. Anterior bulging and spurring have occurred at C4-C5 and C5-C6, along with compression fractures of the C5 and C6 vertebral bodies.

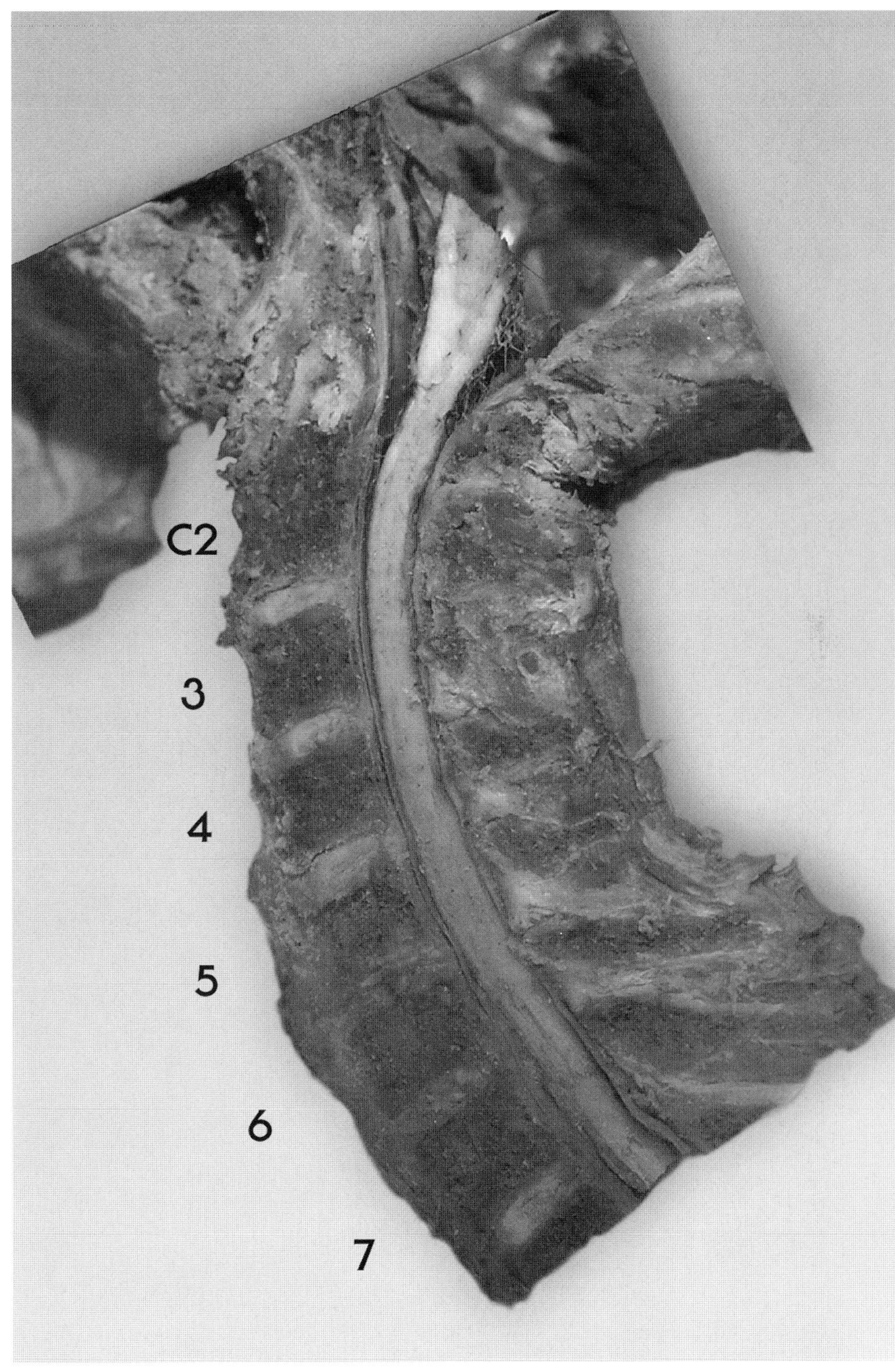

This type of injury is consistent with a fall where the individual lands on their buttocks with head flexing forward violently. (The lumbar damage in this specimen would support this). The main point is the lack of A-P misalignment. All segments except C1 and C2 show very slight stairstepped subluxation; C3 is retro to C4, C4 to C5 to C6 and C6 to C7. However, since the vertebral bodies still share weight-bearing with the facets, disc degeneration has not occurred to a pronounced degree in spite of the traumatic injury.

(A) Compression fractures of anterior vertebral bodies.

(B) Osseous repair and changes indicating old trauma

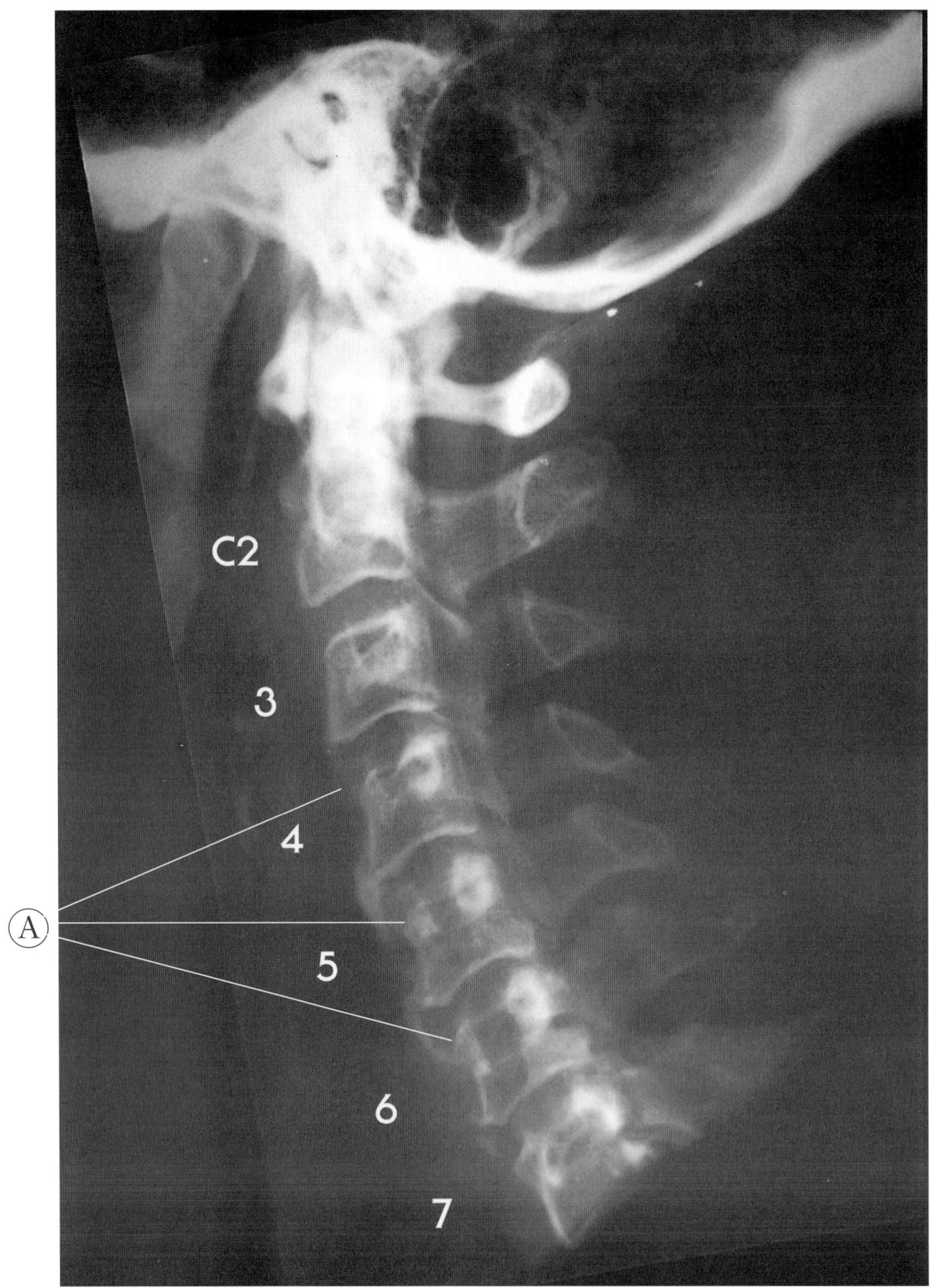

Plates 3-2 A & B
SUBLUXATIONS WITH LORDOTIC CERVICAL CURVE
The modest lordotic curve, despite the signs of trauma and subluxations, has allowed some normal weight bearing.

This specimen shows vertebral canal stenosis at the subluxated portion of the spine and stairstepped retrolisthesis from C3 through C5, with complete retrolisthesis of C6 (to C5 and C7).

(A) The vertebral bodies at C4, C5 and C6 appear to have been anteriorly crushed;

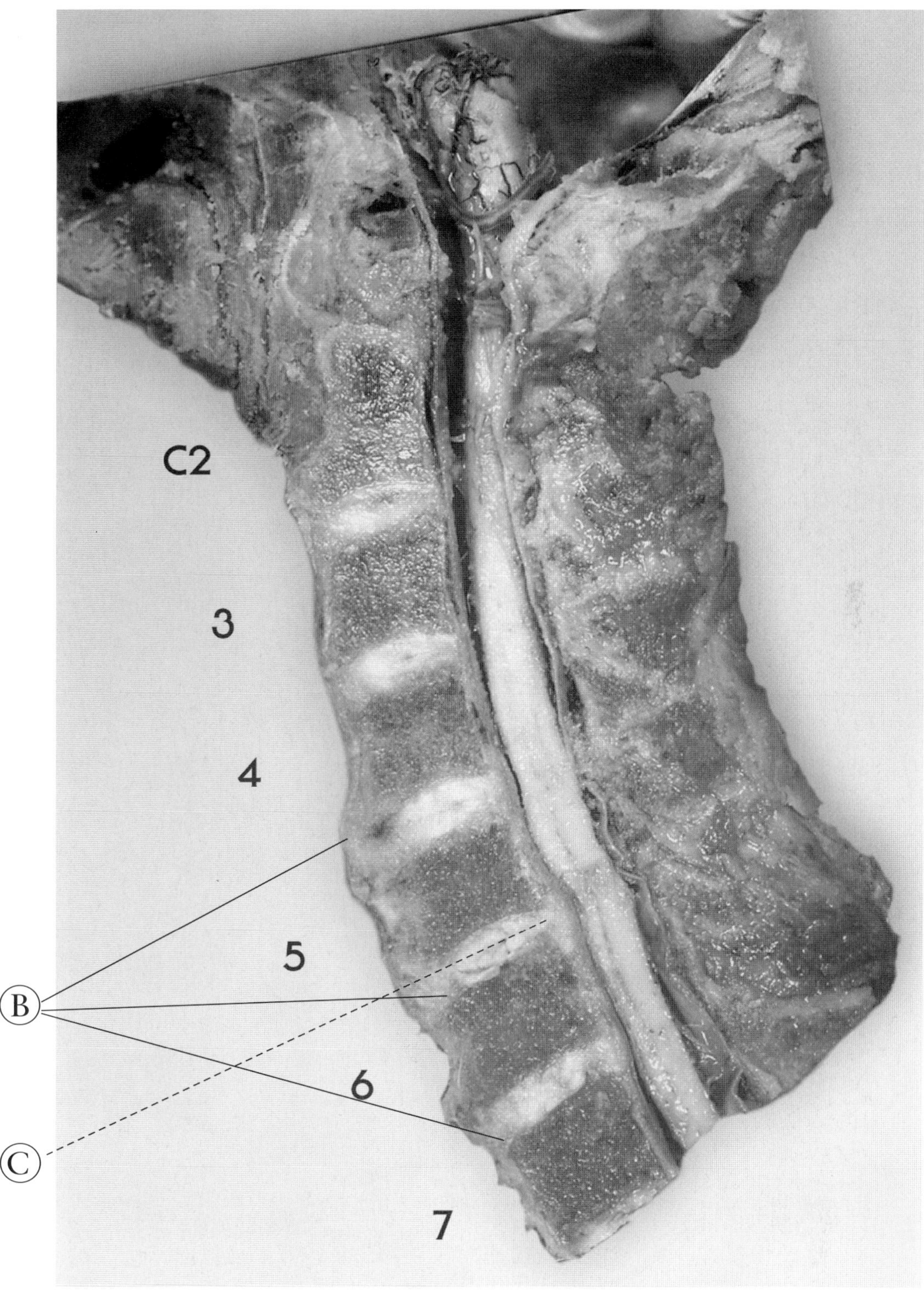

(B) The discs have bulged anteriorly and calcification of the anterior longitudinal ligament has occurred at C4-C5, C5-C6, and C6-C7. A traumatic flexion event such as a head-on collision may have caused these injuries.
In spite of the trauma, the discs are all present and hydrated.

(C) The only significant disc damage is at C5-C6, where tearing and posterior bulging have occurred (Phase II degeneration). The bulge impinges dramatically on the spinal cord, so it was probably of clinical significance to the individual.

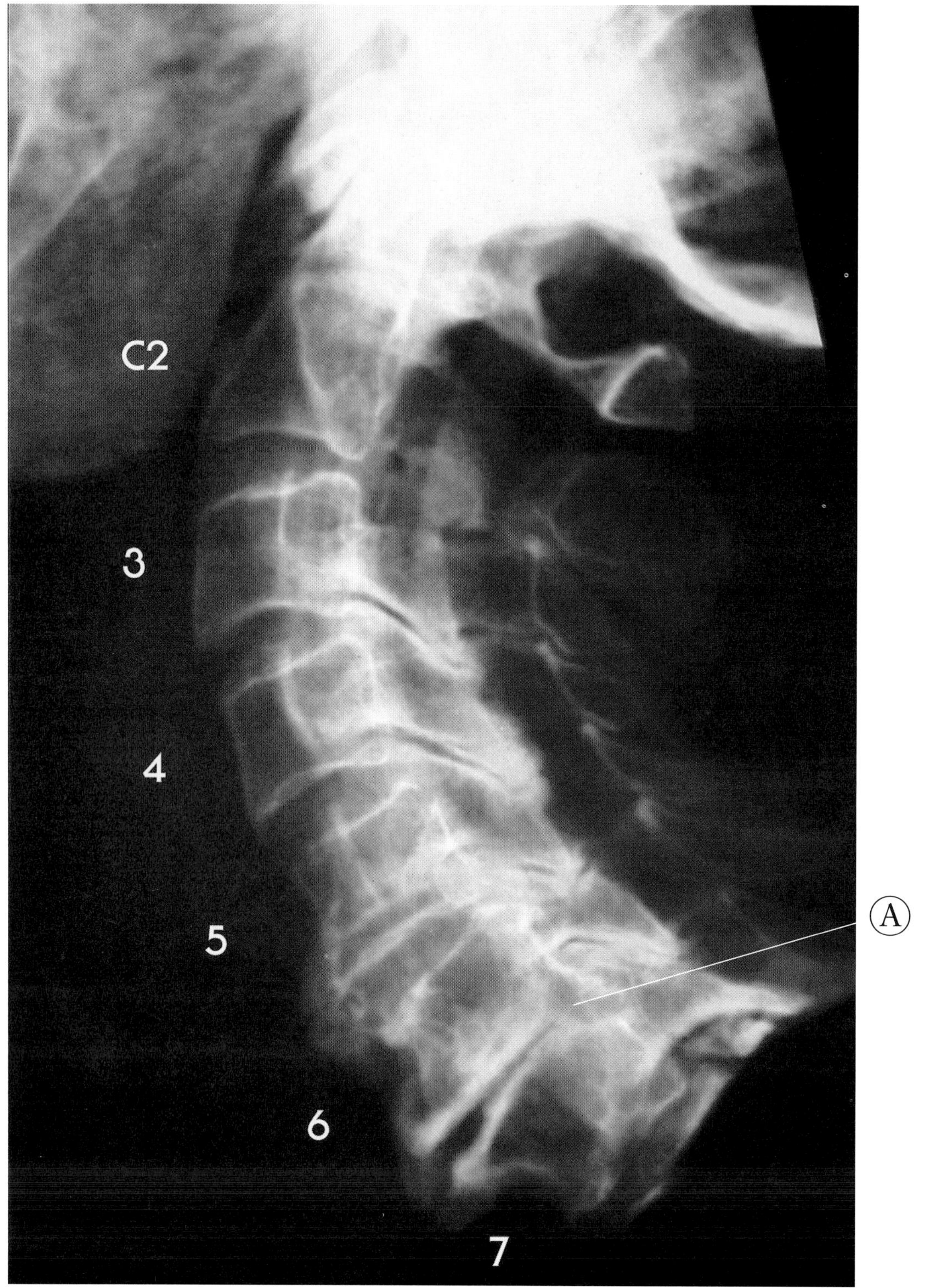

Plates 3-3 A & B
SUBLUXATIONS WITH LORDOTIC CERVICAL CURVE

In this view, the curve is maintained, with the subluxation and damage at each segment with disc bulging clinically insignificant. There are slight subluxations at all levels with loss of posterior disc height at every segment and loss of facetal joint space with eburnation (hypertrophy) of facets. Note that the loss of interspinous space-spinous contact can cause bony changes. This is secondary to the loss of the posterior disc height.

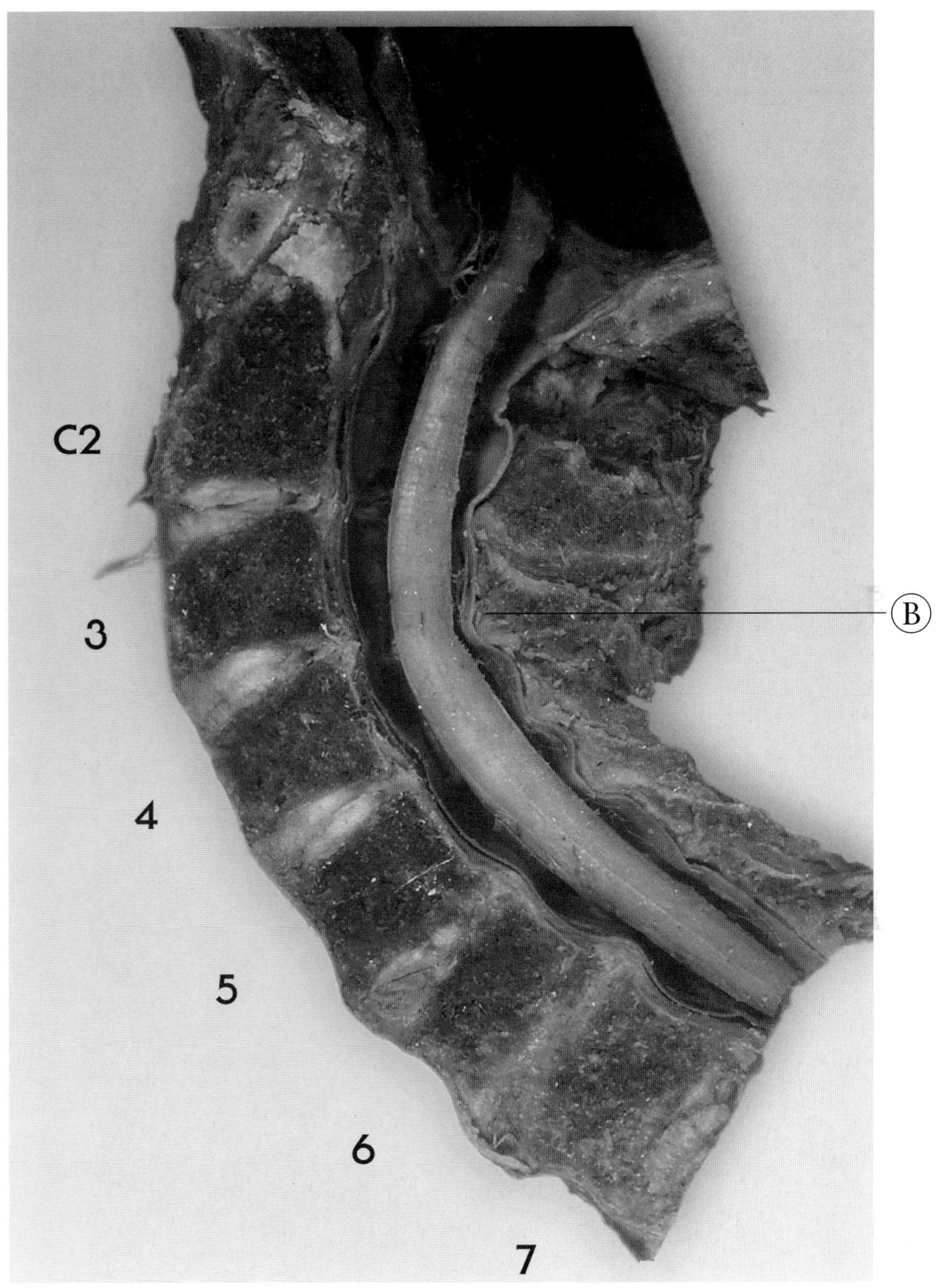

(A) Note: fusion of posterior of vertebral bodies of C6 and C7 forming a permanent protrusion into the vertebral canal.

(B) Ligamentum flavum protrusion and cord contact at C3-4 can be associated with loss of disc height, wedging, and subluxation.

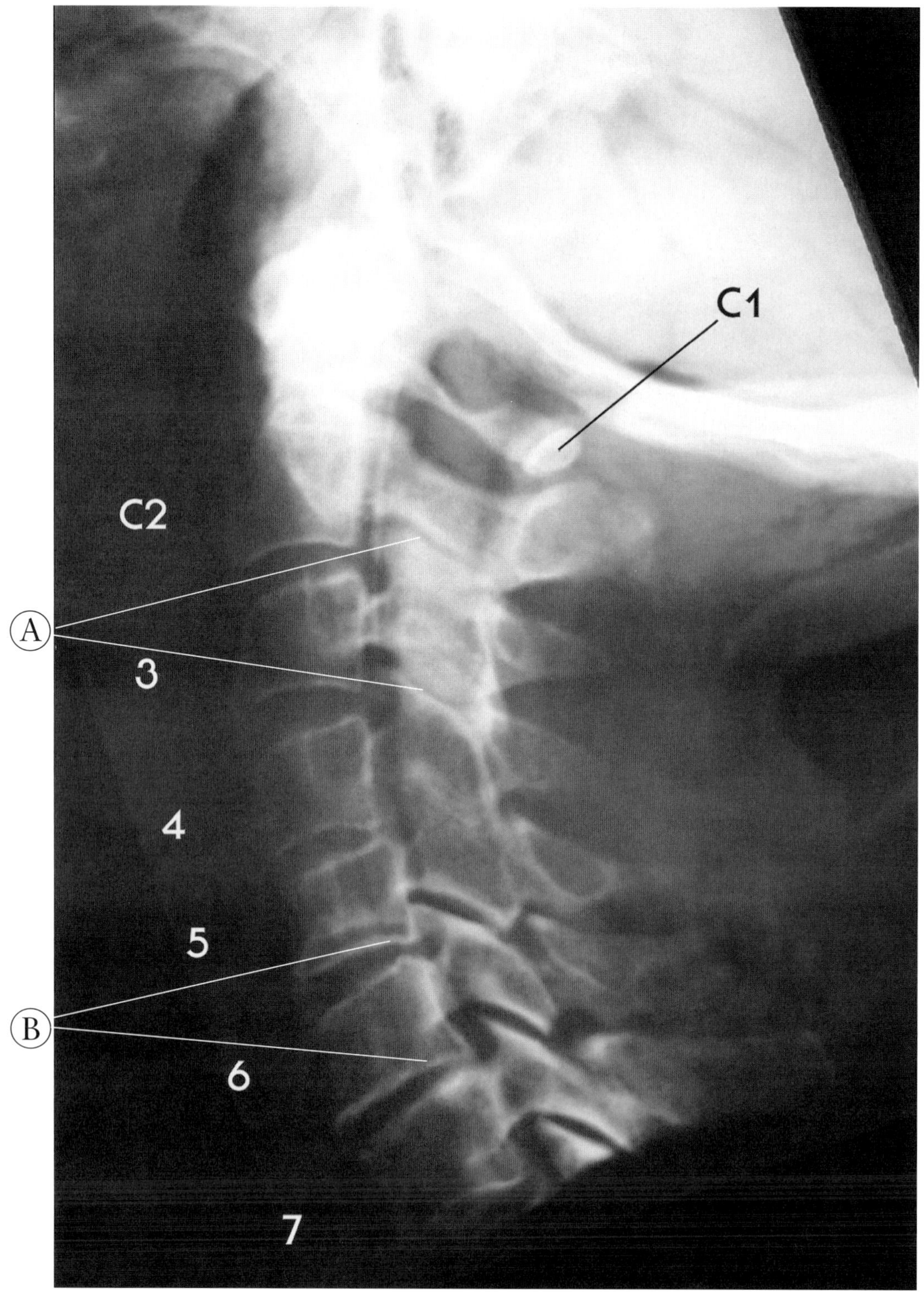

Plates 3-4 A & B
SUBLUXATIONS WITH LORDOTIC CERVICAL CURVE

The curve is somewhat maintained with C1 anterior to C2; C3 retro to C2 with disc tearing; C3-C4 looks all right with slight disc tearing; C5 is retro to C4 (x-ray looks worse) disc tearing with some brown degeneration with loss of disc height; C6 slight retro to C5 with disc tearing and bulging anterior and posterior; C7 retro to C6 with posterior spurring, disc tearing, and brown degeneration, posterior joint changes. The cerebellum and brain stem can be drawn down into the

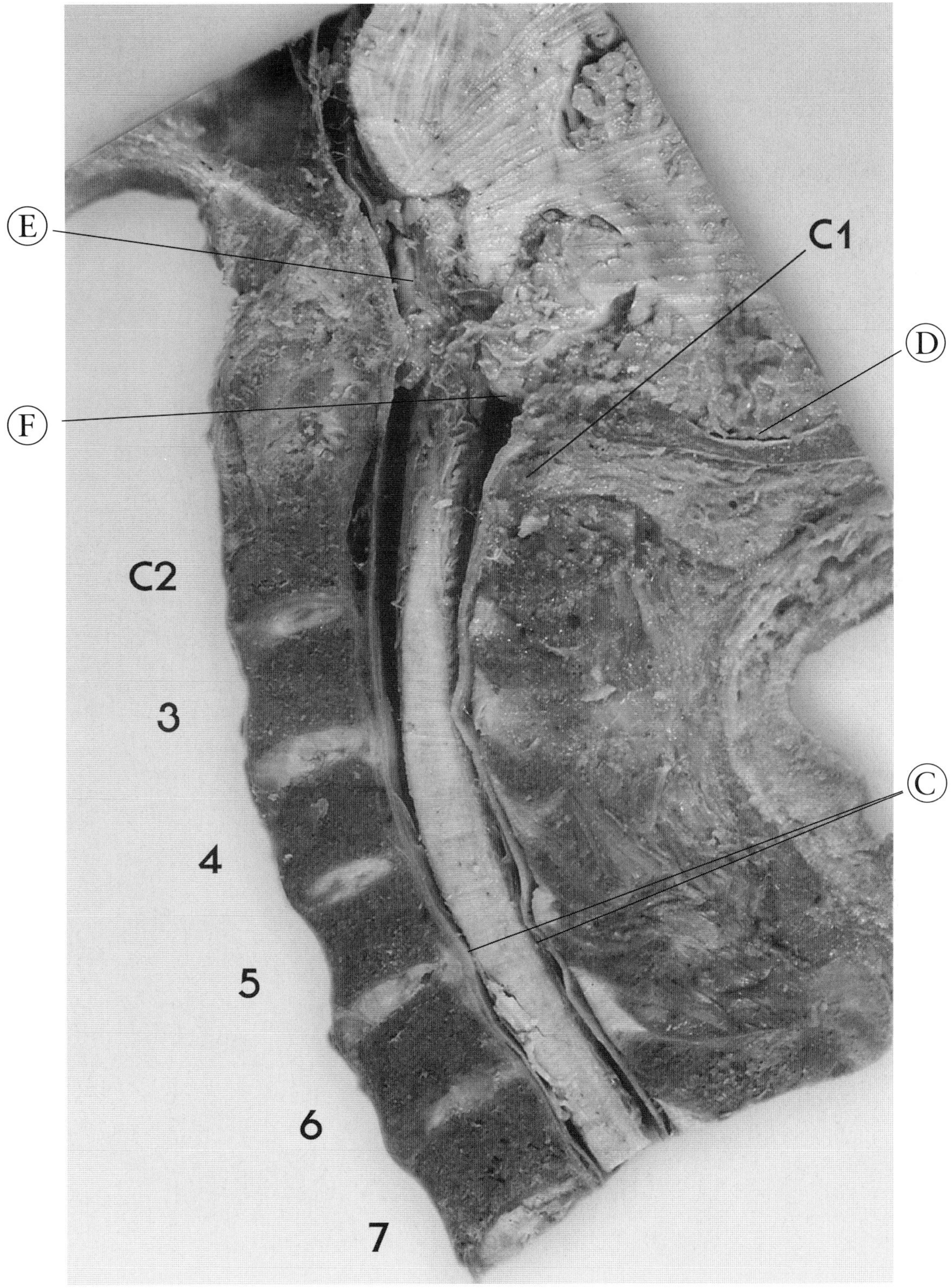

base of the occiput causing arterial compression and cerebellar invagination into the spinal canal.

(A) C2-4 has little curve and loss of facet joint space.
(B) Inferior end plate widening is the hallmark of hyper loading the vertebral body and disc.
(C) Canal stenosis is the result of the widened endplates and bulging disc.
(D) Note cerebellar compression into occiput.
(E) Brain stem contact with the clivus.
(F) Cerebellum invaginating through the foramen magnum.

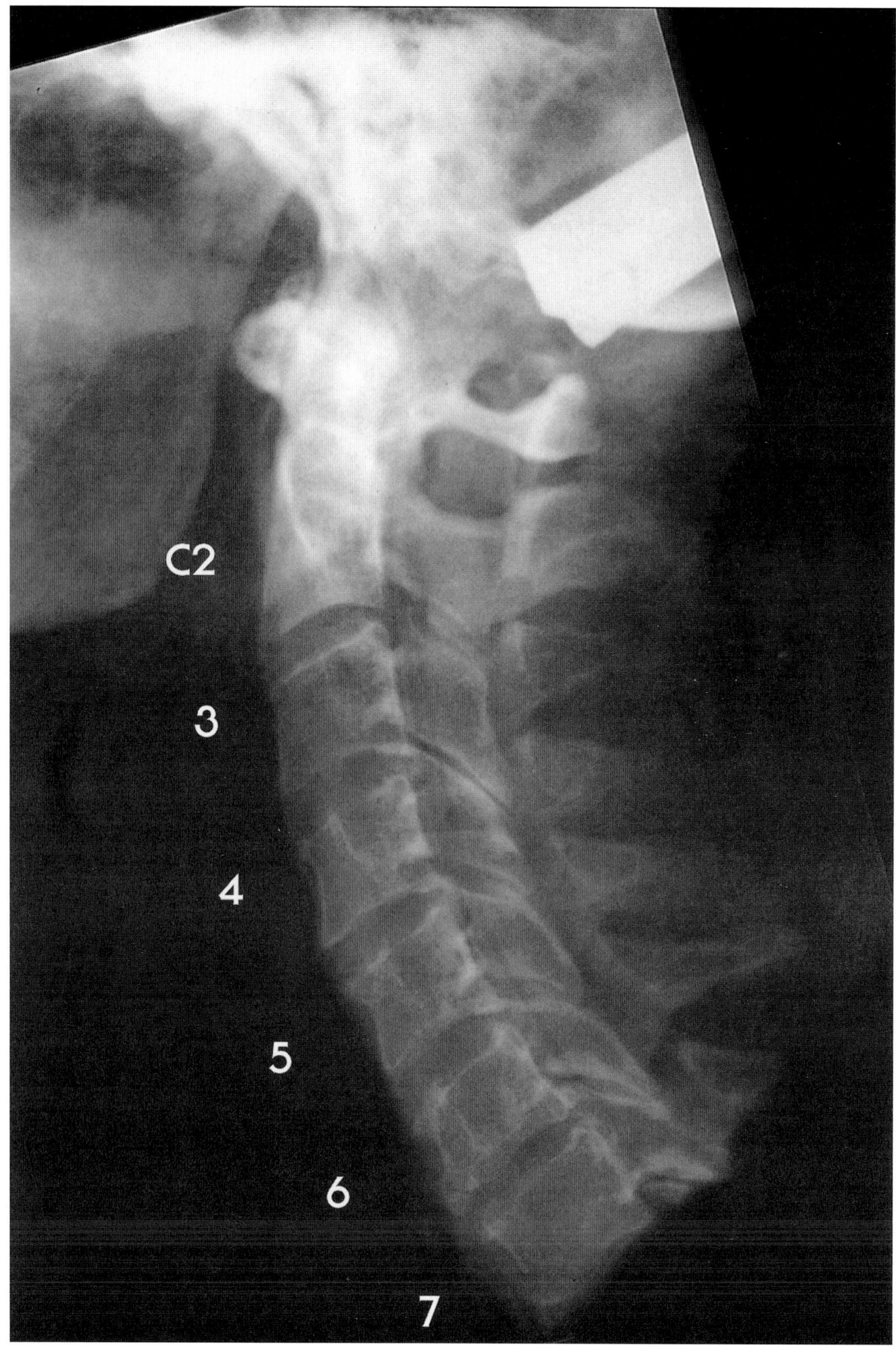

Plates 3-5 A & B
SUBLUXATIONS WITH LORDOTIC CERVICAL CURVE
Minor stairstepped retrolisthesis has occurred which developed posterior spurs and some disc bulging, but the normal lordotic curve has prevented major canal changes.

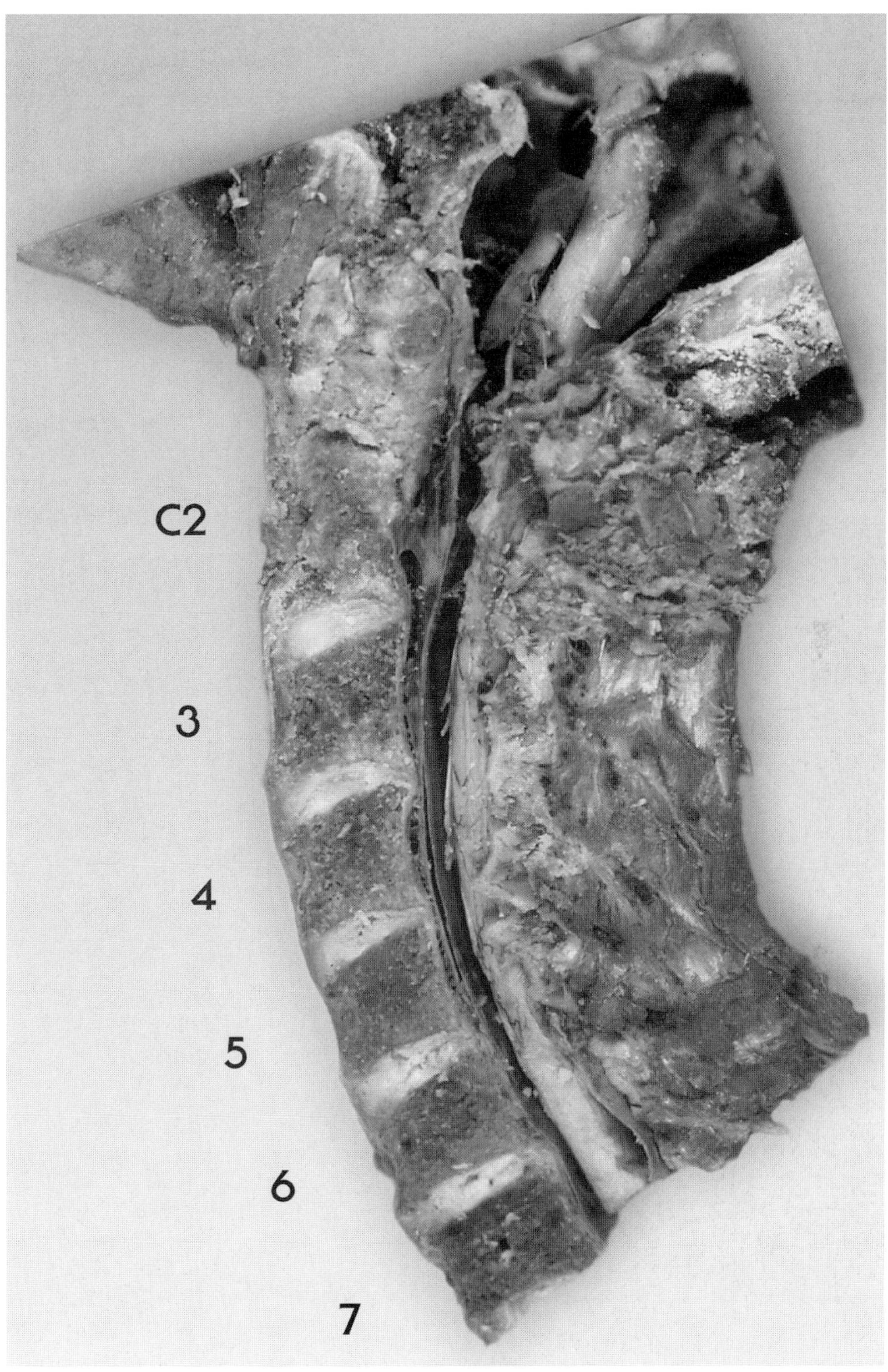

C3 is retro to C4, C4 to C5, C5 to C6, and C6 to C7. Slight posterior bulging and loss of posterior disc height is visible between all segments, and an anterior bulge can be seen at C6-C7. Deformation of the vertebral bodies indicates altered weight bearing beginning at C4.

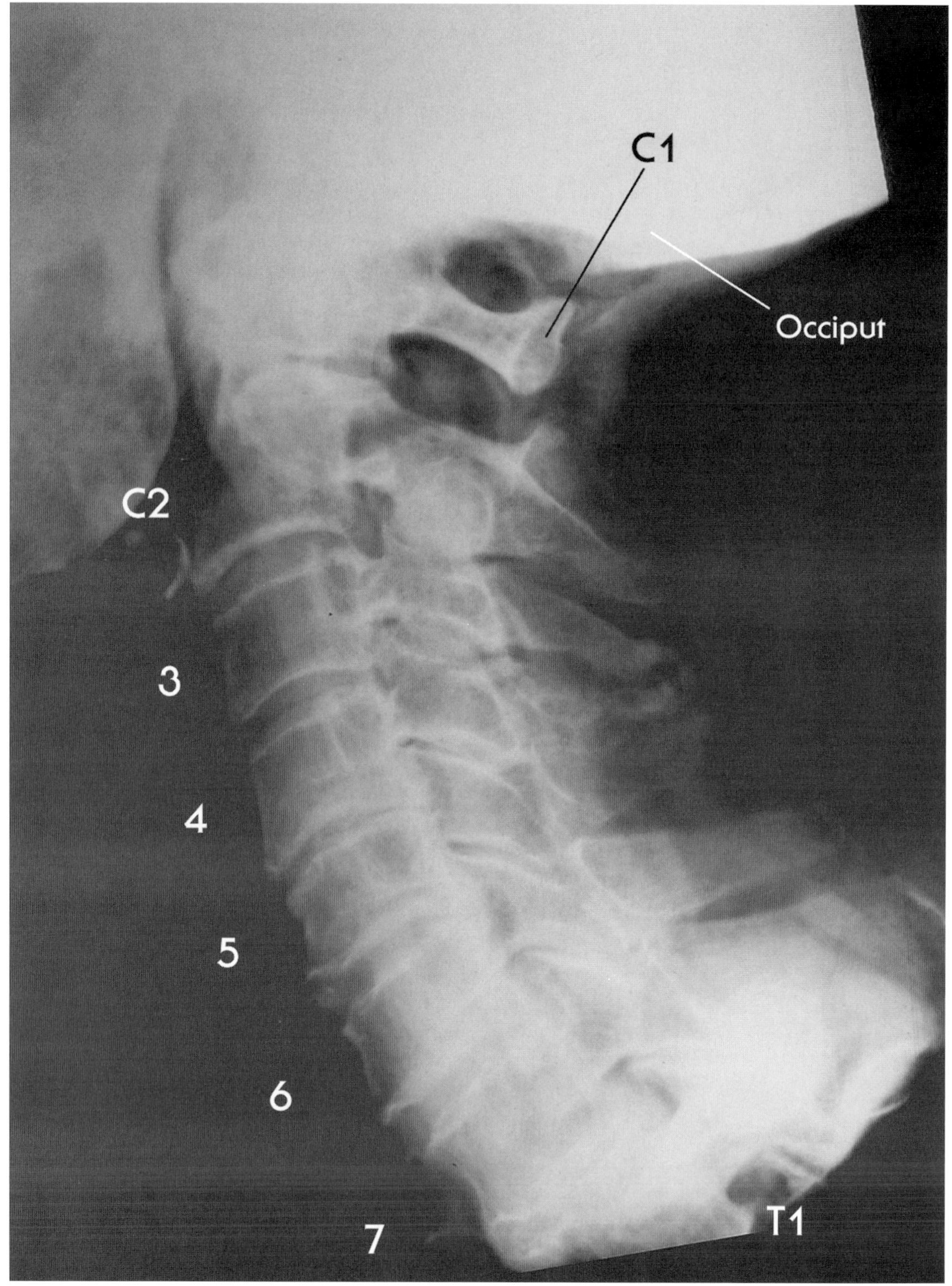

Plates 3-6 A & B
SUBLUXATIONS WITH LORDOTIC CERVICAL CURVE
This specimen shows relatively slight subluxations at every segment, with accompanying disc degeneration. C1 is anterior to the occiput and C2, and C3 is retro to C2 and C4 (complete retrolisthesis). C4 is slightly retro to C5, and C6 is anterior to both C5 and C7 (complete anterolisthesis).

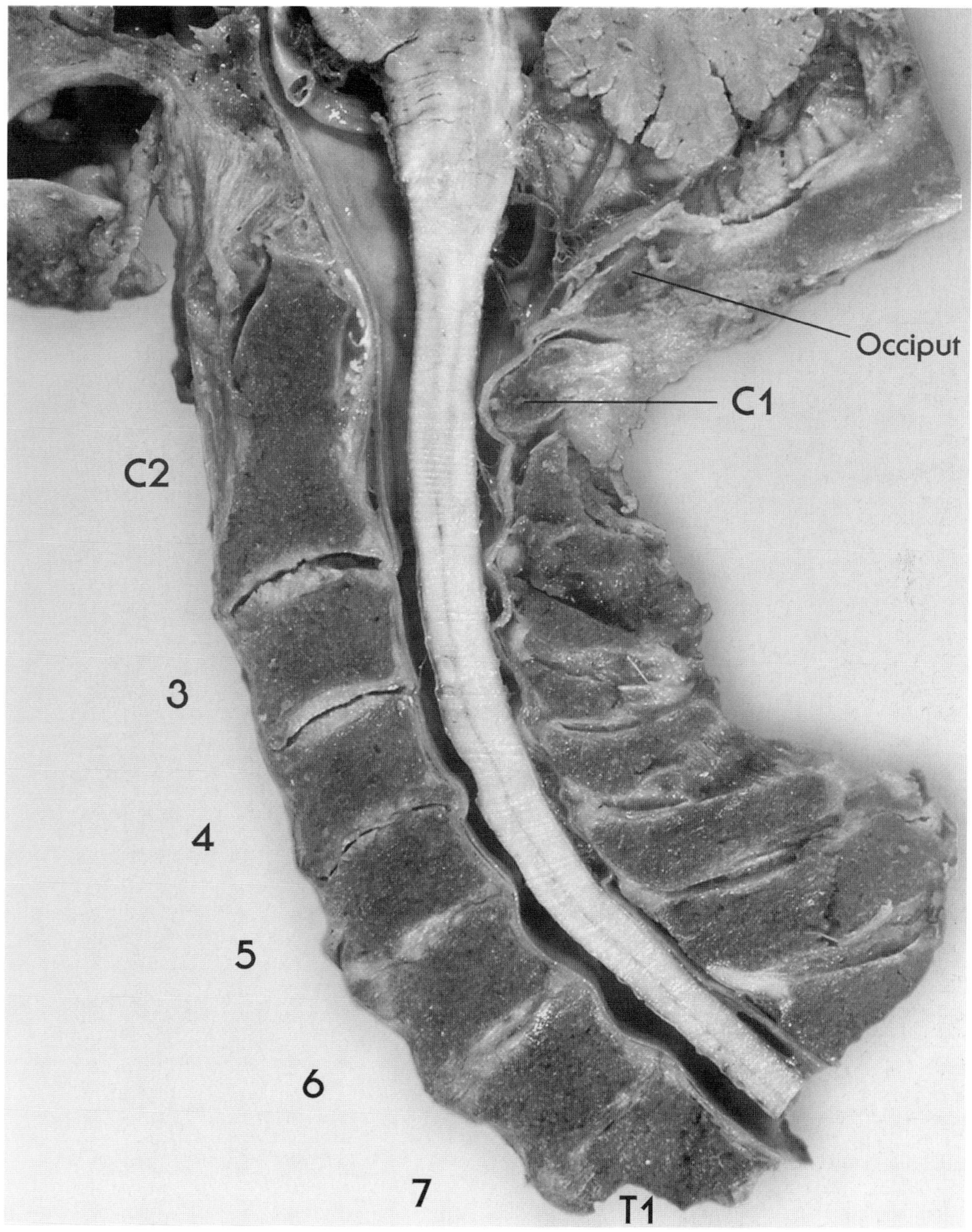

Note that the cervical lordotic curve has been maintained, indicating that the facets are still weight-bearing. Approximation of the spinous processes has occurred with loss of disc height and cavitation. Spurring has occurred in the lower segments, and the canal stenosis is minor. Encroachment on the spinal cord has occurred only at C4-C5 and perhaps slightly at C5-C6, and none of the segments have fused.

Anterior spurring is visible at C4-C5, C5-C6, and C6-C7, and a disc tear can be seen on the X-ray at C3-C4. Disc tears, even prominent ones (e.g., the disc between C2 and C3) may or may not show up on X-ray; however, they do appear on MRIs.

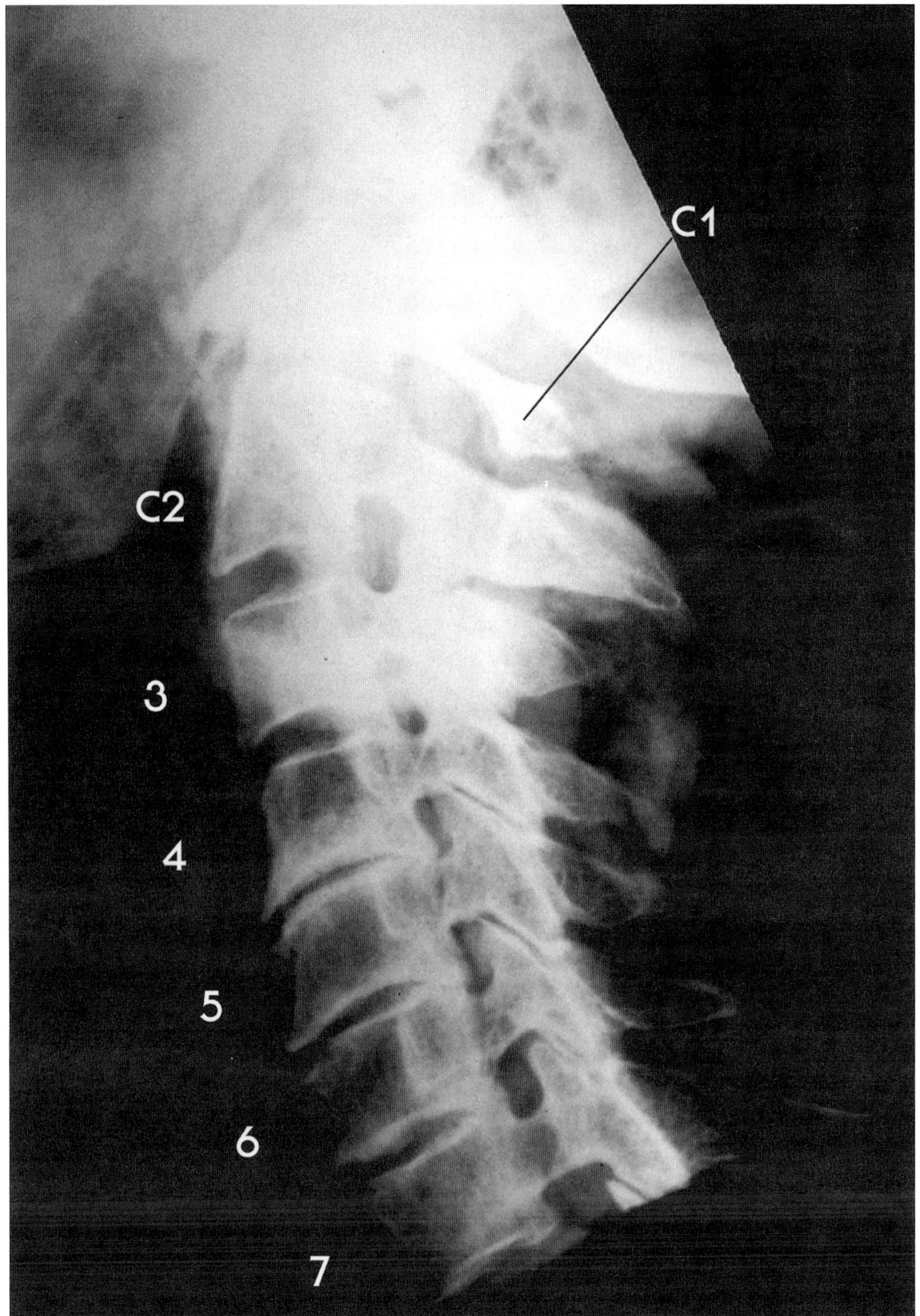

Plates 3-7 A & B

SUBLUXATIONS WITH LORDOTIC CERVICAL CURVE

This specimen has a moderate lordotic curve with significant disc degeneration and spurring at the subluxated segments. There is also cord contact from C3 to C5 with compression of the anterior cord at C4-5.

C1 is anterior; C4 is a complete retrolisthesis to C3 and 5; tearing of C3-4 disc; but near fusion with spurring posterior and anterior; note tearing or fissure of C4-5; C5 retro C6 with tearing

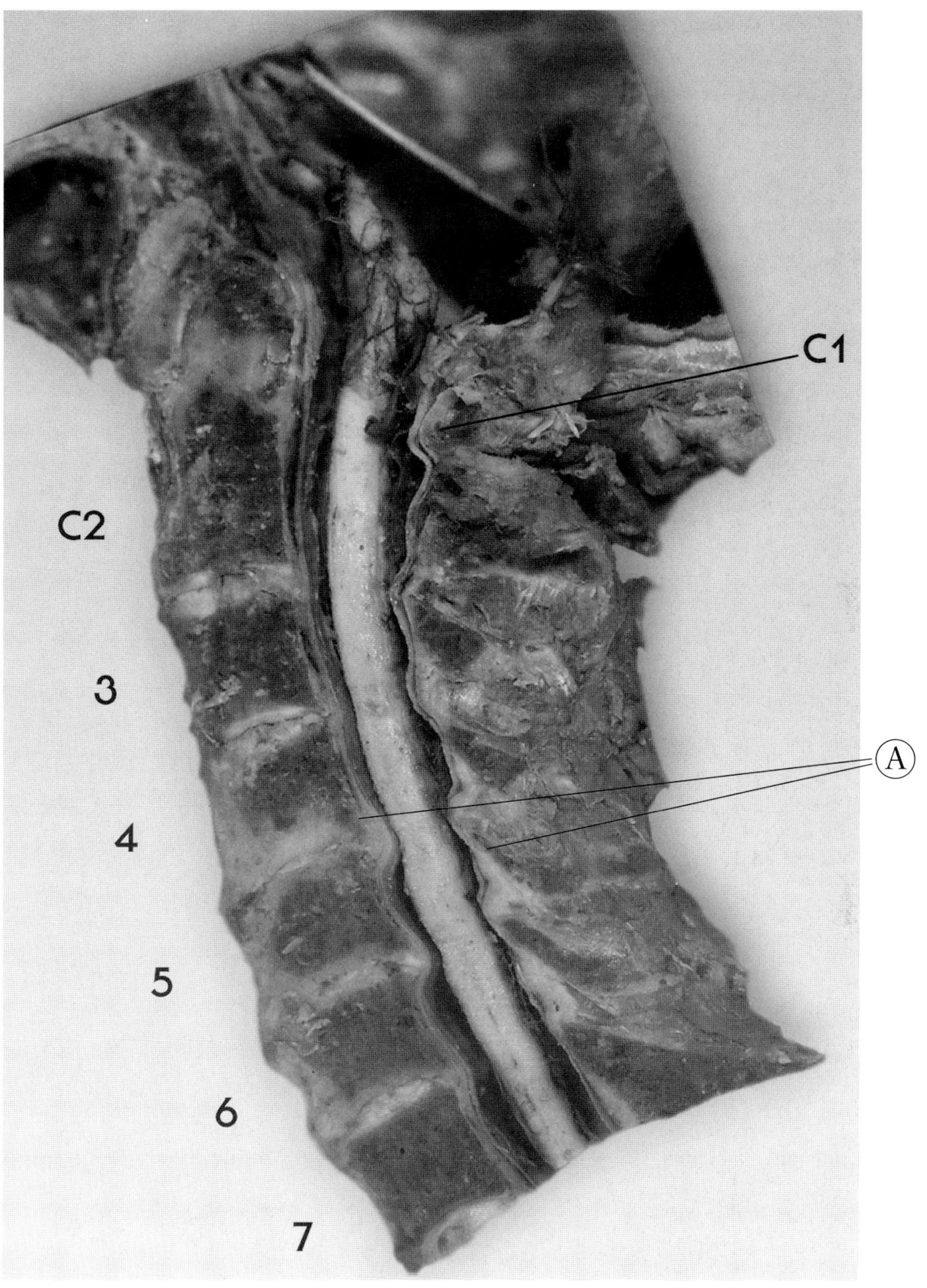

and spurring; C6 retro to C7 with fusion of posterior C6-7 tearing of disc without bulge of C7 superior endplate; moderate canal stenosis with C4-5 disc bulge significant with flexion; also with C5-6 slight significance with flexion.

(A) C4 posterior body retro to C3-5 moves closer to lamina of C5, stenosis is worsened.

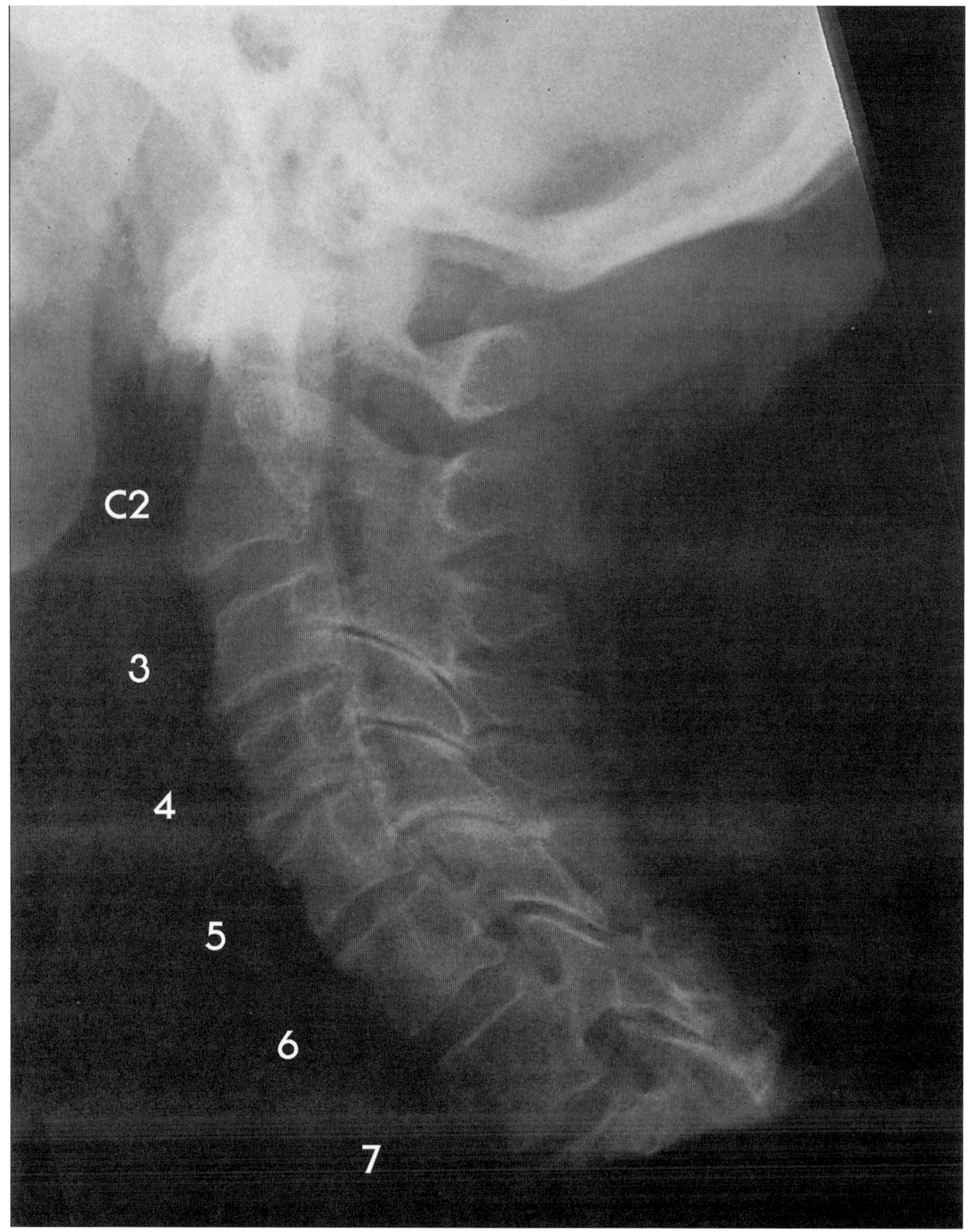

Plates 3-8 A & B

SUBLUXATIONS WITH LORDOTIC CERVICAL CURVE

Most commonly, injuries to the cervical spine occur at the C5-C6 and C6-C7 discs, which have the greatest capability for anteroposterior movement and which, being farthest from the head, are the most vulnerable to whiplash. Occasionally, however, injuries specifically affect the mid-cervical vertebrae and discs.

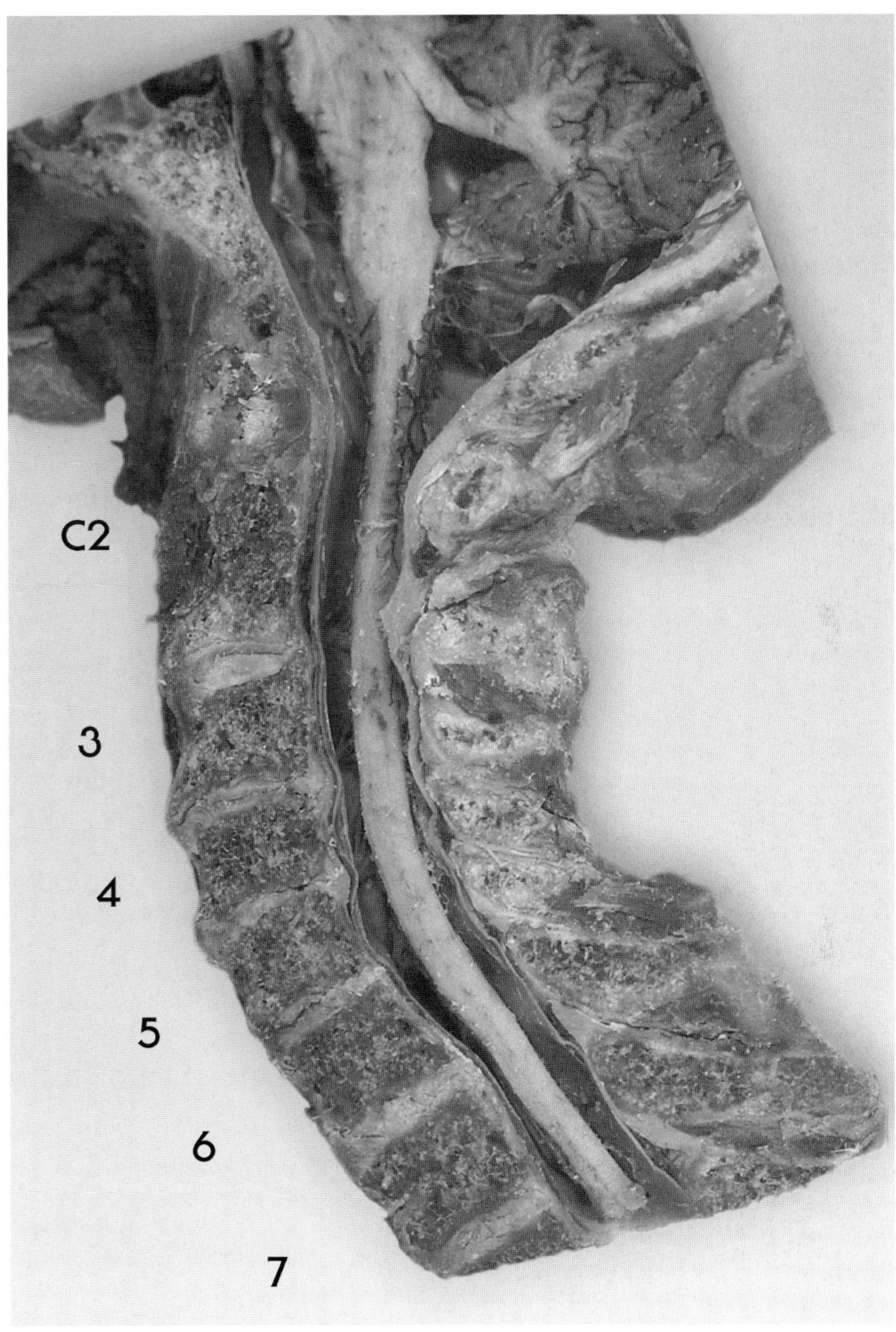

Almost all segments are subluxated; C3 is a complete retro (to C2 and C4), C4 is completely antro (to C3 and C5), and C6 is completely retro (to C5 and C7). Disc tearing and bulging is evident throughout, and is most pronounced from C3-C4 through C5-C6, but because the lordotic curve has been maintained, stenosis of the vertebral canal is minor and the disc bulges do not impinge upon the spinal cord, although close at C6-7 disc. Spinous processes of C4-6 have approximated because of disc height loss and the facets have been affected by the altered weight bearing.

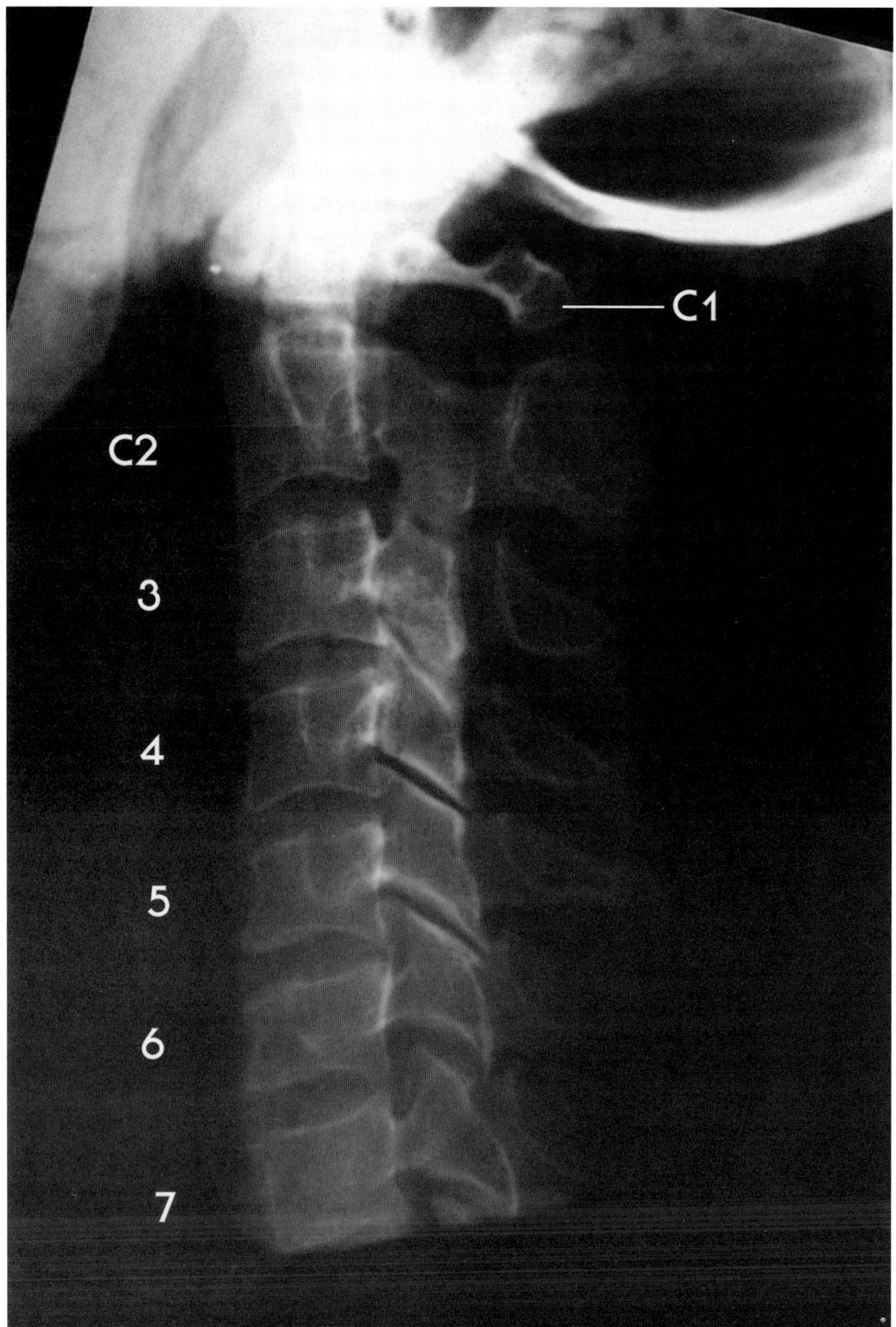

Plates 3-9 A & B
SUBLUXATIONS WITH LOSS OF LORDOTIC CURVE
(Straight or military neck)

This individual shows pronounced straightening of the neck as well as soft tissue and bony changes caused by altered weight bearing. C1 is anterior, C3 is a complete retro (to C2 and C4), C5 is retro to C4, and C6 is a complete retro (to C5 and C7).

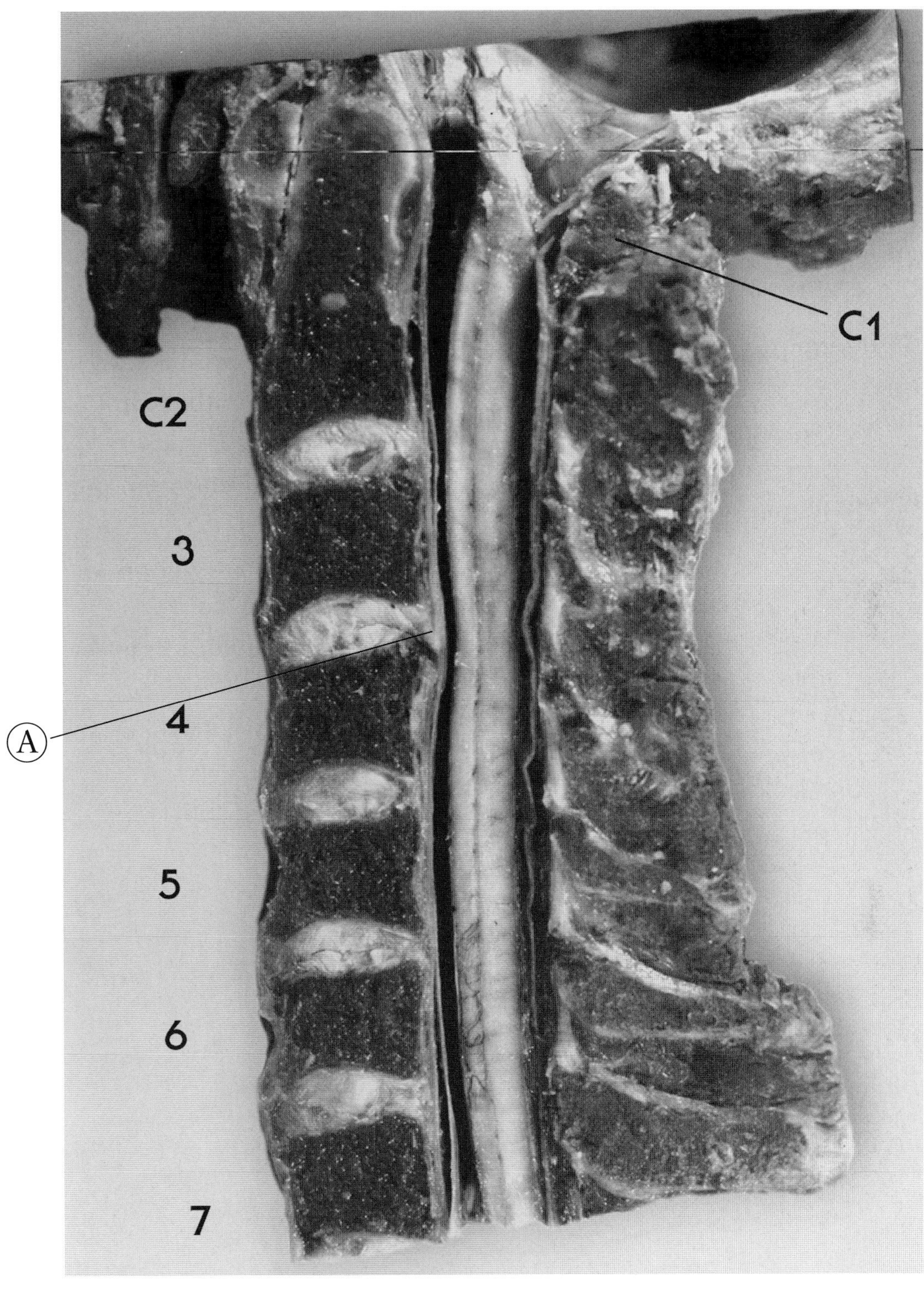

Total loss of the curve usually involves at least one or more complete retrolisthesis.
Disc shearing and bulging occur from C3-C4 downward. Broadening of end plates is evident
below C4, indicating increased weight bearing in the vertebral bodies. Anterior bulging and
end plate deformation at C5-C6 and C6-C7 were probably traumatic in origin.

(A) Note that the relatively slight posterior disc bulge at C3-C4 impinges on the spinal cord.

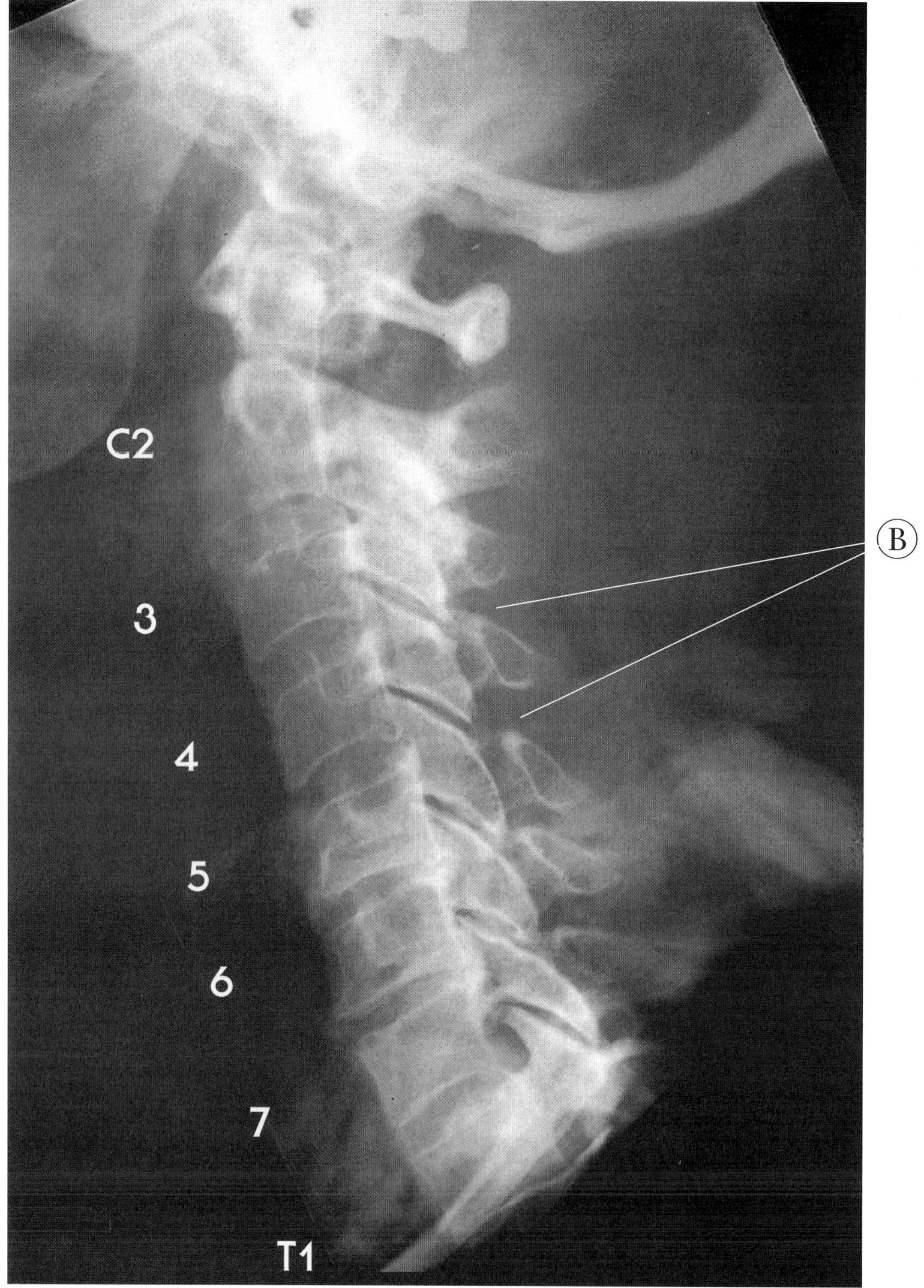

Plates 3-10 A & B
SUBLUXATIONS WITH LOSS OF LORDOTIC CURVE
(Straight or military neck)

This specimen shows a loss of cervical curve with a slight reversal from C4 through C6 with a complete retrolisthesis of C5. C3 is retro to C2, C4 to C3, C5 is a complete retro (to C4 and C6), and C6 is retro to C7. Disc tearing (shear), spurring, and loss of disc height can be seen indicating a long-standing forward alteration of weight bearing.

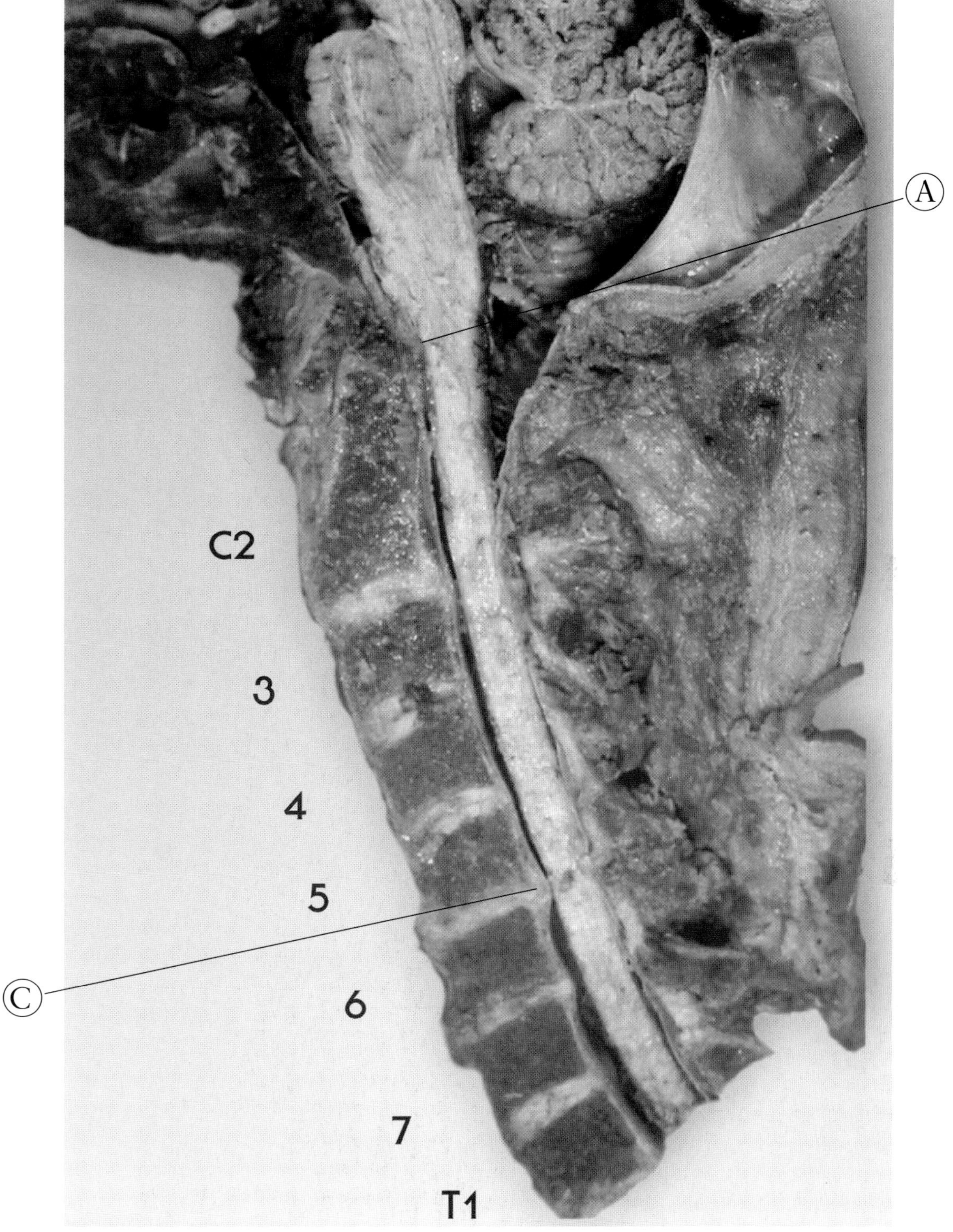

(A) Note that the pons and brainstem are tethered against the posterior surface of the dens and transverse ligament. Introduction of any flexion in the vertebral column will cause further tethering at this point.

(B) Increased interspinous distance indicates lengthening of the canal.

(C) Subluxation and end plate changes in this individual makes the posterior disc bulge at C5-C6 clinically significant. Advanced disc degeneration is evident at the most subluxated and structurally stressed part of the cervical spine.

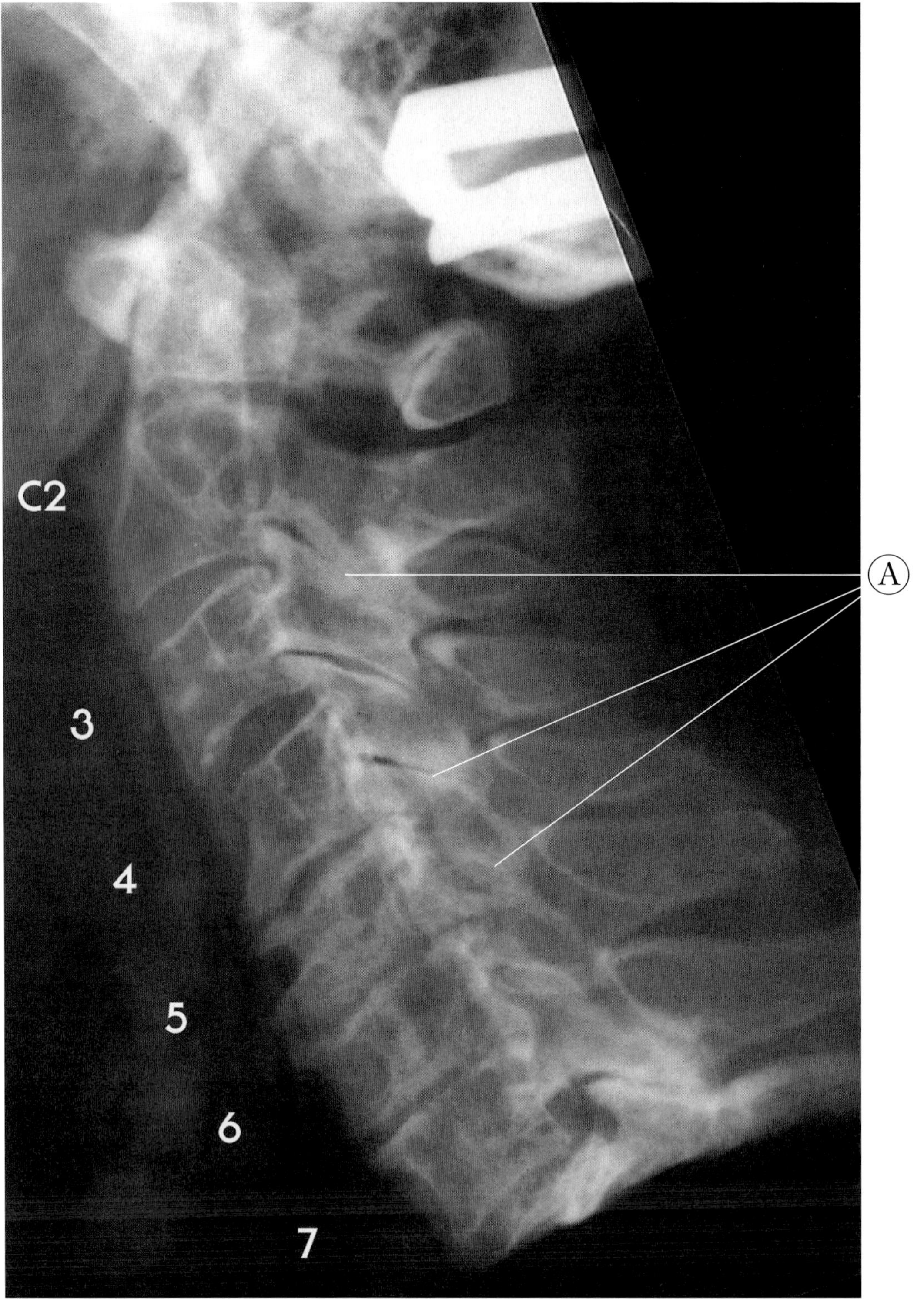

Plates 3-11 A & B
SUBLUXATIONS WITH LOSS OF LORDOTIC CURVE
(Straight or military neck)

Note the canal stenosis from chronic degenerative changes due to subluxation. C2 retro C3 with tearing and bulging of the disc, C3 anterior to C2 and C4; C4 retro to C3 with major vertebral body changes; C5 a complete retro to C4 and C6 with near fusion of C4-5 and

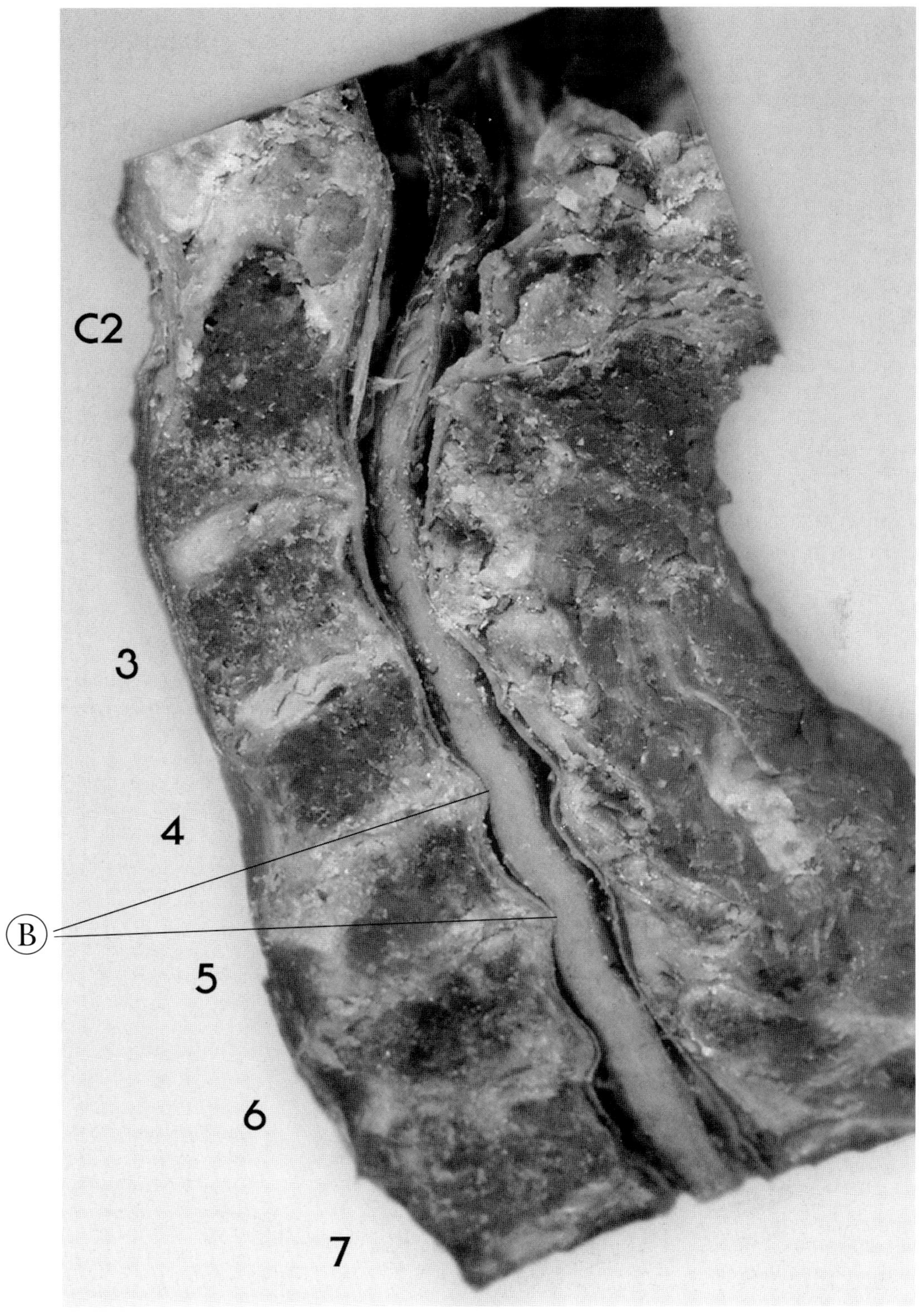

C5-6 with posterior spurring and further stenosis; C6-retro to C7 with tearing near fusion; Note loss of posterior disc height C2-3 with spinous contact and facet jamming and sclerosis. This can also be seen in all the facets due to loss of disc height and altered weight bearing of subluxation.

(A) Facet degeneration
(B) Cord-osteophyte contact

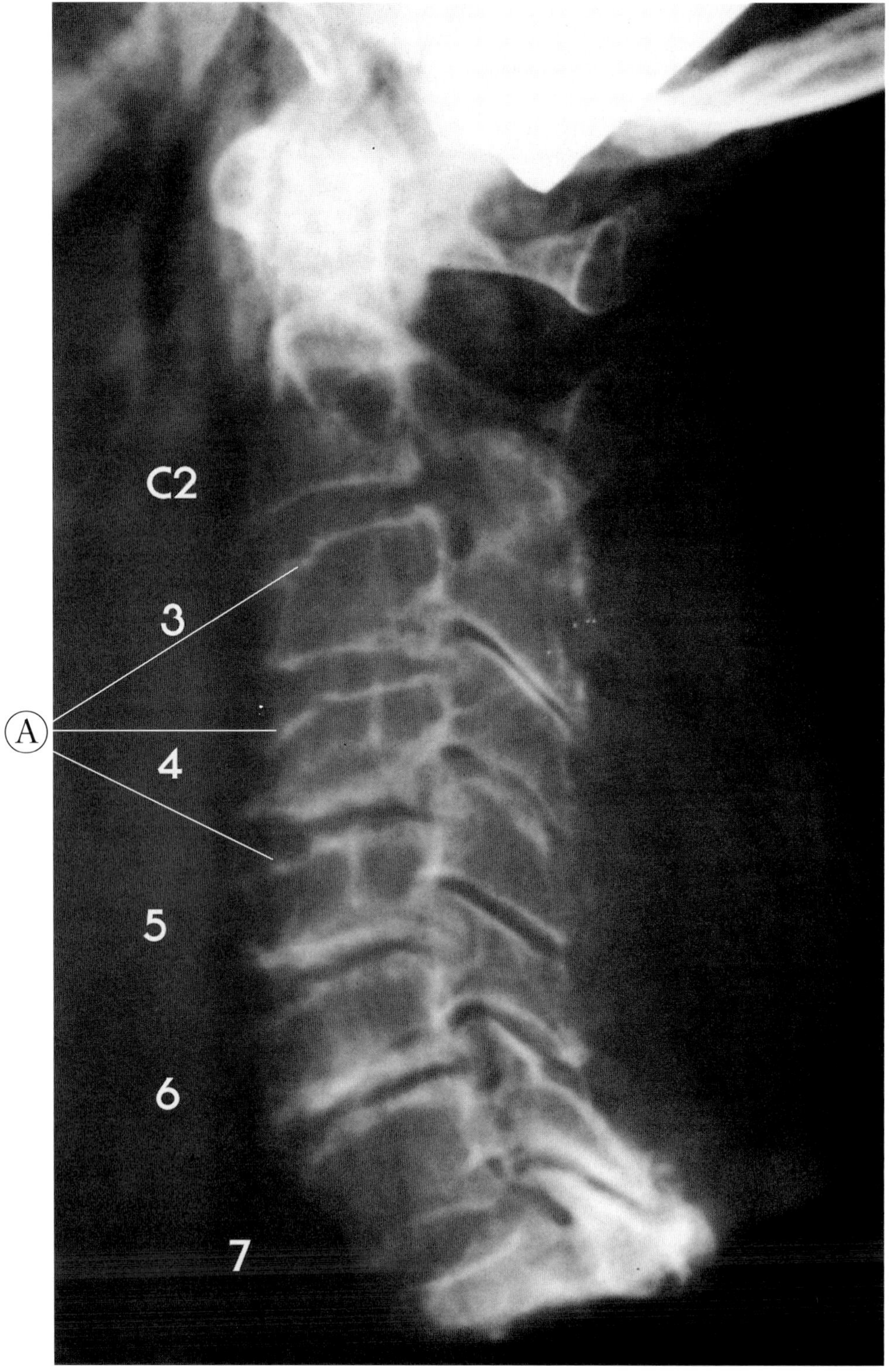

Plates 3-12 A & B
SUBLUXATIONS WITH REVERSED OR KYPHOTIC CURVE
Upper cervical subluxations

This view shows a reversal of the lordotic curve at C2-3. Retro C3 to C2 with disc
tearing and bulging; C4 is a complete retro to C3 and C5 with disc tearing and
wedging; C6 is anterior to C5 with disc tearing and bulging and near fusion

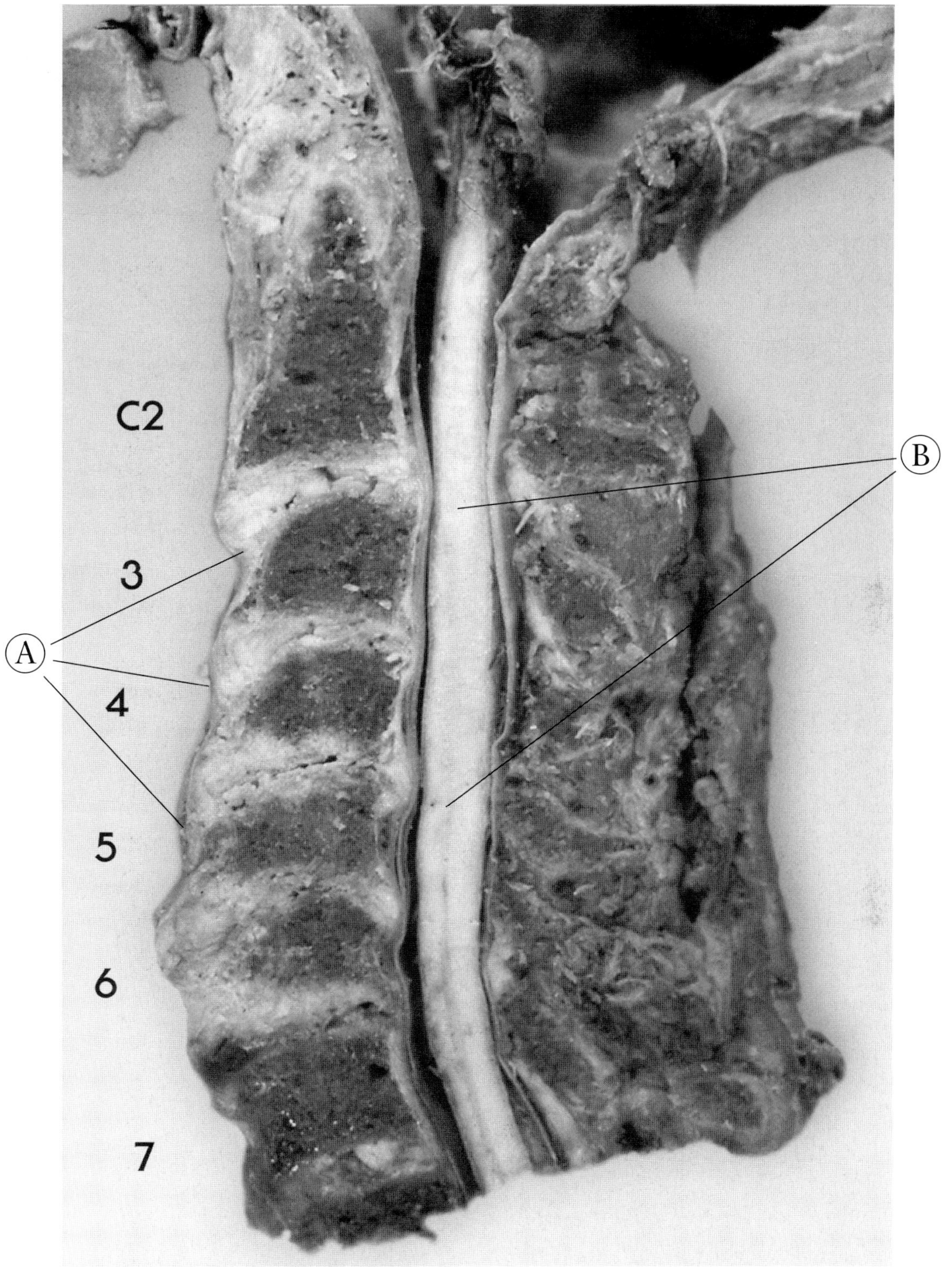

posteriorly.
All discs are torn with anterior spurring and disc bulges posterior. Canal stenosis is due to the subluxations and the resulting alteration of soft and bony tissues.
(A) Small compression fractures of anterior and superior vertebral bodies C3-C6.
(B) Spinal cord and canal contact from C3-C5.

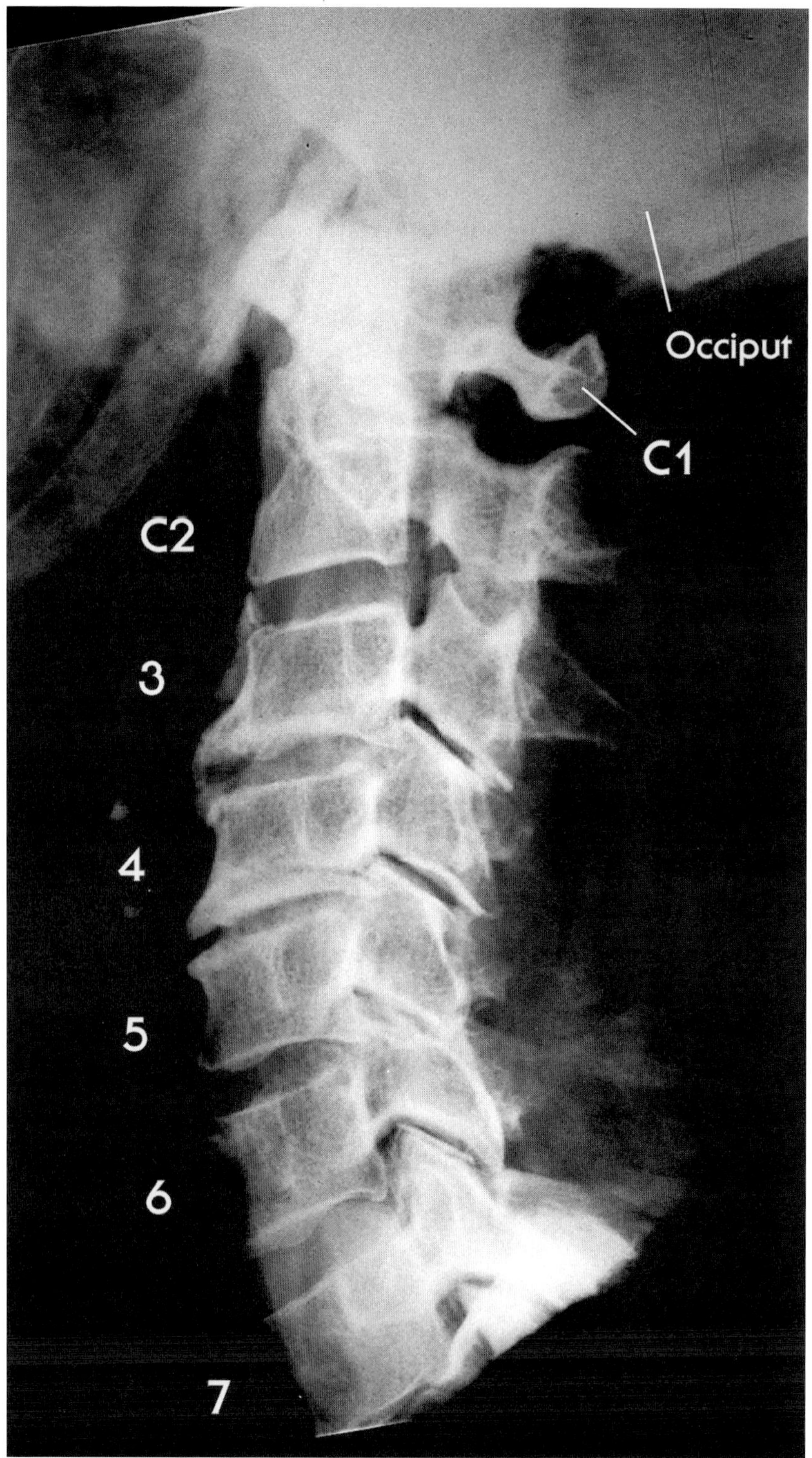

Plates 3-13 A & B
SUBLUXATIONS WITH REVERSED OR KYPHOTIC CURVE
Upper cervical subluxations
This specimen shows a reversal of the lordotic curve at C3 with stenosis of the vertebral canal at the subluxated segments, which makes the relatively minor disc bulges at C3-C4, C4-C5, and C5-C6 clinically significant.

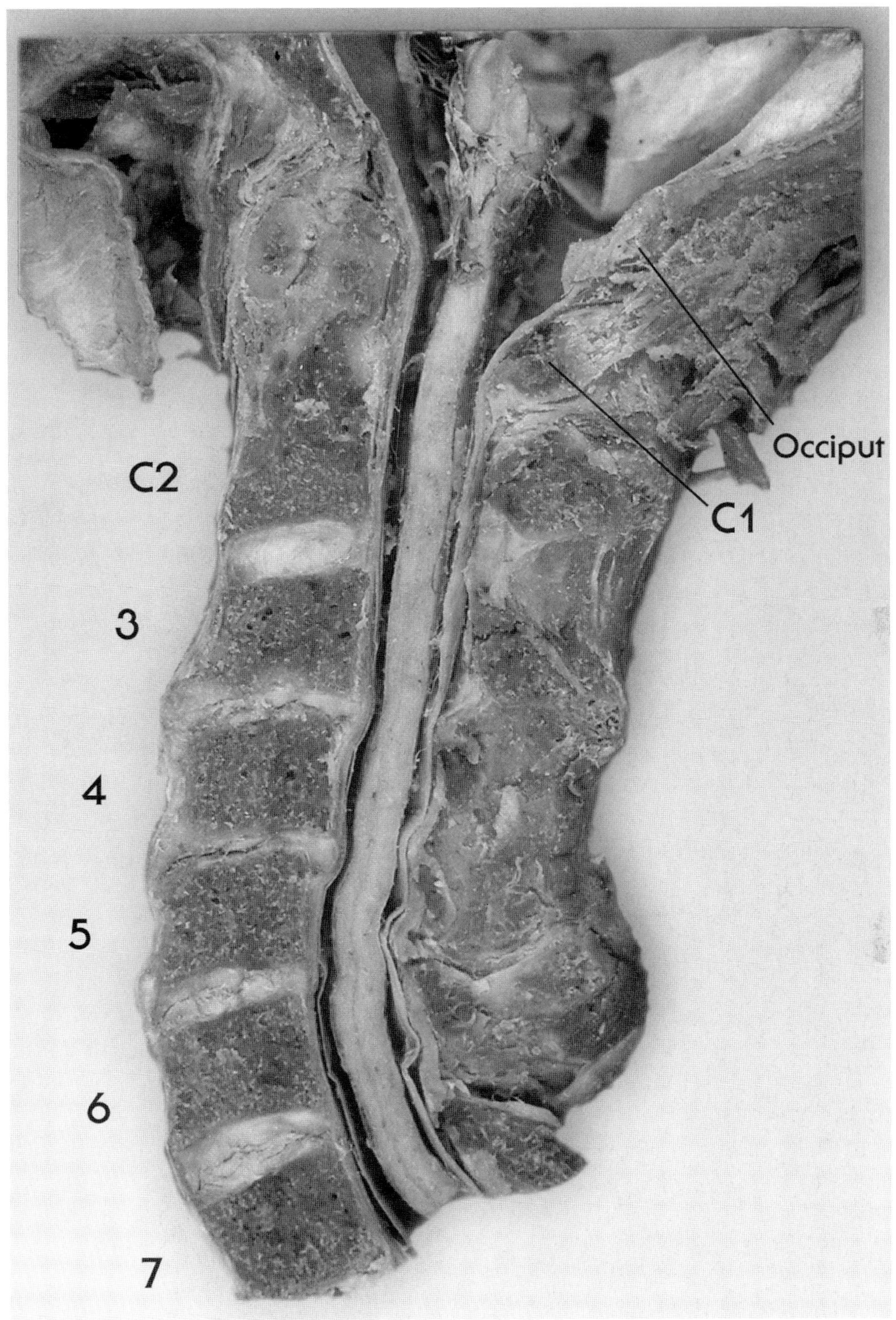

Gapping at the facets indicates that weight bearing has been transferred to the vertebral bodies in the mid cervicals. C1 is anterior to the occiput and C2. C3 is a complete retrolisthesis to C2 and C4. Bulging and tearing of the C3-4 disc have occurred. C5 is retro to C6, with a slight loss of disc height. A posterior disc bulge is visible at C5-6 with cord contact. C6 and C7 are nearly aligned with normal canal shape and size. The subluxated vertebrae probably have interfered with the central nervous system.

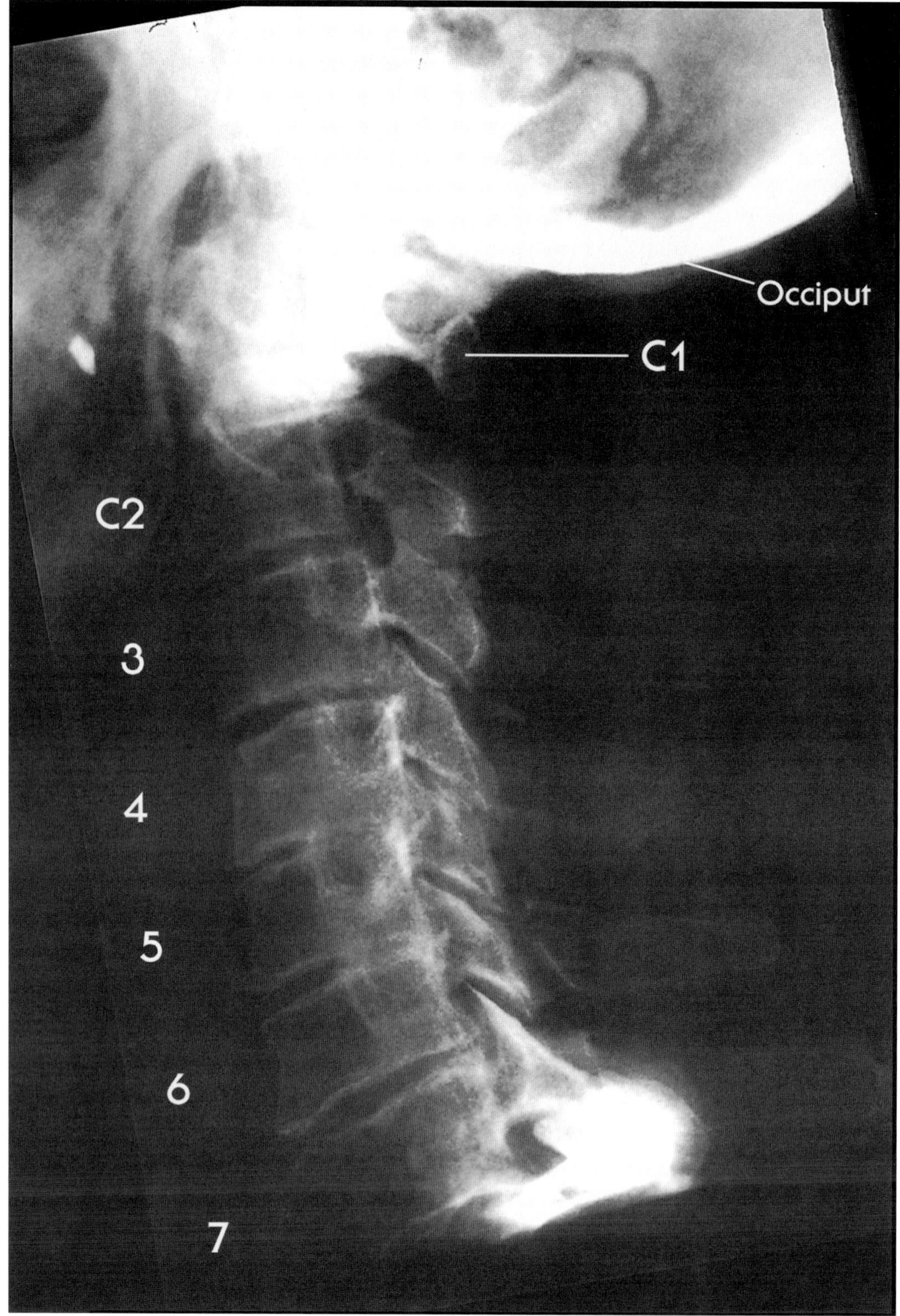

Plates 3-14 A & B
SUBLUXATIONS WITH REVERSED OR KYPHOTIC CURVE
Upper cervical subluxation

This individual suffered degeneration in all of his cervical discs due to subluxation of every segment. C1 superior on the dens and anterior to the posterior rim of the foramen magnum and the C2 spinous process contacting the dorsal surface of the spinal cord. C3 is a complete retrolisthesis with a reversal of the lordotic curve at this level. In addition, it appears that C1 is anterior to the occiput and C2.

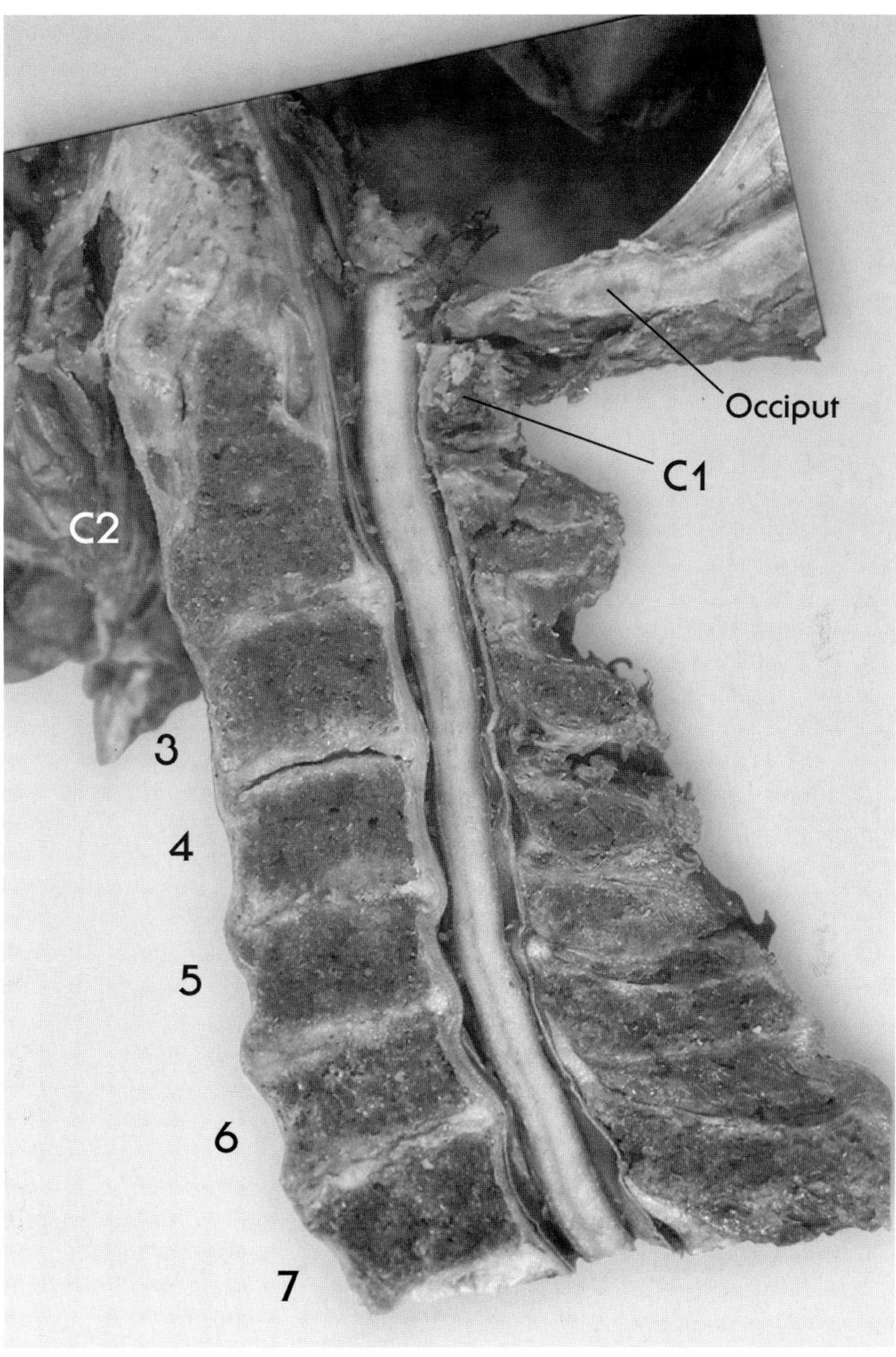

The degree of posterior bulging and spurring from the subluxations has resulted in acquired stenosis. The spinal cord is tractioned against the anterior wall of the vertebral canal, with contact on the cord. C3 is a complete retro to C2 and C4 with reduced disc height, tearing and posterior bulging, and with a cavitated disc at C3-4. C4 is retro to C5 with spurring and partial fusion at C4-5. C6 is retro to C5, and has partially fused with it posteriorly. C7 is retro to C6; the disc has collapsed, but fusion has not yet occurred. All of the discs are bulging posteriorly, and anterior bulging occurs from C3-4 through C6-7.

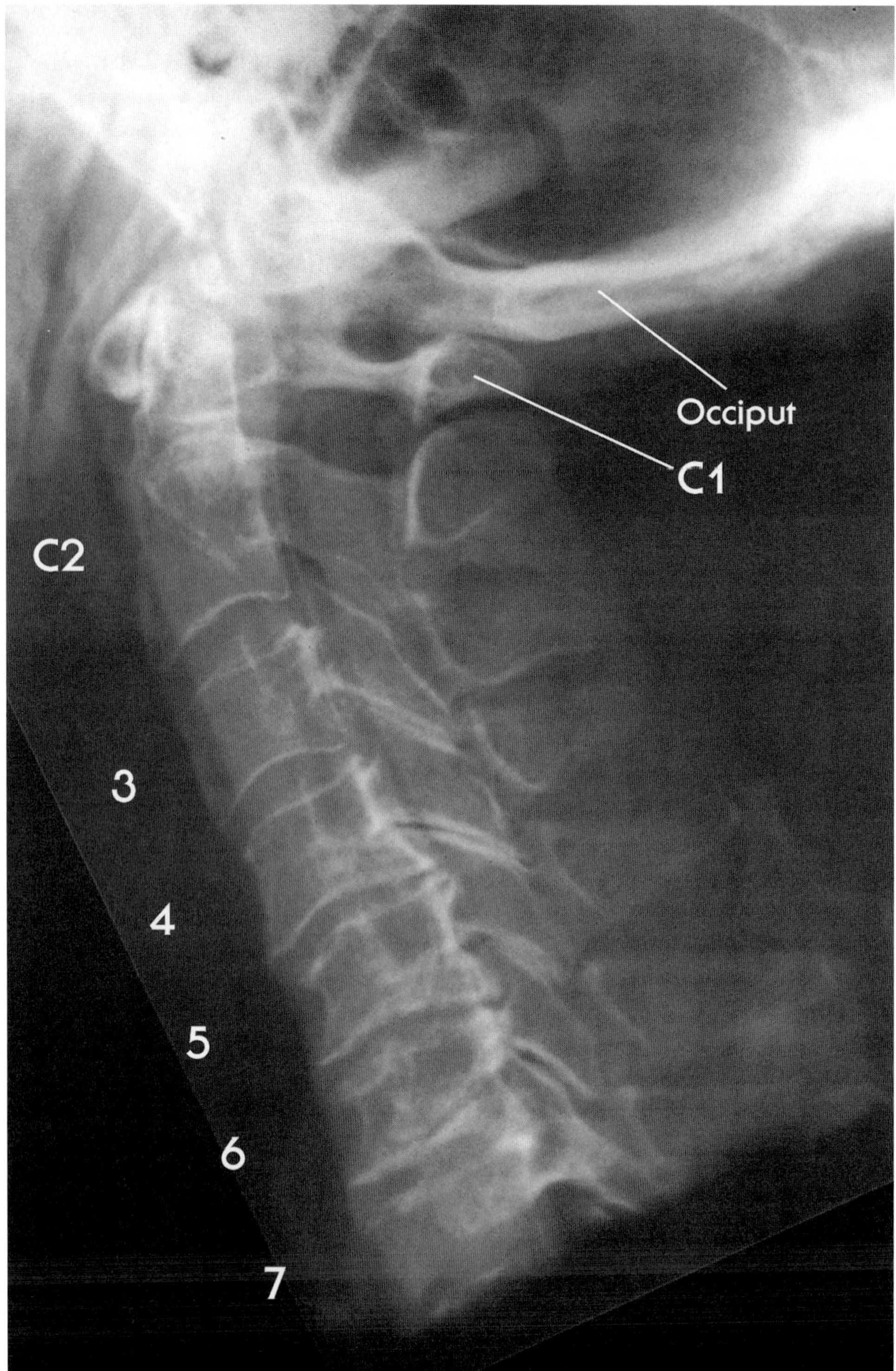

Plates 3-15 A & B
SUBLUXATIONS WITH REVERSED OR KYPHOTIC CURVE
Mid-cervical subluxations

Shown here is an interesting occiput C1/C2 relationship. C1 is anterior to the occiput and the posterior arch has become weight bearing. C2-3 looks good, with a good disc. C4 is retro to C3 with disc narrowing posterior and just a hint of anterior brown degeneration with significant endplate changes. C5 retro to C4 with disc tearing, necrosis, and moderately significant posterior spurring with cord impingement.

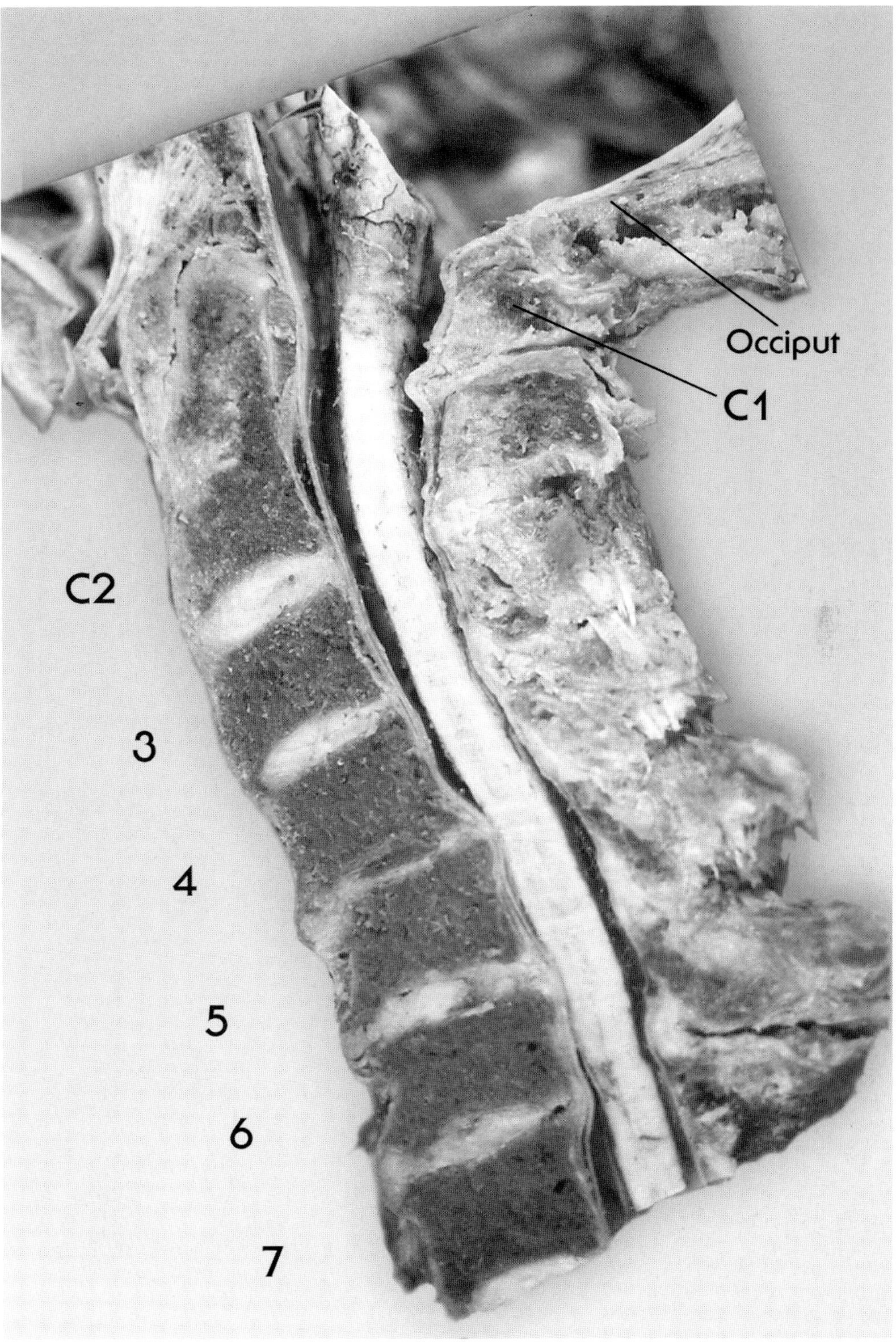

Note increased endplate thickness on the X-ray, which gives the appearance of a bulging disc in the specimen. C6 is a complete retrolisthesis to C5 and C7. Spinal cord contact and compromise from subluxation, posterior spurring, and significant DJD with disc bulging of C5 & 6; C6-7 looks significantly degenerated with minor bulge but near fusions - not seen on X-Ray.
Note facet jamming C3 to C6 - where is cartilage on facets? Loss of disc height causes facet sclerosis and shortening of the canal.

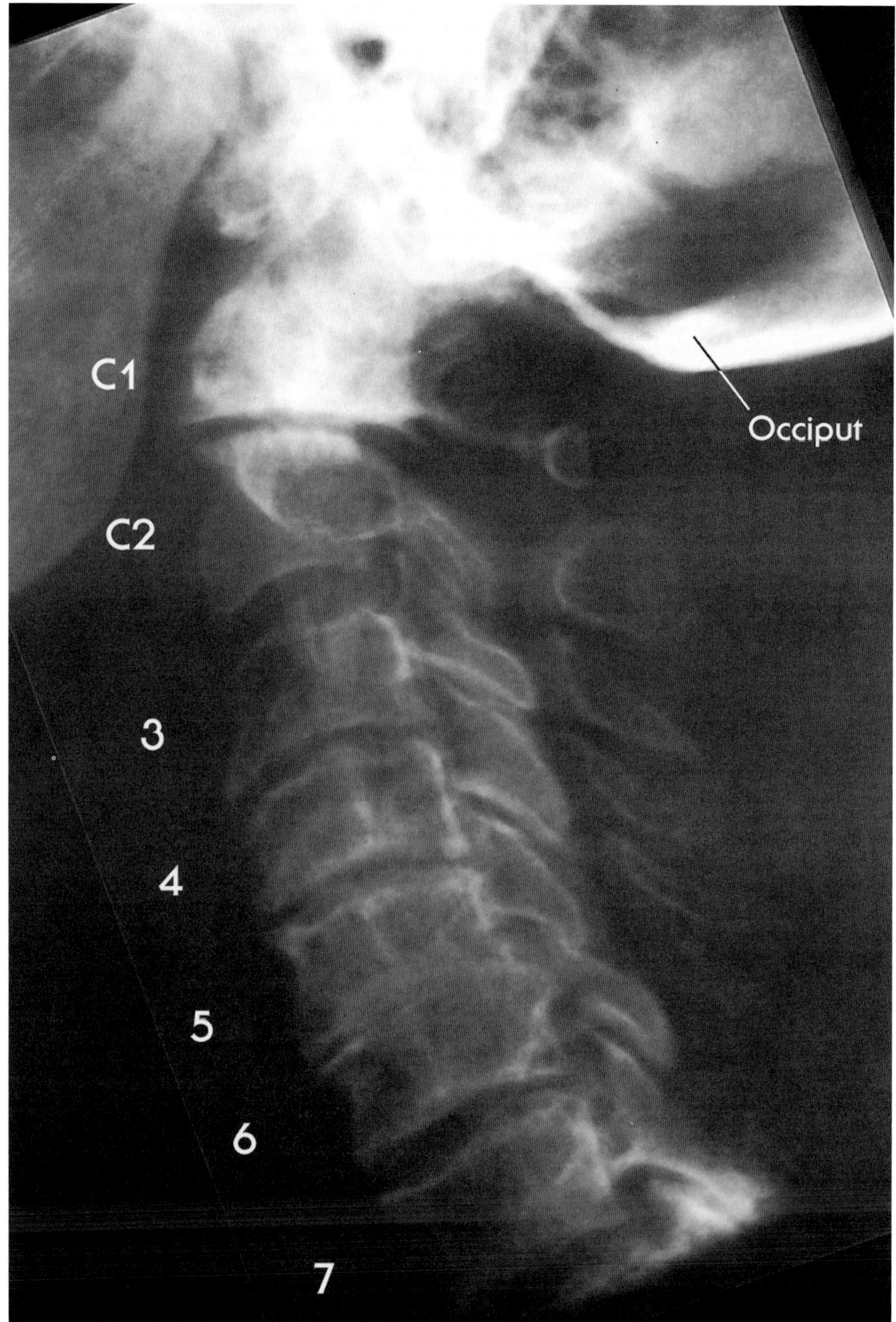

Plates 3-16 A & B
SUBLUXATIONS WITH REVERSED OR KYPHOTIC CURVE
Mid-cervical subluxations

C1 anterior to occiput and C2; C2 & C3 look aligned but facets show altered weight bearing; C4 retro to C3 and C5 retro to C4 with disc tearing of C3-4 and C4-5 with posterior spurs and loss of disc height; fusion of C5 and C6; C6 is a complete retrolisthesis to C5

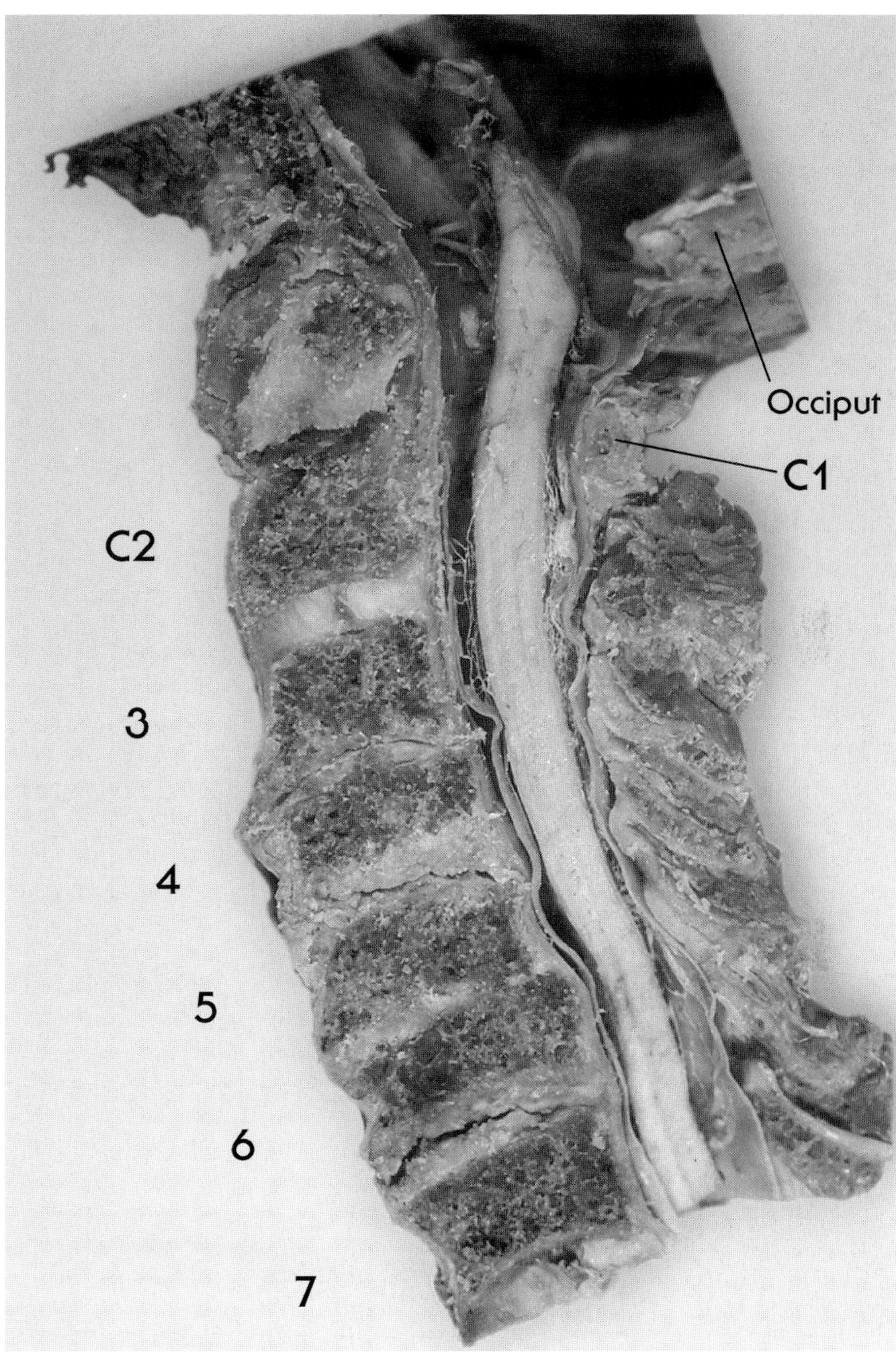

and C7 with tearing of C6-7 and posterior bulging, significant canal stenosis from subluxation and the expected degenerative changes.
Note: vertebral body diameter of C4-5 & 6 compare to C2 and C7; significant cord compression and canal stenosis at C6 and C7.

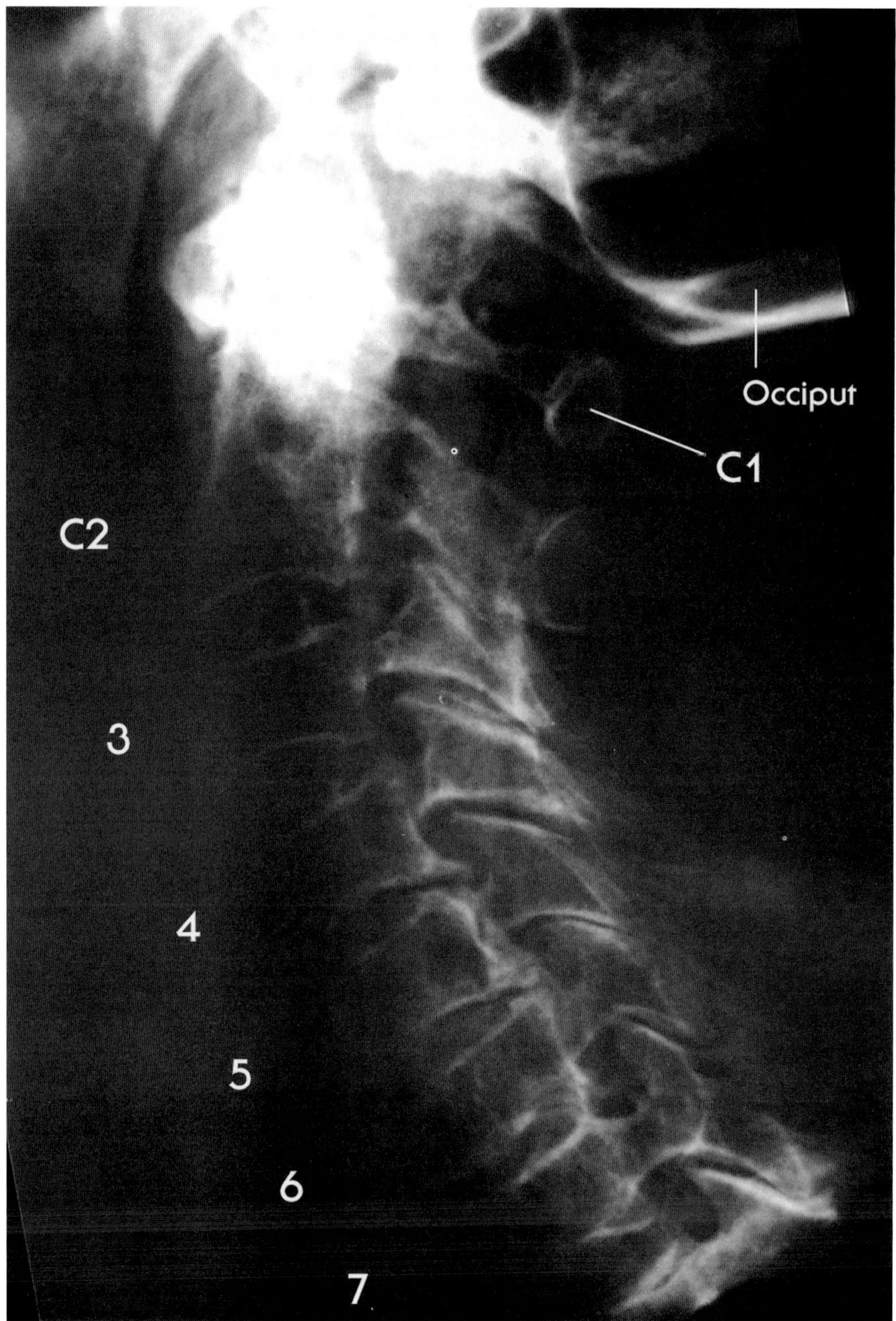

Plates 3-17 A & B
SUBLUXATIONS WITH REVERSED OR KYPHOTIC CURVE
Lower cervical subluxations

In this specimen there is a reversal of the curve at C6 but the lordotic curve in the upper cervical area is maintained and well-hydrated discs have persisted. Hypertrophy of the facets in this region indicates that they suffered altered weight-bearing function.

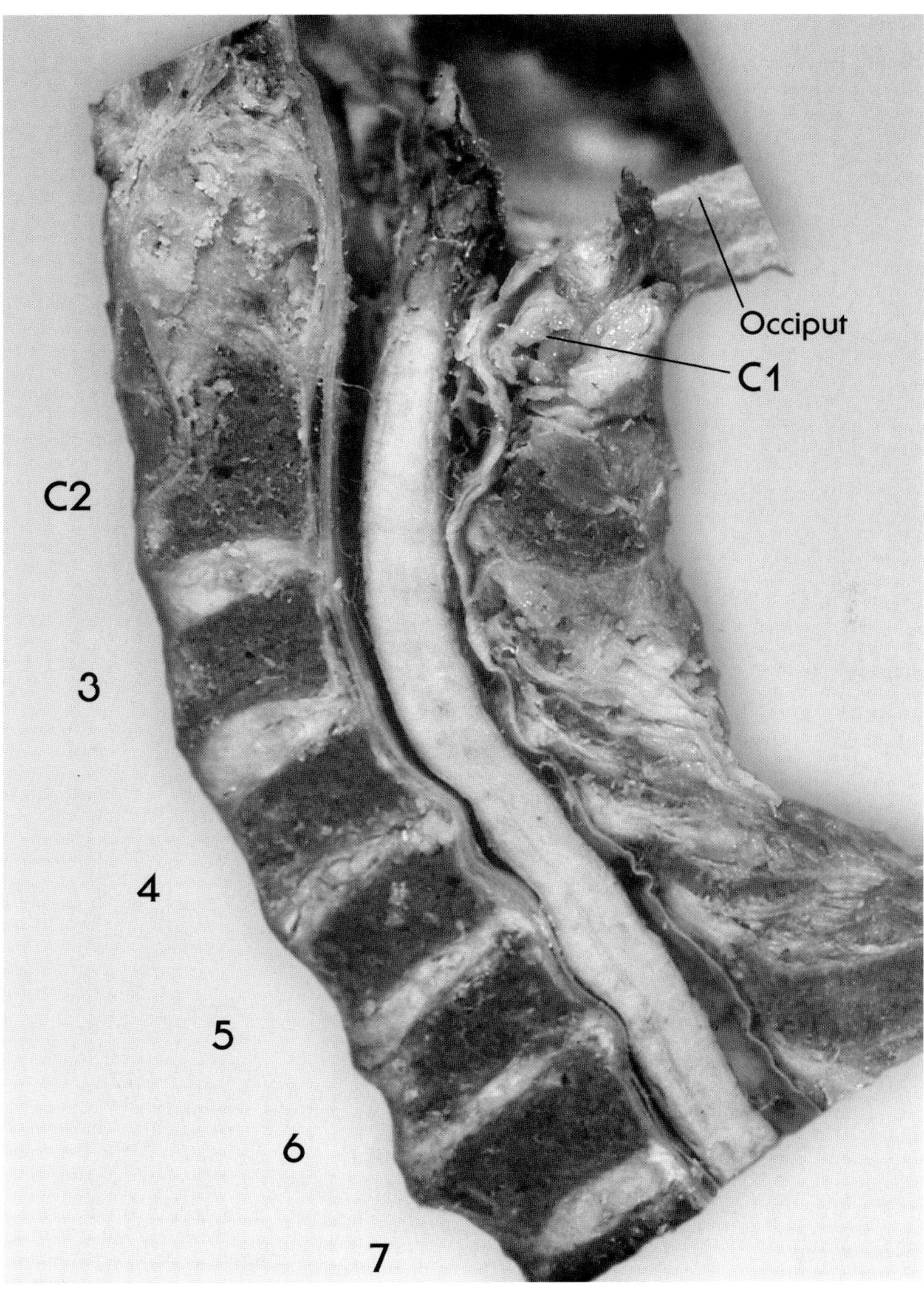

C1 is anterior to the occiput and C2, C3 is retro to C2, C4 is retro to C3, C5 is retro to C4 and C6 shows a complete retrolisthesis to C5 and C7. Bulging, spurring, loss of disc height, and disc tearing have begun to develop at C4-C5 and C5-C6. Note canal stenosis and spinal cord impingement beginning at C4-C5. C6-C7 shows significant loss of disc height with bulging and spurring anteriorly and posteriorly. The whole disc appears to have collapsed (there is no visible line of shear). Note impingement on the spinal cord, which is tethered against the anterior surface of the vertebral canal at this level.

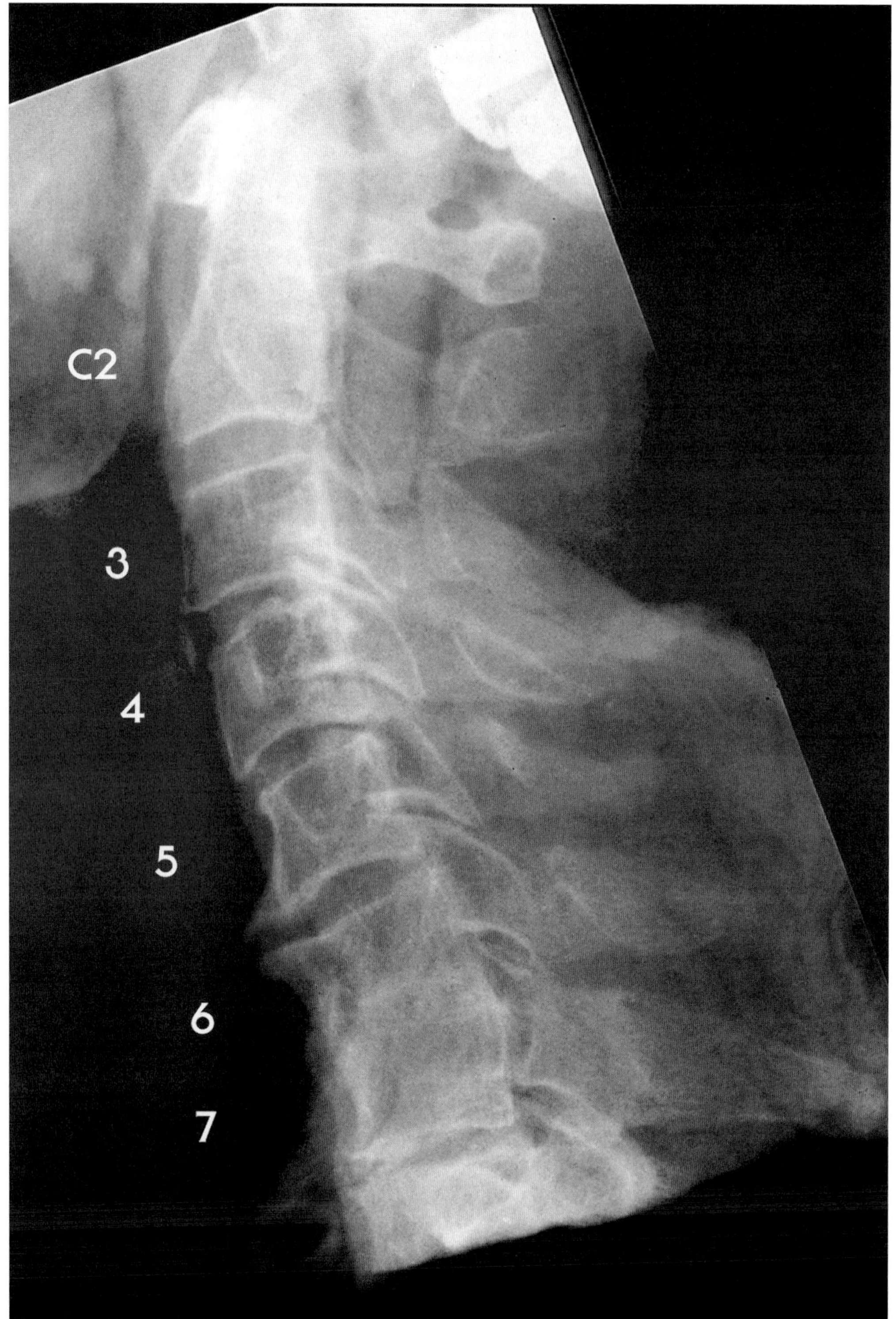

Plates 3-18 A & B
SUBLUXATION WITH REVERSED OR KYPHOTIC CURVE
Lower cervical subluxations

This specimen has a reversal of the lordotic curve at C6-C7 with significant cord compromise from C3-C7. The space behind cord at C5-7 and compression of cord into anterior canal wall C5-C7 are due to tractioning. Moderate congenital stenosis.
Note C2 and C7 canal size; these levels are near normal and reduced in diameter.

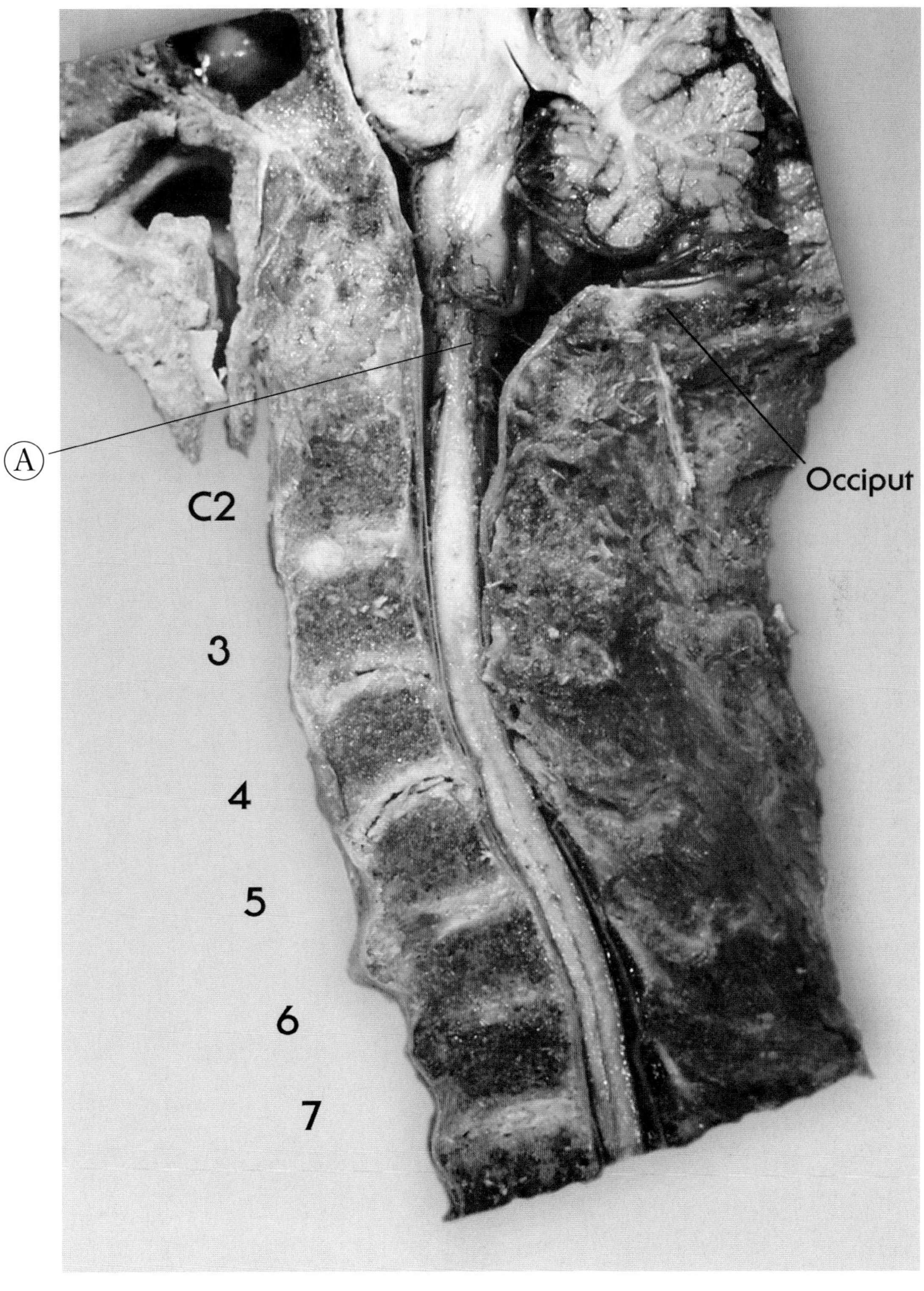

There C2 is aligned with C3 with a healthy disc; C3 is stepped behind C4 - or C4 is anterior to C3 with disc tearing and bulging of C3-C4; C4 is retro to C5 with tearing and bulging; endplate changes are moderate; C5 is anterior to C6 (and C4); C5 has become a complete antrolesthesis; C6 is retro to C5 with significant endplate changes; note the necrotic (brown) tissue in C5-6 disc, also the disc material all the way out between "spurs" of C5 and C6. C6-7 fused with C7 retro to C6

Note reduced pontine flexure and the brainstem is well below occiput.

(A) Brainstem

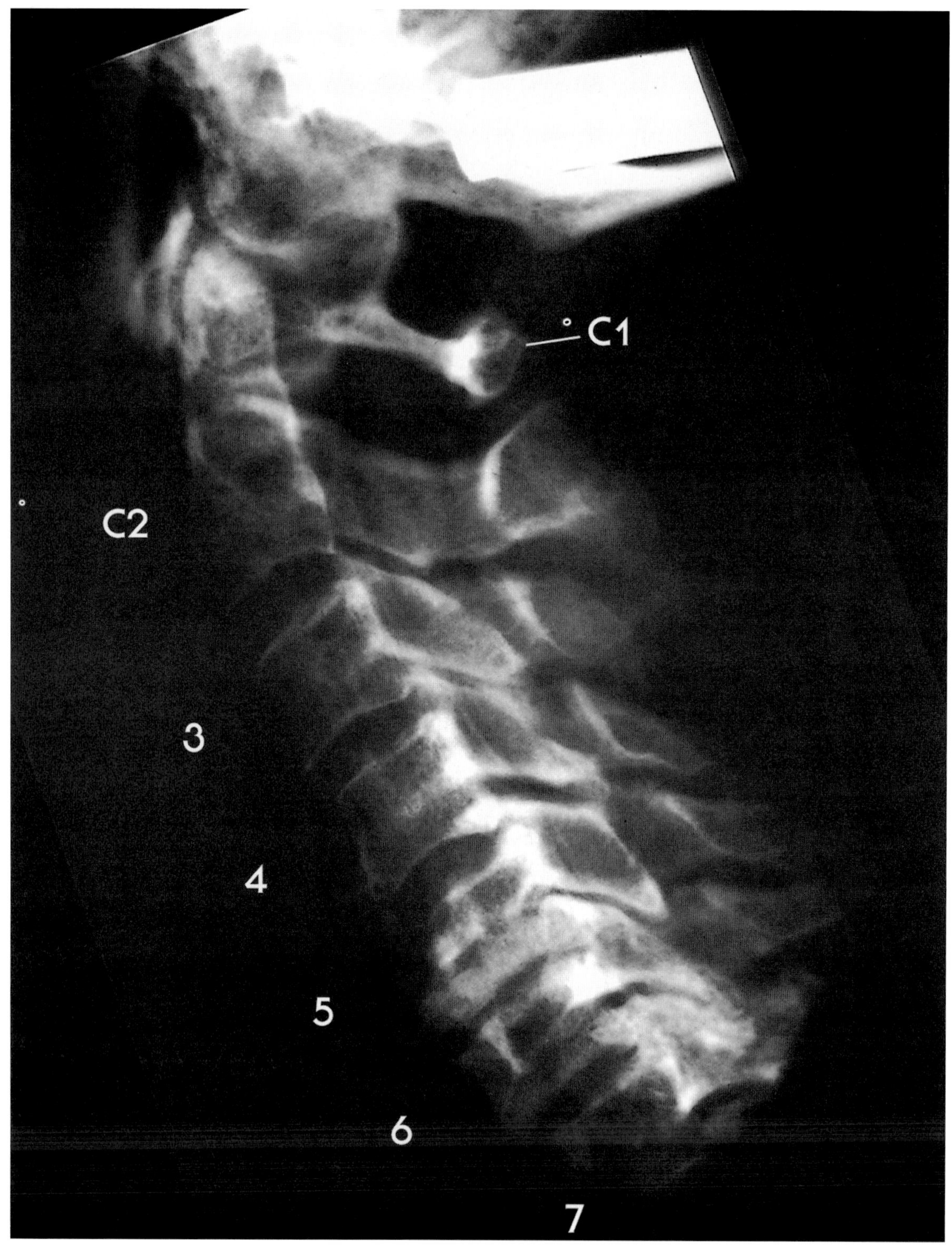

Plates 3-19 A & B
SUBLUXATIONS WITH REVERSED OR KYPHOTIC CURVE
Lower cervical subluxations

In this individual, the C2-C3 disc is normal, but C4 is retro to C3 with a visible line of shear in the disc. C5 shows complete retrolisthesis (i.e., is retro both to C4 and C6), with a shear line and posterior spurring at the C4-C5 disc and complete fusion at C5-C6. C7 is retro to C6 with pronounced loss of disc height, disc shearing, and posterior spurring.

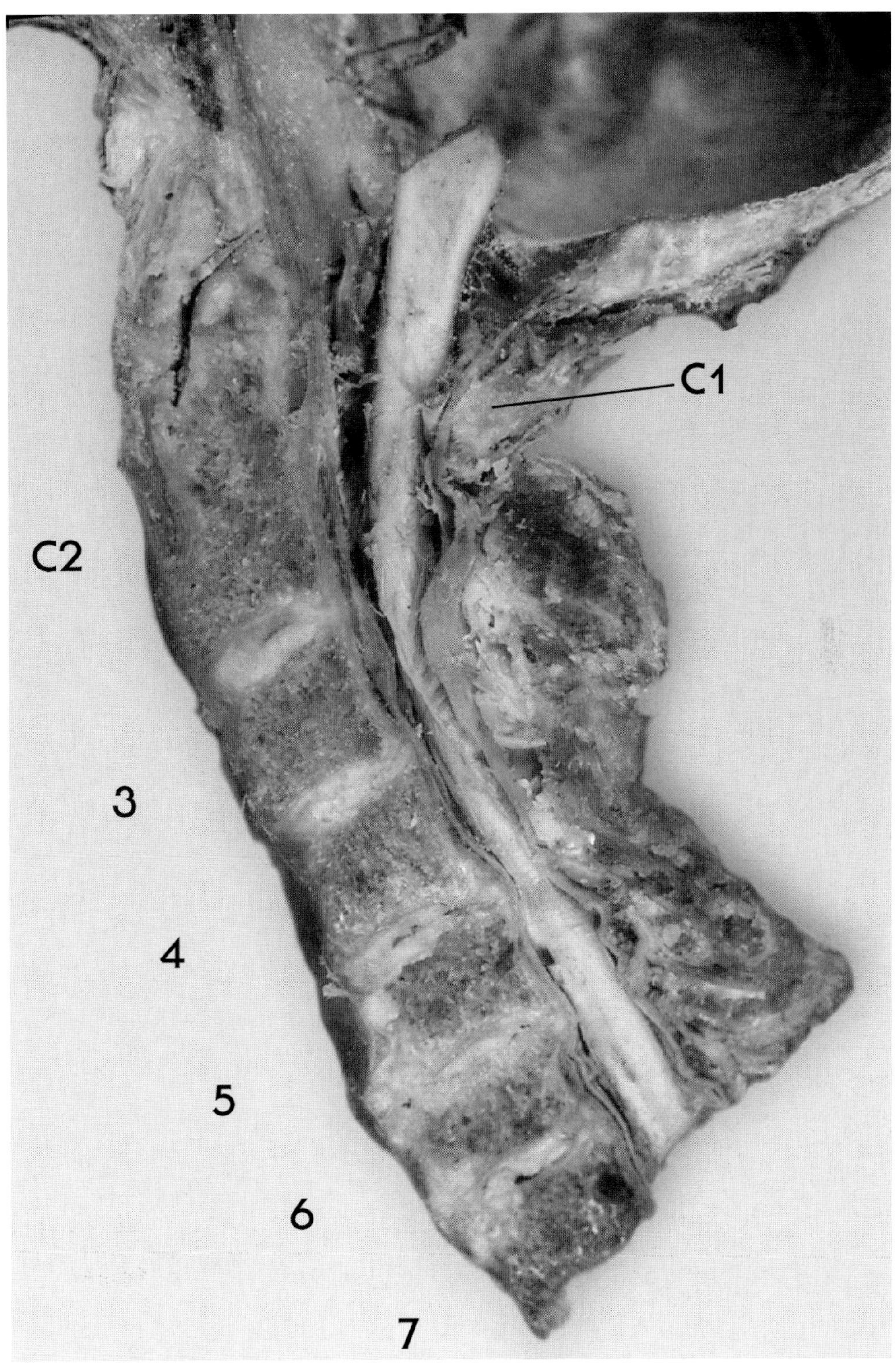

(Note: in MRIs disc shear appears as a black line through the disc.) At the level of C2, the spinal cord rests in a spacious vertebral canal; however, at C4 through C7 the broadened end plates of the vertebral bodies have resulted in canal stenosis (narrowing) to the point where the spinal cord is actually compressed. This probably had clinical significance for the individual.

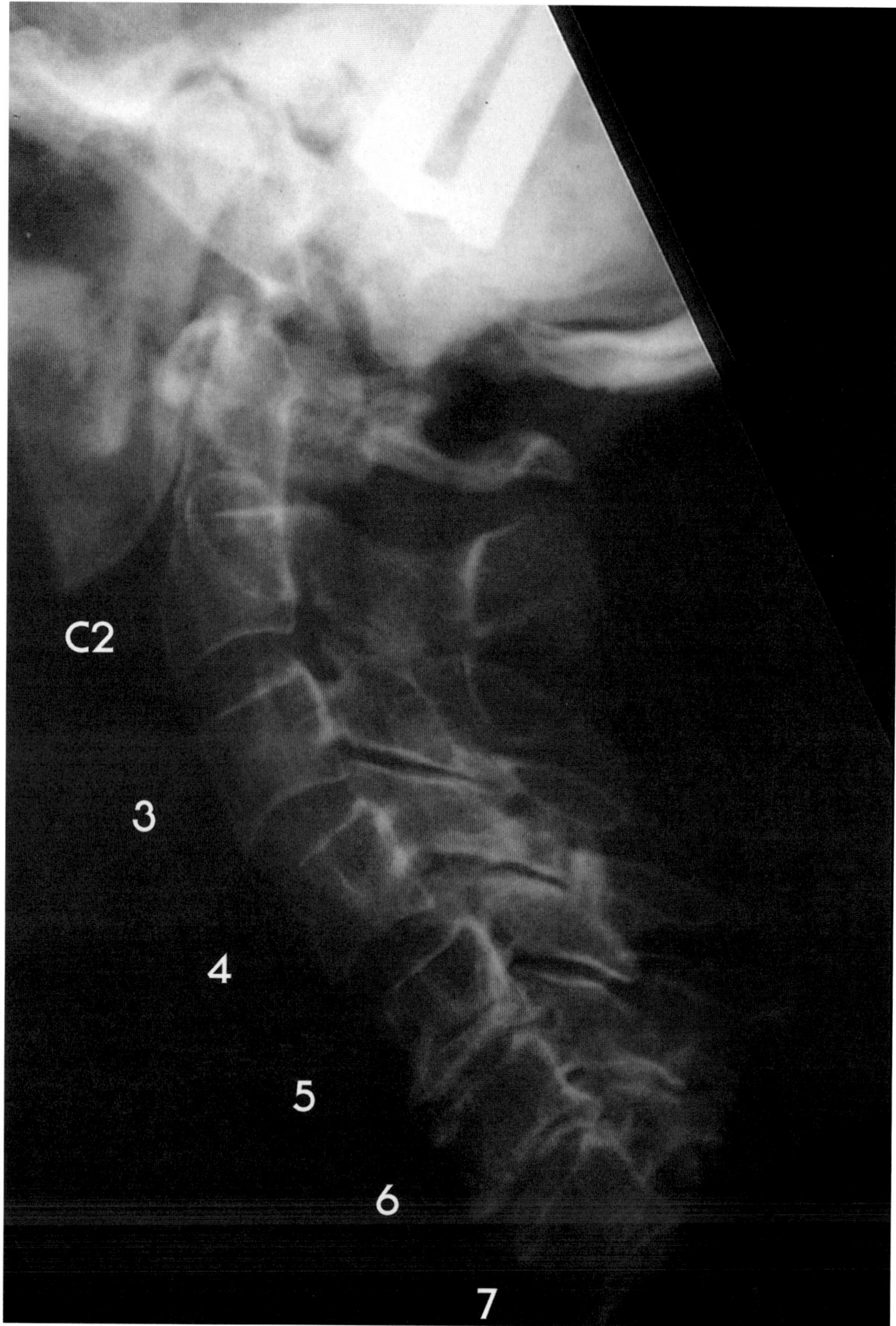

Plates 3-20 A & B
SUBLUXATIONS WITH REVERSAL OR KYPHOTIC CURVE
Lower cervical subluxations

This person evidently sustained an injury which severely affected her lower cervical spine several years before her death, and a second, lesser trauma which altered her upper cervical spine shortly before her death.

Note the almost normal lordotic curve from C1 through C4, with a dramatic straightening and reversal of the at the C5-C7 level. C3 shows a complete anterolisthesis (C2 and C4), and

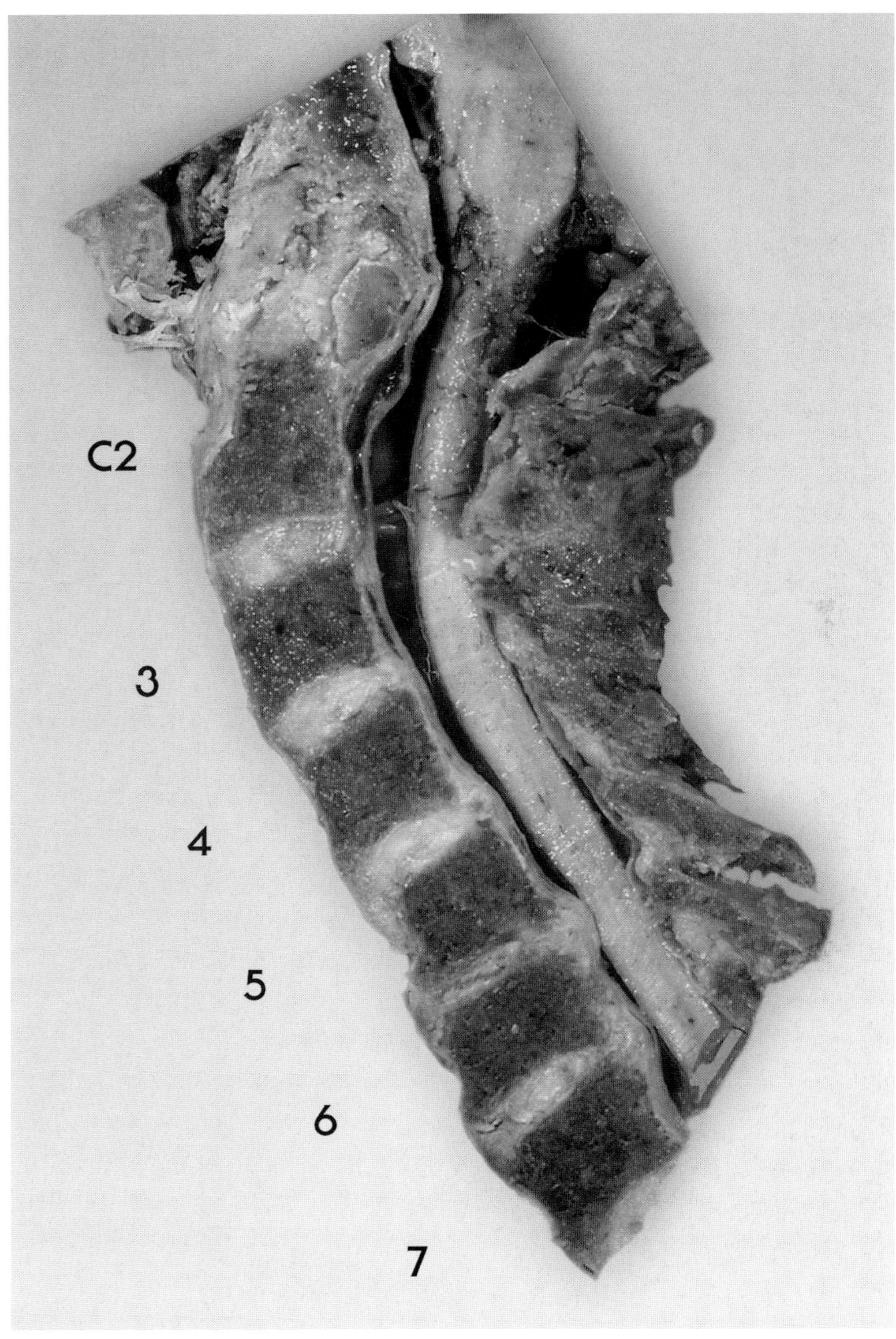

C4 is anterior to C5. However, the C2-C3 and C3-C4 discs show only slight degeneration. Despite slight disc bulging, the vertebral bodies have not yet begun to change shape.
In the lower spine, C5 is completely retro (to C4 and C6) and C6 is completely antro (to C5 and C7). The C5-C6 disc has significant degeneration, showing dramatic loss of height, anterior and posterior bulging, and alteration of the shape of the vertebral bodies to accommodate altered weight bearing. The C6-C7 disc has sheared and bulged posteriorly, and has lost height posteriorly. The posterior bulge at C5-C6 is pressing into the spinal cord. The disc below it appears to be touching, but not yet deforming the cord.

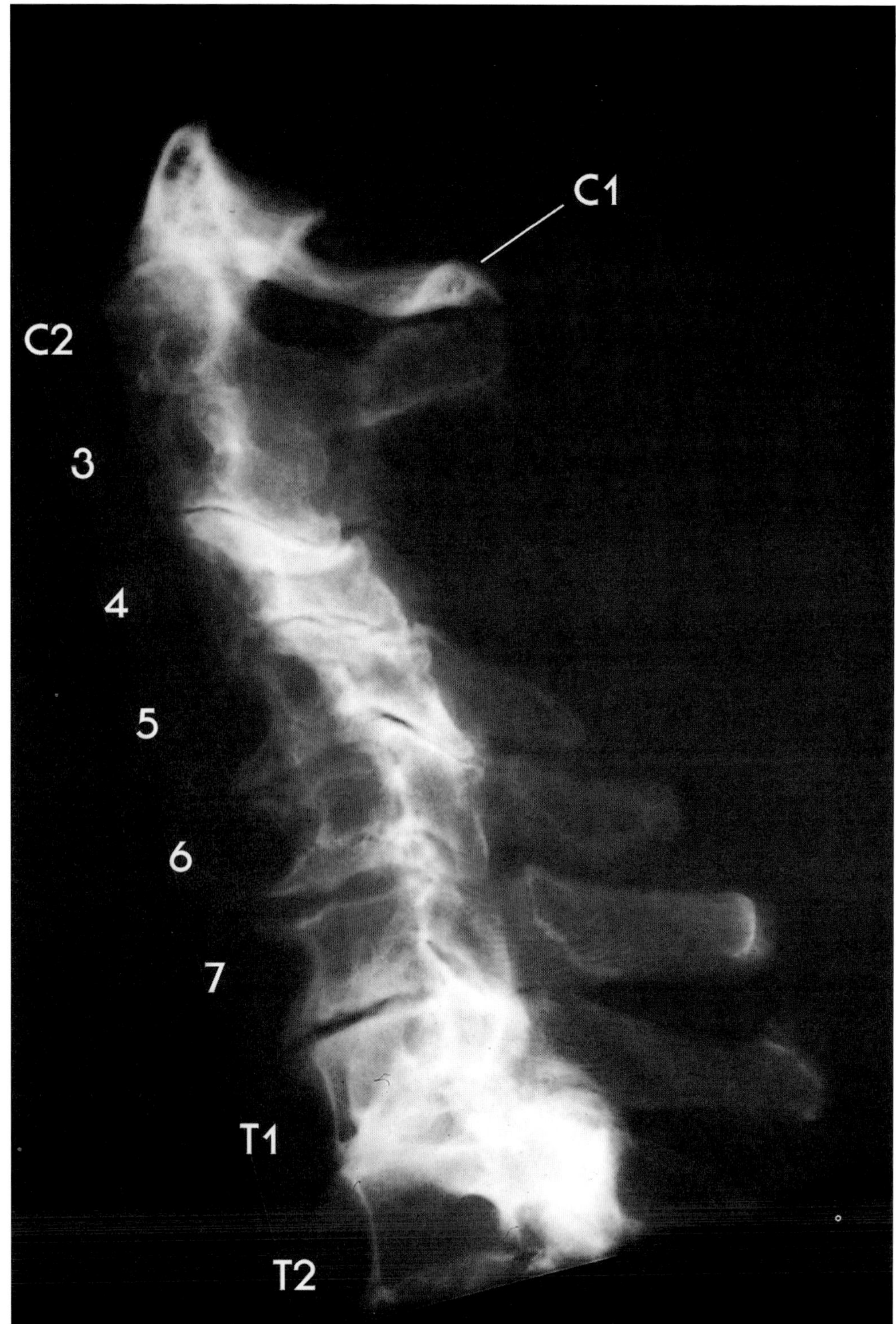

Plates 3-21 A & B
SUBLUXATIONS WITH REVERSED OR KYPHOTIC CURVE
Mid-cervical subluxations

In this specimen a reversal of the lordotic curve is present from C4 through C7. Canal stenosis has occurred, but the individual originally possessed a large vertebral canal as seen at the C2 and T2 levels. However, the cord is tethered against the anterior surface of the canal starting at C4. This is an extreme example of the spinal cord deforming to the shape of the spinal canal.

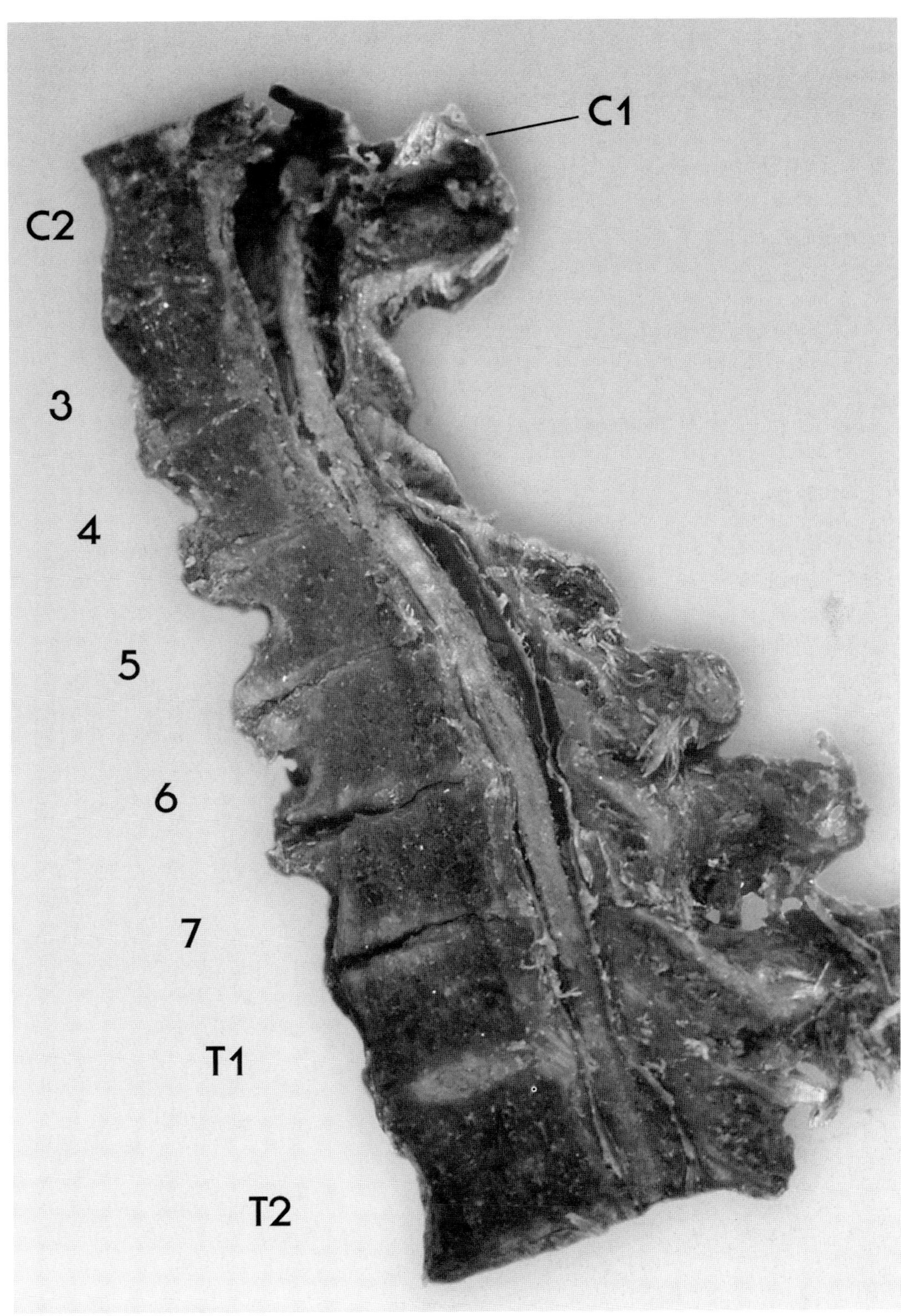

Note that a pseudo-joint has formed between the posterior arch of Atlas and the spinous process of C2. (The spinous processes of C3, C4 are missing because they were rotated out of the midsaggital plane when the specimen was cut.) C3 is retro to C2, C4 is retro to C3. C5 is retro to C4, C6 is a complete retrolisthesis (to C5 and C7), and C7 is retro to T1. The C5-6, C6-7, and C7-T1 discs have completely degenerated, but the vertebrae have not yet fused. Anterior spurring is pronounced, but posterior spurring does not appear significant except at C6-7. Note that the T1-2 disc is not subluxated, and appears to be fully hydrated.

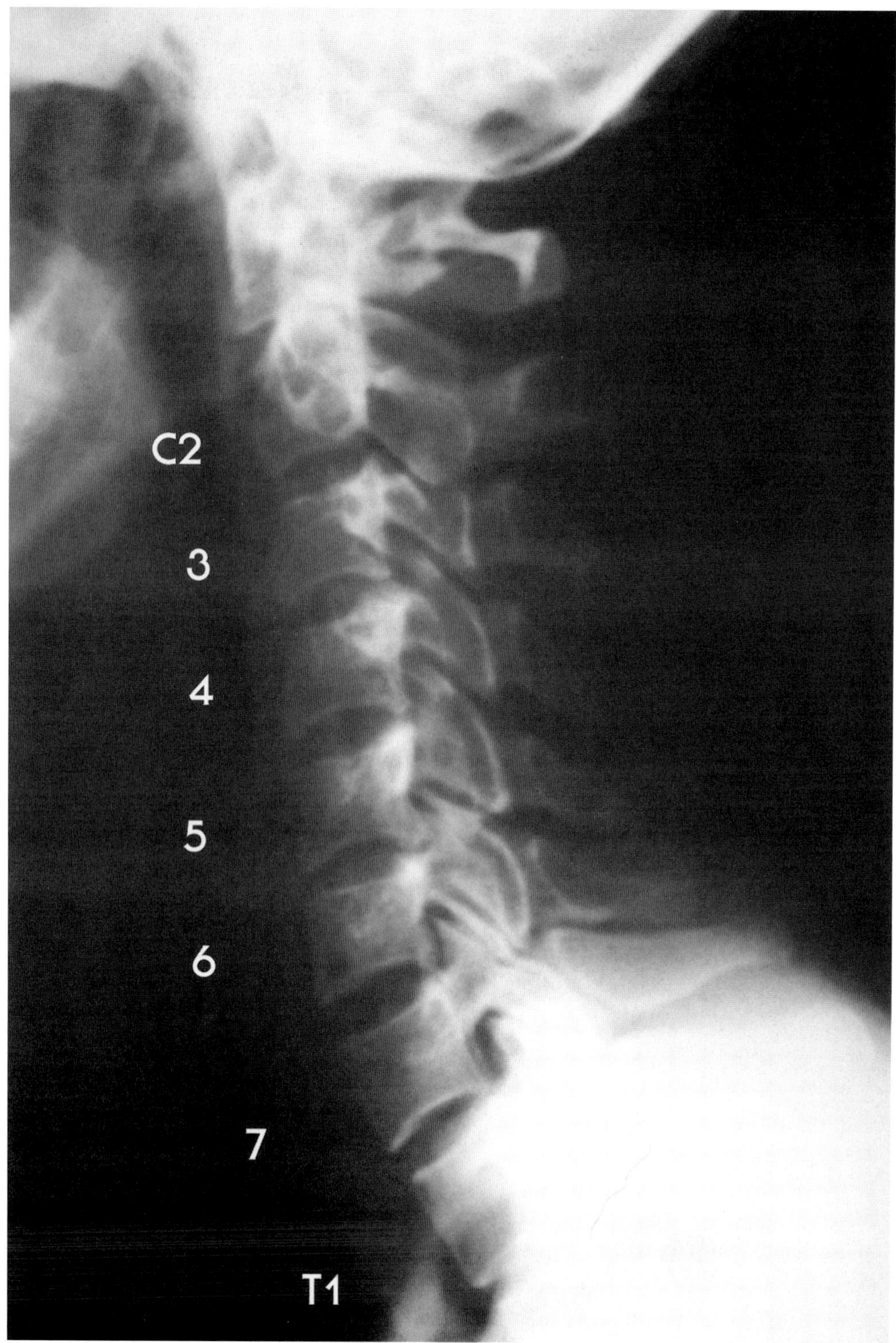

Plates 3-22 A/B
SUBLUXATION WITH REVERSAL OR KYPHOTIC CURVE
An X-ray and MRI comparison.
This is a lateral cervical X-ray and mid-sagittal cervical MRI of the same person. This shows a reversal of the lordotic curve. There is a retrolisthesis of C3 to C2, C4 to C3 and C4-5, the later pair form a posterior apex of the "kyphosis" or kyphotic curve.
Note the brainstem and spinal cord have straightened, and there is close contact at the C5-C6

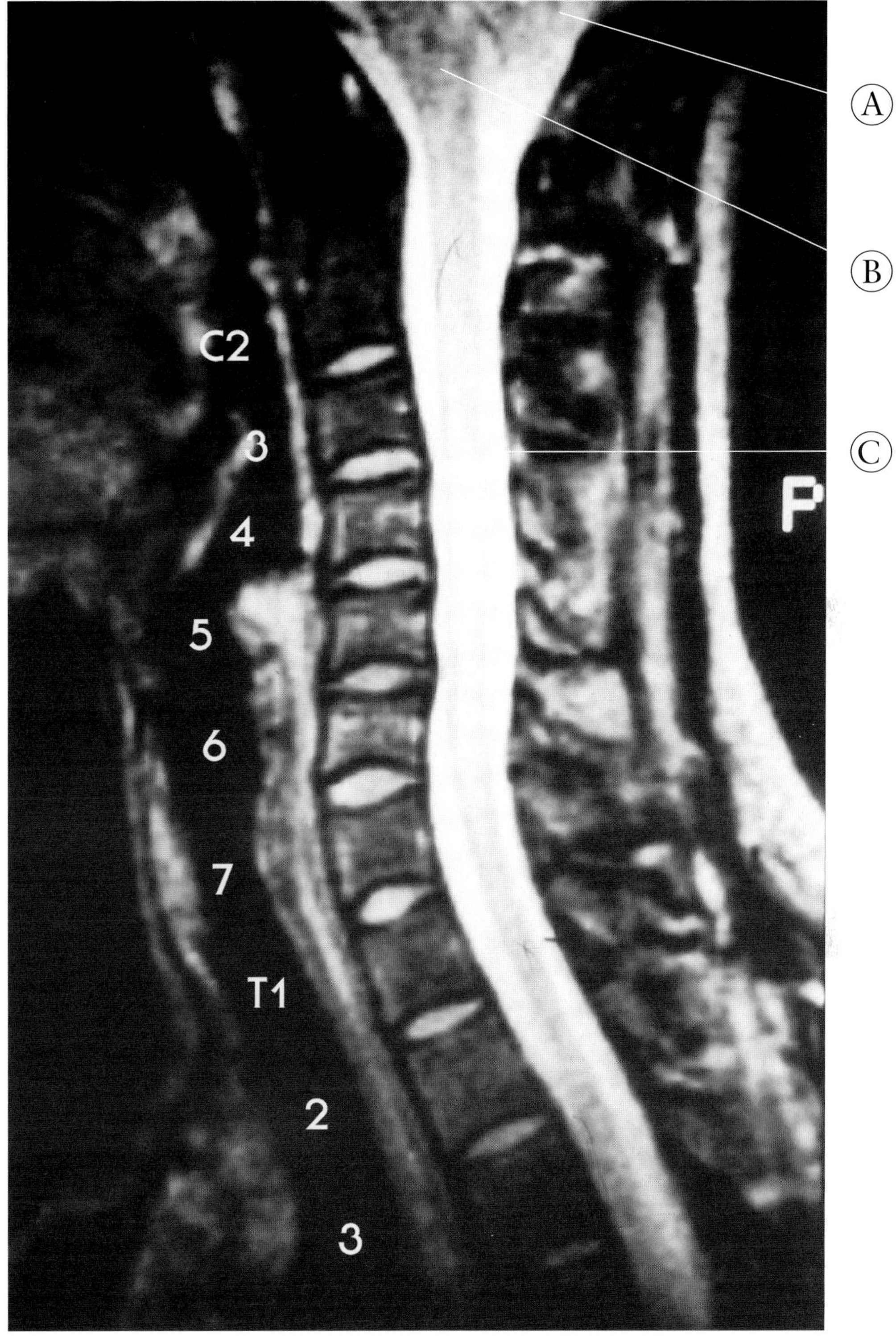

level and direct contact at T3 and T4. The cerebellum has contact with the posterior inferior occiput, in the neutral position. Flexion and an increase in canal length will add to this deformity
(A) Cerebellum
(B) Brainstem
(C) Spinal cord

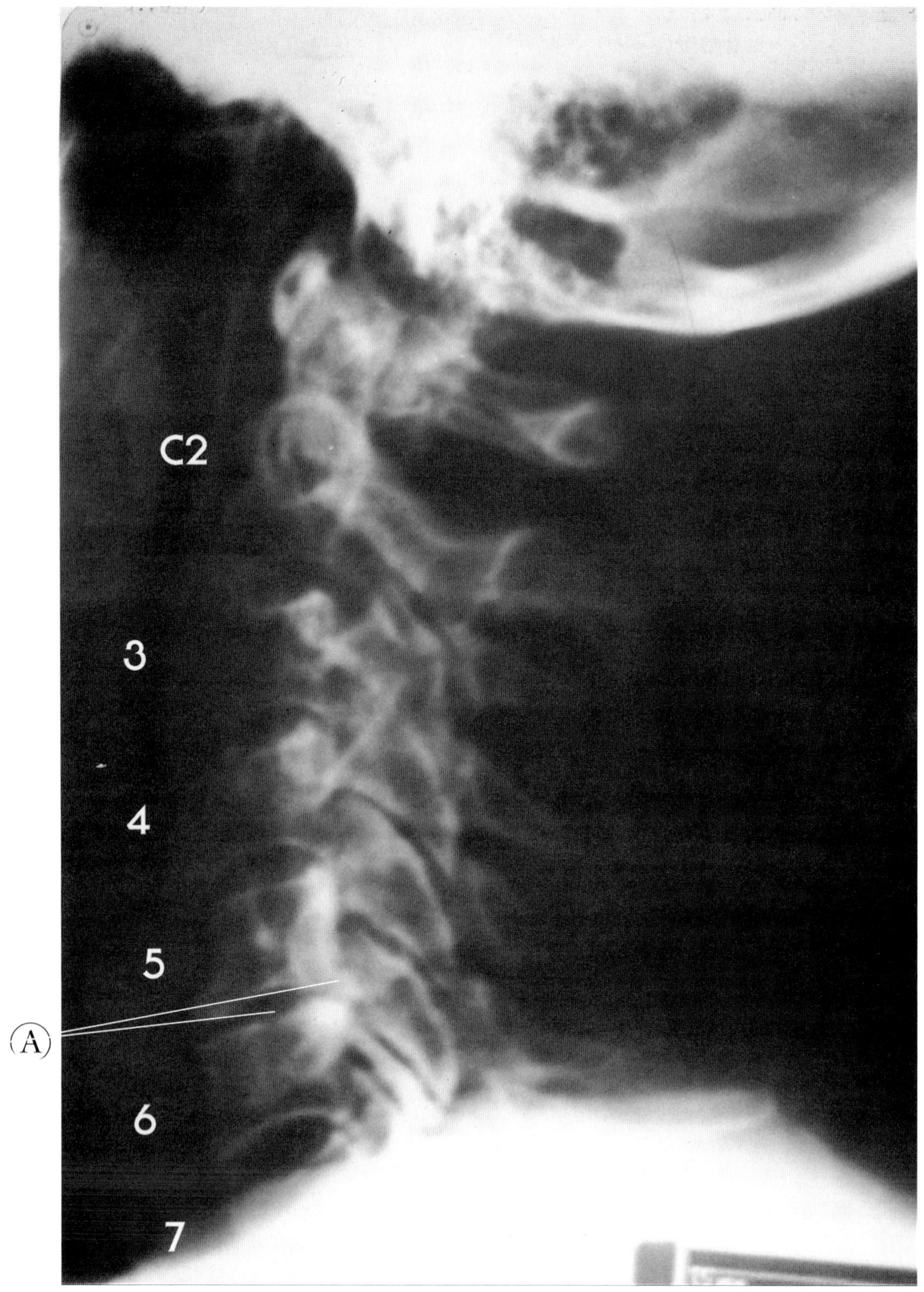

Plates 3-23 A/B
SUBLUXATION WITH REVERSAL OR KYPHOTIC CURVE
An X-ray and MRI comparison.
This pair of images is the lateral cervical X-ray and MRI of the same person. The spinal
cord is moved to the anterior portion of the canal, and has close contact with the C5-C6
osteophytes and disc. Ligamentum flavum at C6-C7 is bulging into the canal, partly from

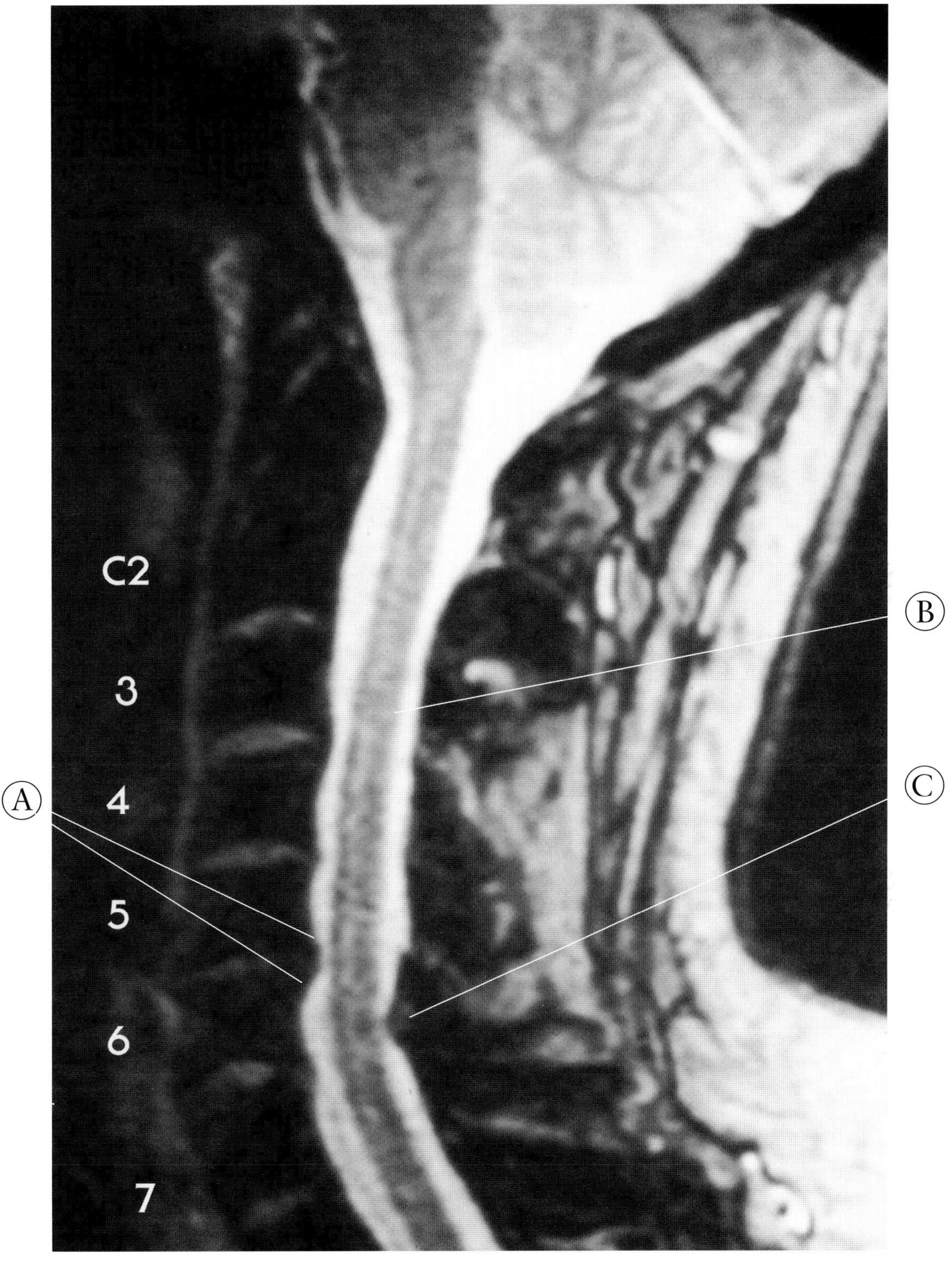

the loss of disc height and vertebral misalignment. The collective loss of disc height in the vertebral column can partly relieve cord tension by decreasing canal length.
(A) C5-6 osteophytes
(B) Spinal cord
(C) Ligamentum flavum between C6 and C7.

CHAPTER FOUR

Subluxations Of The Thoracic Spine

Discussion

The way in which the ribs are attached in the thoracic region of the spine makes it significantly different from the cervical and lumbar regions. Each rib articulates with a transverse process to a set of demifacets on the same vertebra and to the adjacent inferior vertebral body. The ribs between T2 and T10 also attach to the disc between demifacets, and have the appearance of three small joint complexes. These include two small synovial joints and an intervening fibrous joint where it contacts the disc. In **Figure 4-1** the rib-disc articulation is seen at the T1-2 disc. Subluxation can alter any or all of these articulations, just as it alters intervertebral discs and facets.

The combined effects of these complex rib articulations with the vertebrae and the extensive network of supporting ligaments and muscles give the thoracic spine the quality of being a single functional unit. This is called the rib cage. The head, rib cage, and pelvis comprise the three masses of the axial skeleton. The connecting, and much more mobile, cervical and lumbar columns can buckle when these masses are displaced. The head can displace relative to the thoracic spine, and the thoracic spine can displace relative to the pelvis. Many different terms have been used to describe the events that generate common subluxation complexes. The primary subluxation complexes can occur in the thoracic spine itself as a result of various

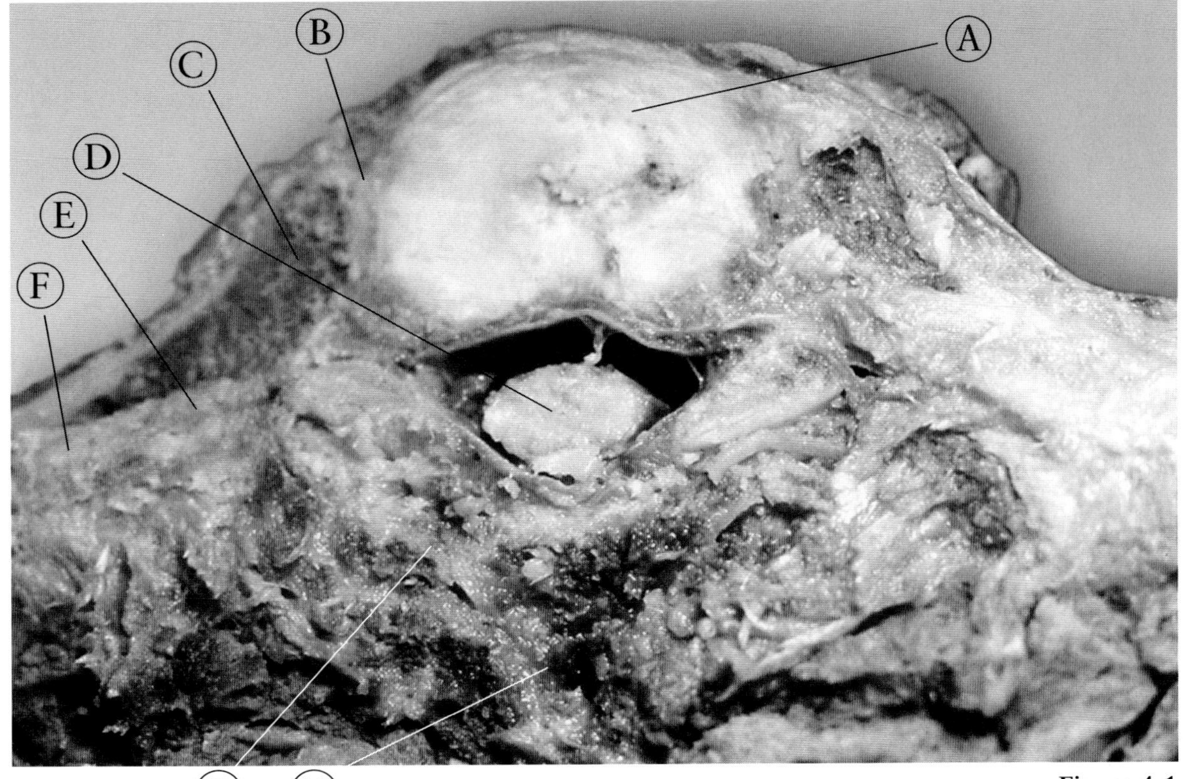

Figure 4-1

This is an axial view of the second ribs articulating with the T1-2 disc. These are costo-vertebral joints.

(A) Disc
(B) Costo-vertebral joint
(C) Rib
(D) Spinal cord
(E) Costo-transverse joint
(F) Transverse process
(G) Lamina
(H) Spinous process

Illustration of thoracic spine with sympathetic chain, showing orientaton of Figures 4-2 and 4-3.

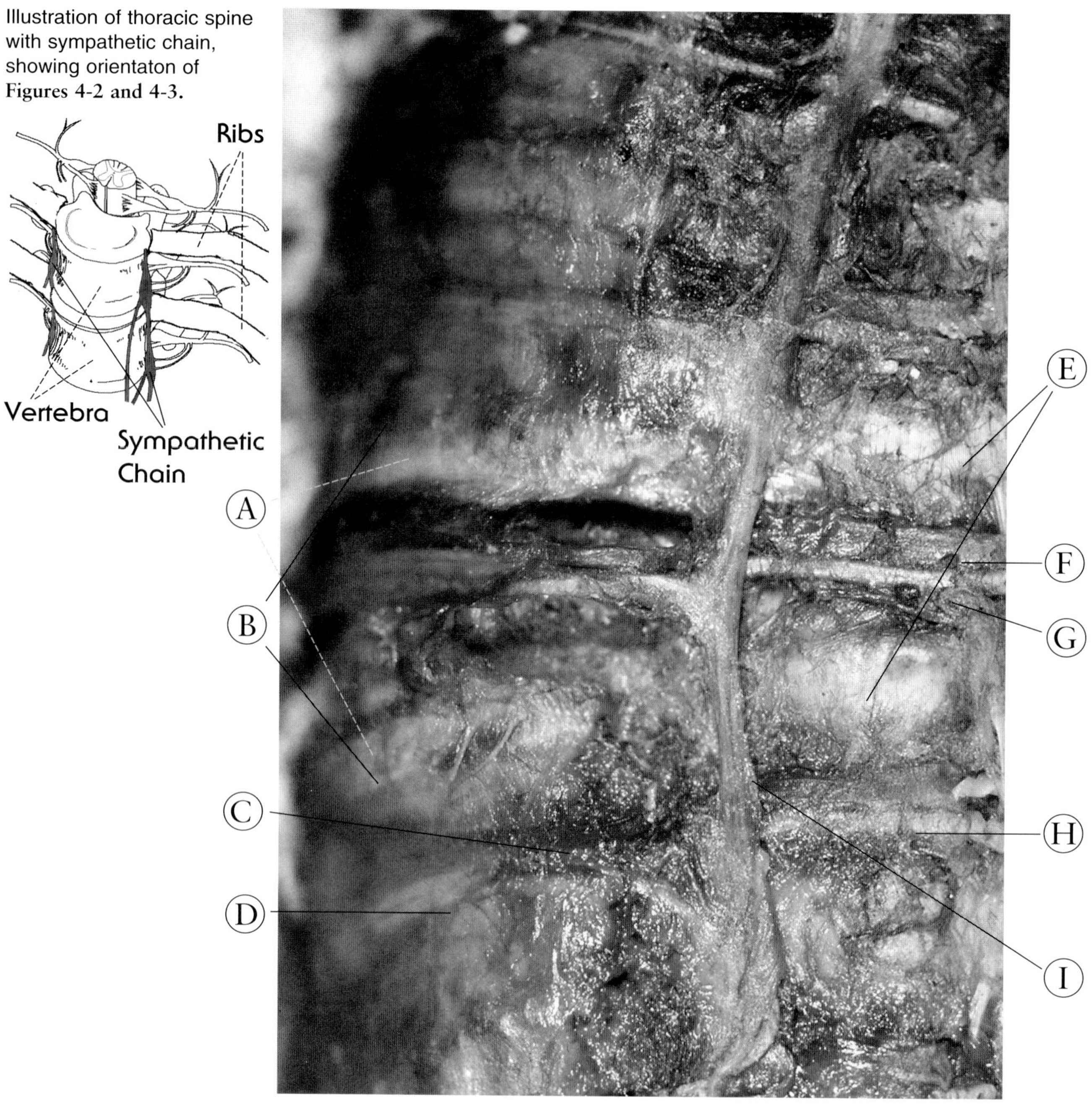

Figure 4-2

THORACIC SPINE ANTERIOR VIEW WITH SYMPATHETIC CHAIN AND RIB-SPINE RELATIONSHIP

Here is an anatomical proximity of the extra spinal nervous system to the costo-vertebral joints. The sympathetic chain can be immediately anterior to the costovertebral joints. Costo-vertebral subluxation and the resulting degenerative joint changes are concomitant with vertebral subluxation and the degenerative changes at those joints. Costo-vertebral subluxation and the sclerosis and inflammation can cause significant pathology to the autonomic nervous system.

(A) Endplates
(B) Discs
(C) Intersegmental twig arteries
(D) Anterior rami of nerve root
(E) Ribs
(F) Intercostal vein
(G) Intercostal nerve
(H) Intercostal artery
(I) Sympathetic chain

traumas. Rib articulations are all posterior structures, and provide increased structural support in that area. The anterior aspect, comprised of the vertebral bodies and discs of the thoracic spine, is therefore more vulnerable to change than the posterior aspect, where anterolesthesis and retrolisthesis of the thoracic vertebrae occur, altering the shape of the vertebral canal. Even though I did not have the means to depict or study them in detail, I have to acknowledge the lateralesthesis and rotational subluxation complexes. More detailed anatomical studies in this area are needed.

The vertebral canal is considered to be a posterior structure, but anterior changes of the thoracic spine can indeed affect the canal, ribs, and other posterior structures. More importantly, they can affect the neural contents, the spinal cord, and nerve roots. In the thoracic spine,

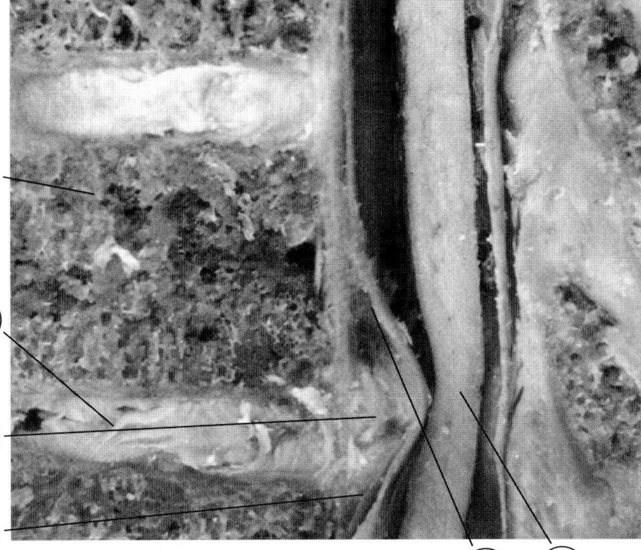

Figure 4-4

This a posterior disc herniation at the T9-10 level. The disc has pushed the posterior longitudinal ligament and thecal sac into the spinal cord.

  (A) Vertebrae
  (B) Disc
  (C) Herniation
  (D) Posterior longitudinal ligament
  (E) Thecal sac
  (F) Spinal cord

there is an extra-spinal nervous system component to consider. The sympathetic chain in the thoracic spine is at or near the costo-vertebral joints, (**See Figure 4-2**). The integrity of the sympathetic chain is at risk when these joints are subluxated. Chronic degenerative changes have been observed to alter the nervous tissue of the sympathetic chain. There can be a variation between individuals as to the location of the chain. In **Figure 4-2**, the sympathetic chain is over the costo-vertebral joints and in **Figure 4-3** the chain is oriented over the costo-transverse joints.

One of the most common postural patterns in our society is anterior weight bearing or displacement of the head anterior to the rib cage or shoulders, usually characterized by loss of the cervical curve. This has an important implication for the thoracic spine. Over time, the weight of the head carried habitually in an anterior position can create a deforming force on the thoracic spine and cause increased kyphotic curvature. The condition appears gradually and becomes worse over a period of time, so the patient may not be aware of pain or discomfort, only an increasing perception of stiffness and lack of flexibility.

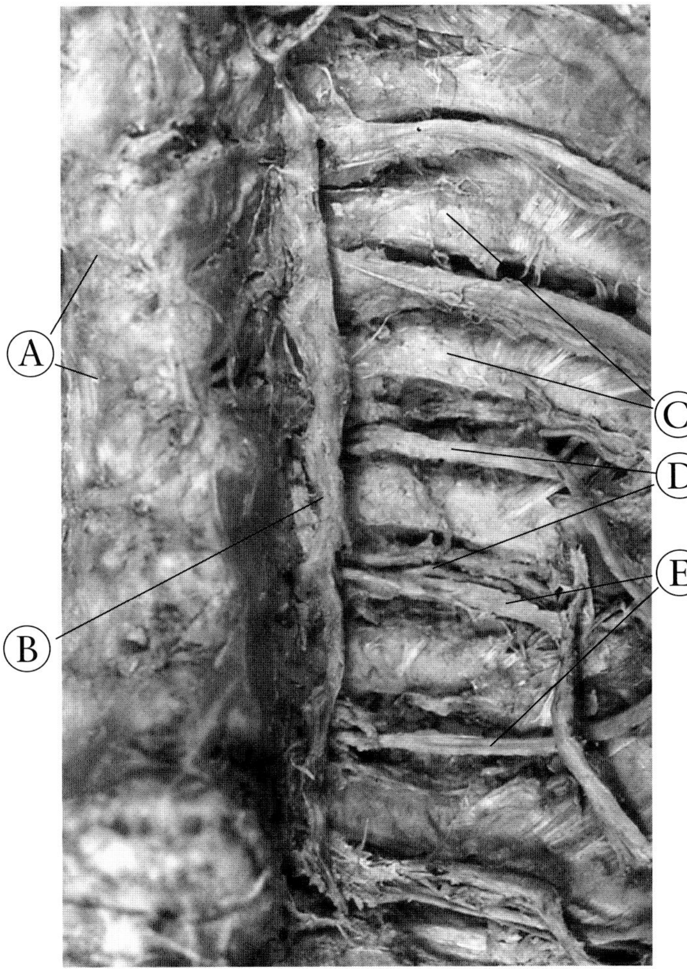

Figure 4-3

  (A) Discs
  (B) Sympathetic chain
  (C) Ribs
  (D) Intercostal nerves
  (E) Intercostal neurovascular bundles

Vertebral bodies in the thoracic spine sometimes are compressed anteriorly more than posteriorly, making them wedge-shaped. The added posterior stability that the rib articulations and the network of ligaments provide to the transverse processes, canals, and pedicles may retard posterior crushing during certain kinds of trauma. It should also be noted that the thoracic spine is much less susceptible to posterior spurring than the cervical and lumbar spines.

Posterior herniation of the thoracic discs does occur. **See Figure 4-4**, a T10 disc. It should be noted that the lower the thoracic disc herniation, the lower the neurological involvement. Since the conus medularis ends at T12 or L1, the disc herniation at T11 could affect the neurons of the legs or even the bladder.

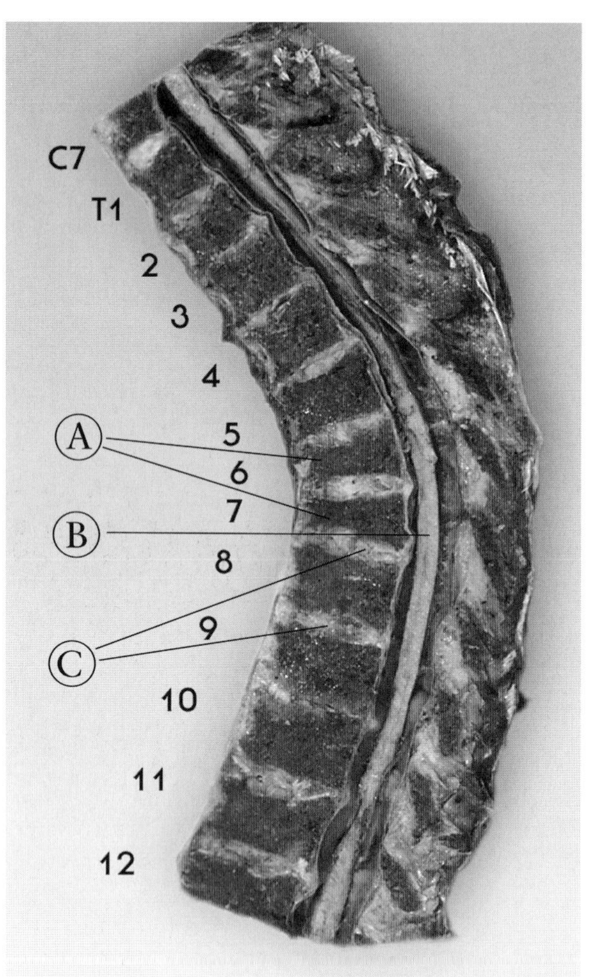

Figure 4-5
HYPERKYPHOSIS OF THE THORACIC SPINE.

The thoracic vertebrae 6 and 7 have compression fractures with more anterior height loss. The result is an anterior translation of the spinal cord to the anterior wall of the canal.
Note cord contact from T5 to T7.
  (A) Compression fractures
  (B) Spinal cord
  (C) Discs

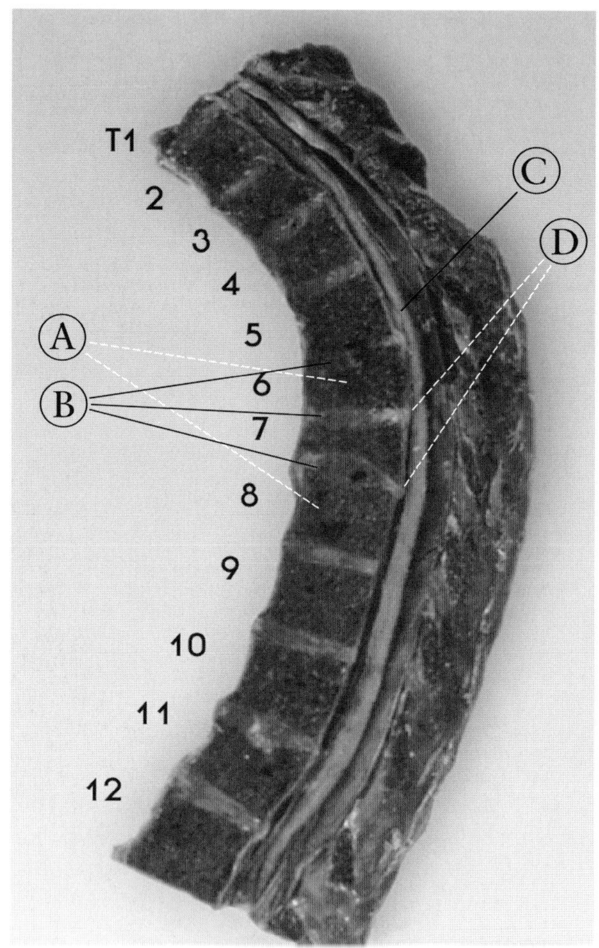

Figure 4-6
HYPERKYPHOSIS AS A RESULT OF OSTEOPOROSIS

Compression fractures of T6 and 7 have increased the kyphotic curvature. Note the spinal cord contact with the canal wall from T1 to T7 and small disc protrusions into the cord.
  (A) Vertebrae
  (B) Discs
  (C) Spinal cord
  (D) Disc protrusion

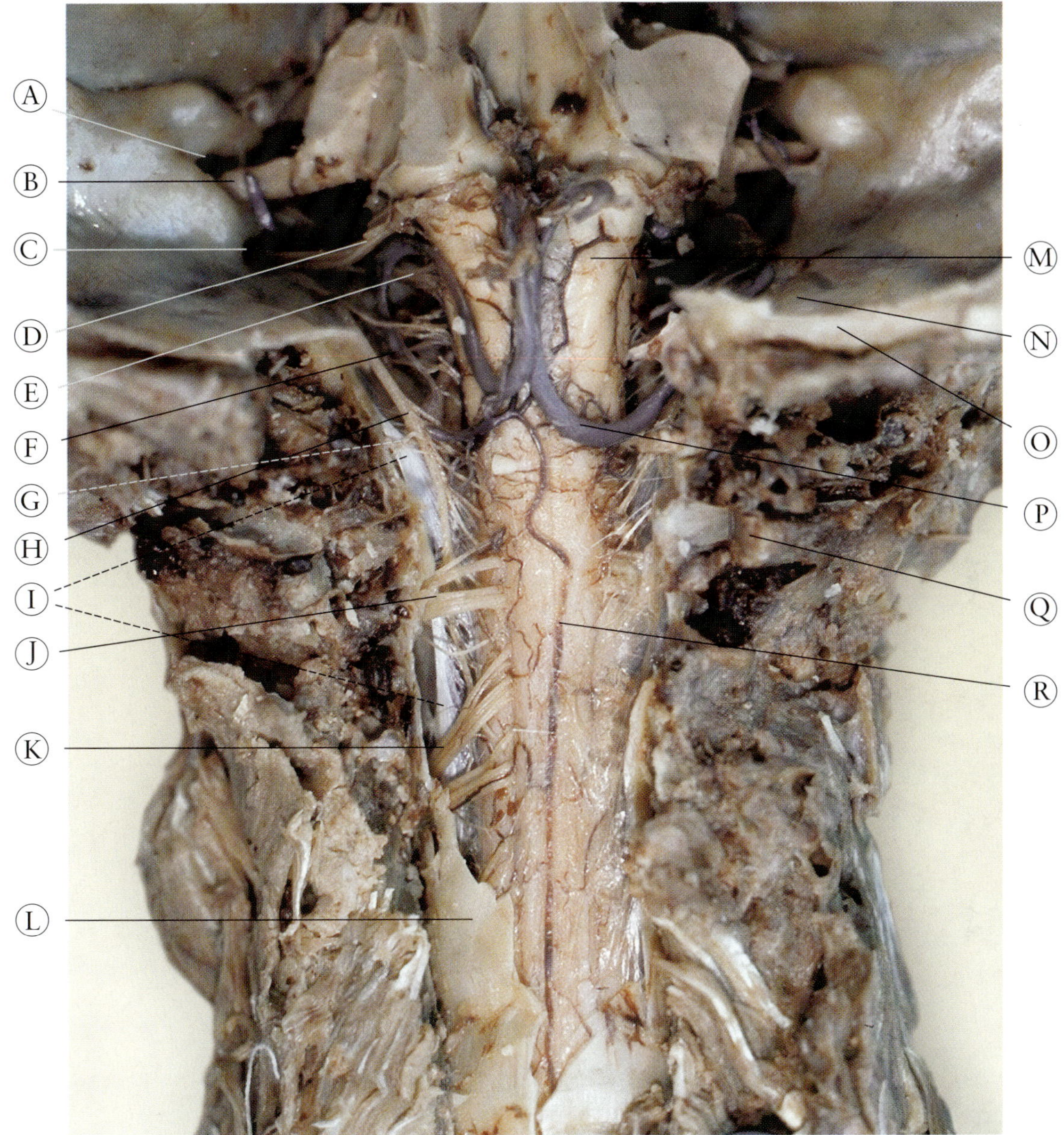

Color Plate 1 (same as Figure 1-5)
NORMAL ANATOMICAL RELATIONSHIPS, continued

Same specimen as Figure 1-4 with occiput opened and cerebellum removed, with the skull in the neutral position relative to the neck.

(A) Internal Auditory Meatus
(B) Acoustic Nerve(VIII)
(C) Jugular Foramen
(D) Glossopharyngeal Nerve(IX)
(E) Vagus Nerve(X)
(F) Hypoglossal Nerve (XII)
(G) C1 nerve rootlets
(H) Spinal Accessory Nerve (XI)
(I) Dentate Ligament
(J) C2 Nerve rootlets
(K) C3 Nerve rootlets
(L) Thecal sac (dural side)
(M) Brainstem
(N) Cerebellar Fossa
(O) Occiput (cut edge)
(P) Inferior Cerebellar Artery
(Q) Arch of Atlas
(R) Dorsal Spinal Artery

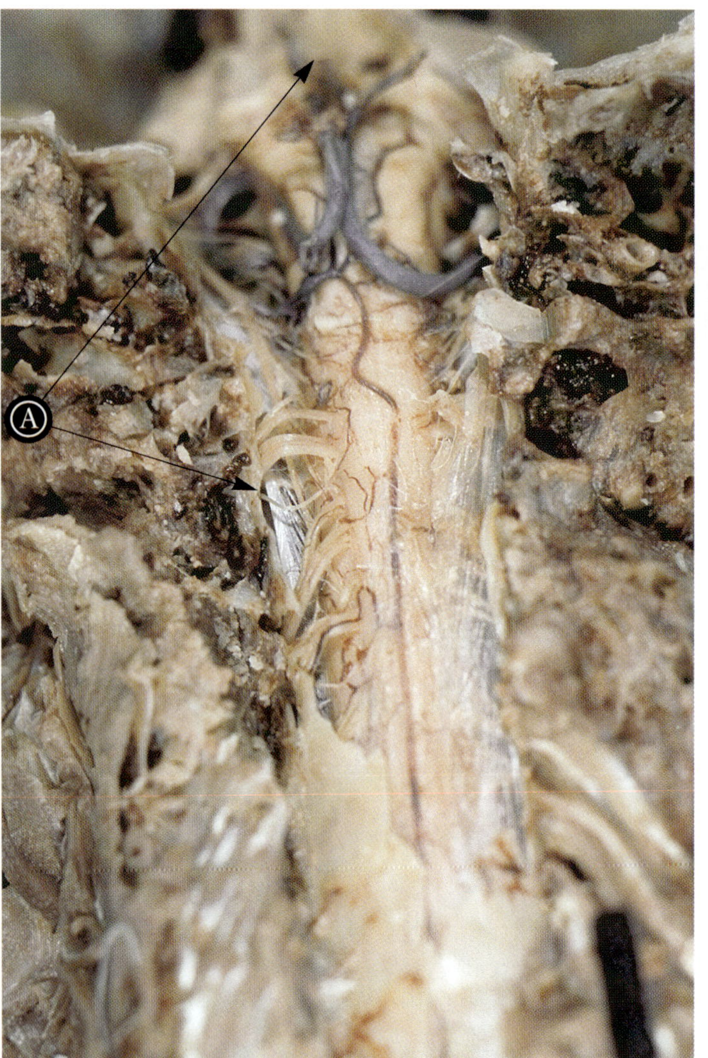

a.

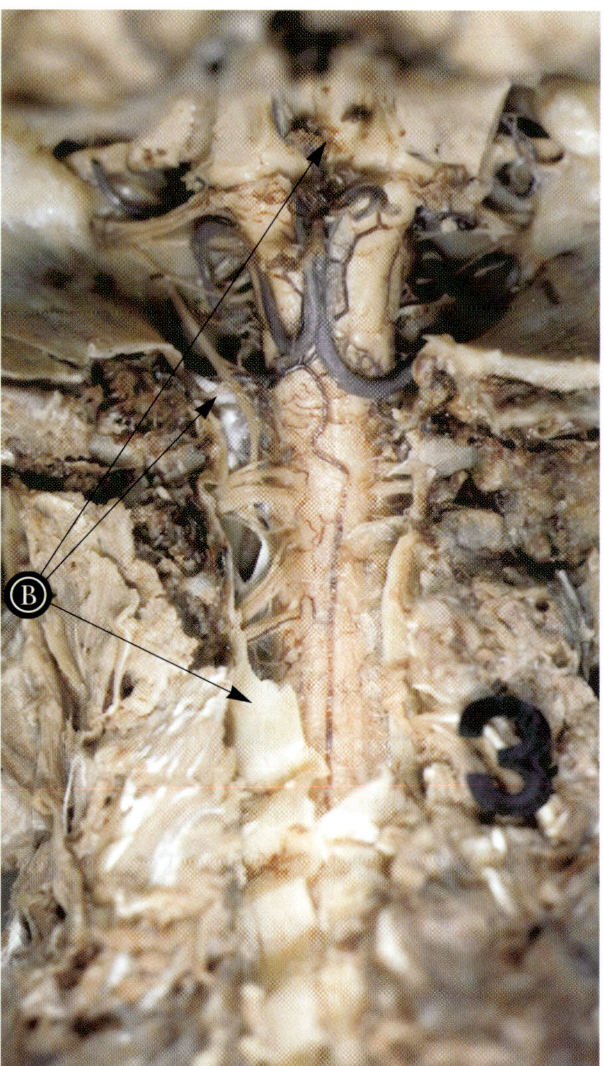

b.

Color Plate 2 (Same as Fig. 1-6)

EFFECTS OF HEAD FLEXION AND EXTENSION ON THE CENTRAL NERVOUS SYSTEM

(a). Flexion(head tipped forward) increases the distance between the occiput and the coccyx, therefore lengthening the neural canal and the stretching the cord and brainstem.

  (A) Note stretching of the dentate ligament and the movement of the brainstem down toward the occiput. Note positions of Dentate Ligament, Brainstem, Base of Occiput, Arch of Atlas (refer to **Fig.** 1-5 for keys to anatomical structures)

(b). Extension (head tipped backward) decreases the distance between the occiput and the coccyx, shortening and relaxing the cord and brainstem.

  (B) Note the relaxed left dentate ligament, the folded, relaxed dura mater (thecal sac), and the distance of the brainstem from the occiput. Note positions of Dentate Ligament, Brainstem, Base of Occiput, Arch of Atlas, Thecal sac.

COMPRESSION FRACTURES

With traumatic or osteoporotic compression fractures, the thoracic kyphotic curvature increases (**See Figure 4-5**), pulling (tractioning) the spinal cord into the anterior portion of the canal and up against the vertebral bodies. Any structural defects such as osteophytes or disk bulges will have more severe clinical implications this deforming compression fracture pattern. **Figure 4-6** shows how disc bulging and posterior spurs of thoracic vertebra 5, 6, and 7 have made impressions in the spinal cord.

The thoracic spinal cord gives rise to ventral nerve roots which are the motor and efferent (outgoing) nerve pathways for the viscera. The anterior spinal artery lies in close proximity, supplying blood to the neurons of the ventral horns where visceral and somatic motor neurons are found in close proximity. Hypoxia of this neural tissue and the exact clinical results are not known. The dramatic results by some chiropractors can be attributed to changing the vascular condition of the spinal cord. Further studies are recommended.

Tractioning of the cord can lead to an inflammatory condition that results in fibrous adhesions inside and outside the thecal sac involving the cord and nerve roots. **Figure 4-7** shows the cord (in the anterior compartment of the canal, indicating tethering) with nerve roots dropping down toward their intervertebral foramen. They are enmeshed in the dense, fibrous network that commonly results from chronic inflammation. This fibrous mass can trap nerve rootlets proximal to the nerve roots, so that certain positions and actions could create more severe inflammation and tractioning. Further, the increase in kyphosis leads to an overall increase in canal length and length of the cord itself, and can affect the entire middle portion of the thoracic spinal cord.

Over a period of time, in the absence of compression, tethering results, causing a decrease of neural conductivity. Studies show that an initial period of irritation and increase in sensitivity and conductivity of the nervous tissue is followed by a drop in conductivity that results in a loss of all impulses. This must correlate with loss of visceral and motor function. This is a significant factor in the chronic, debilitating postural changes that afflict many people in Western society.

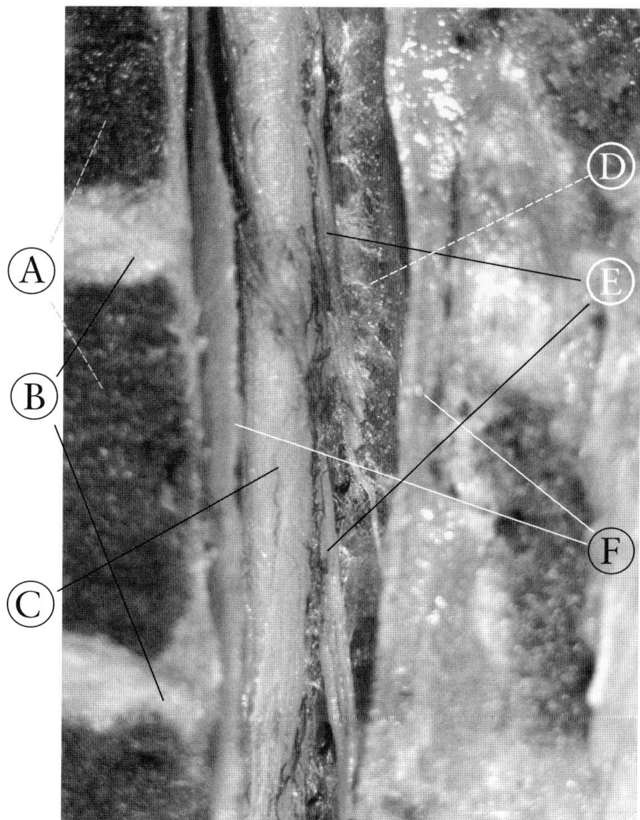

Figure 4-7
SUBARACHNOID ADHESIONS.
Adhesions in the subarachnoid space are common when the spinal cord is tethered
Note the nerve rootlets in the adhesions.

(A) Vertebral bodies	(D) Subarachnoid
(B) Discs	adhesions
(C) Spinal cord	(E) Nerve rootlets
	(F) Thecal sac

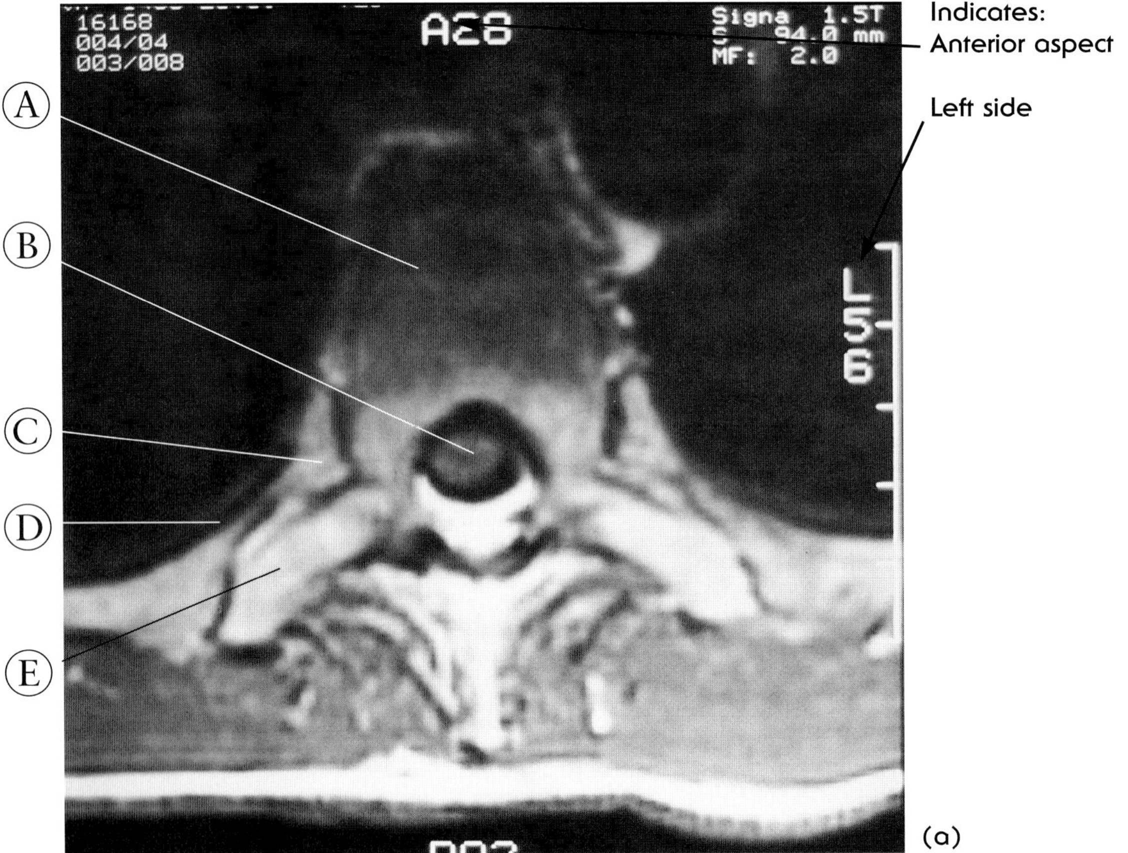

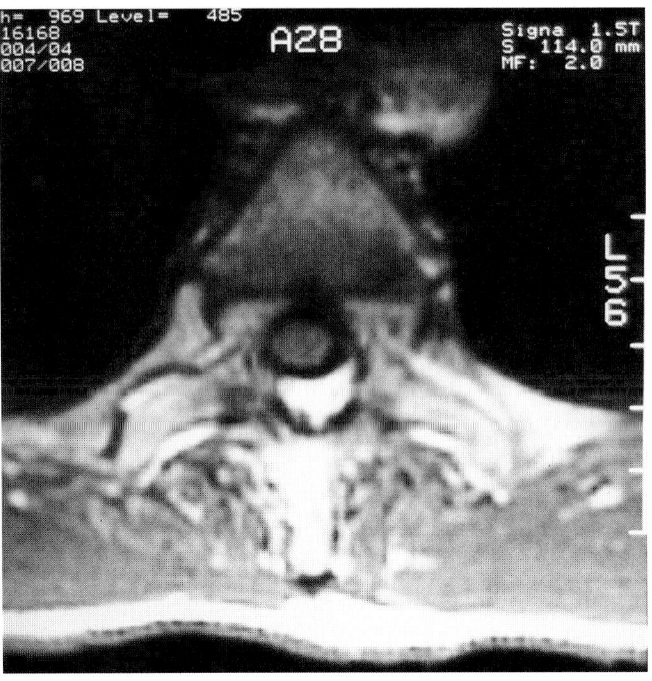

**Figures 4-8 A & B
Thoracic Spine: MRI Axial Views
of Tethered Spinal Cords**

(A) Vertebral body
(B) Spinal cord
(C) Rib head
(D) Neck of rib
(E) Transverse process

(a) Note the spinal cord-canal contact even in the recumbent position, giving the patients relief. Because of gravity, these studies indicate spinal cord pre-tension in the neutral position. The relaxed spinal cord should be in the posterior or bottom part of the canal. Adverse physiological tension will result in flexed positions.
(b) Long-term forces over time will change the shapes of all the tissues.

ANTERIOR WEIGHT BEARING

Anterior weight bearing is a very common condition, and is a by-product of our postural habits. What Americans consider normal posture is, from the human body's point of view, not normal at all. We sit in chairs, get in and out of cars, sit in cars, and spend hours reading, studying, or staring at a computer screen with our heads inclined forward, cantilevered into space. Evolutionarily speaking, these are not "normal" human activities. They are recently acquired, and often mandatory postural situations that are having a profound effect on our spines.

In most people, sitting increases the curvature of the thoracic spine because most desk or computer work, and even watching TV, causes the head to go forward relative to the thoracic spine, thus reducing cervical curvature and increasing thoracic kyphosis. This causes long-term malpositioning and tethering of the spinal cord, which can be associated with visceral, primarily cardiovascular problems.

Loss of ligament and joint integrity causes soft tissue changes. These have gotten different names – Marie-Strumpel, non-marginal osteophytes, spondylosis – it is all the same degenerative process. The result is altered weight bearing leading to altered bone. There are many different mechanisms of injury and ways to lose normal weight bearing. The severity increases with time. The degree of subluxation and chronic neurological distress due to overall postural changes are significant health conditions. Duration and magnitude of the distress on the nervous system are the major factors.

CHAPTER FOUR — EXPANDED TABLE OF CONTENTS
Atlas of Subluxations of the Thoracic Spine

SECTION I:
Subluxations with a normal thoracic curve (1 pair)

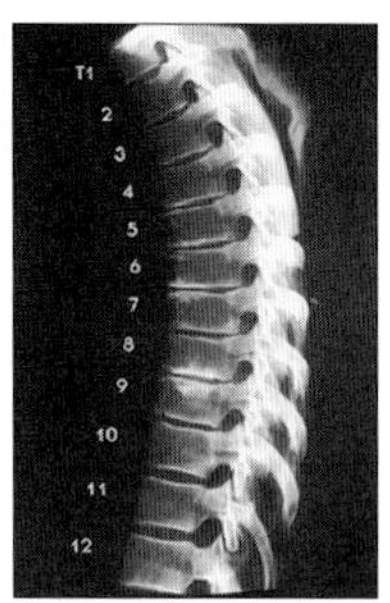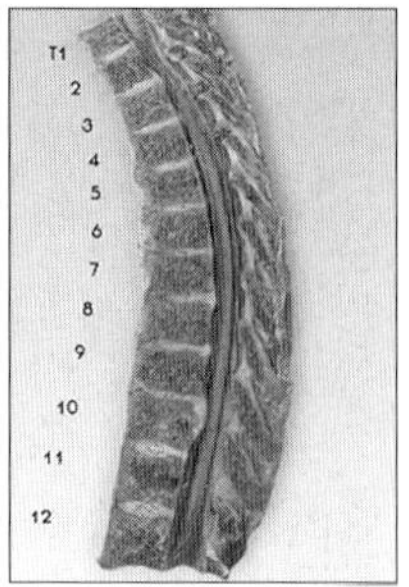

Plates 4-1 A & B
SUBLUXATIONS WITH A NORMAL KYPHOTIC
CURVE
This shows the thoracic spine with minor compression
fractures and multiple disc herniation.
Pg. 86-87

SECTION II:
Subluxations with a reversal of the upper curve (3 pairs)

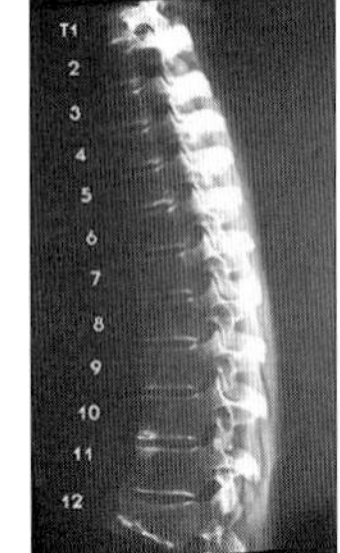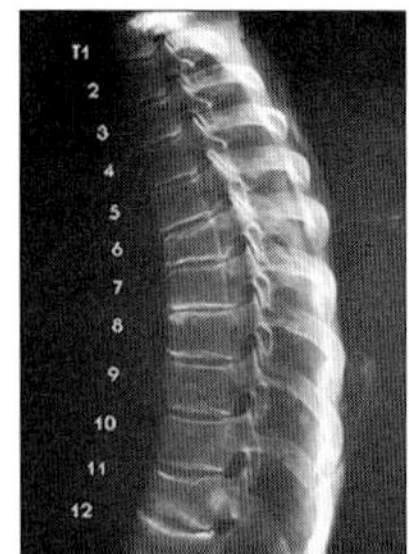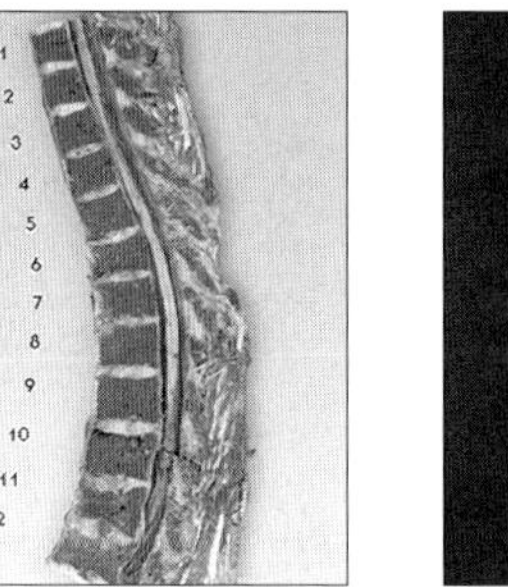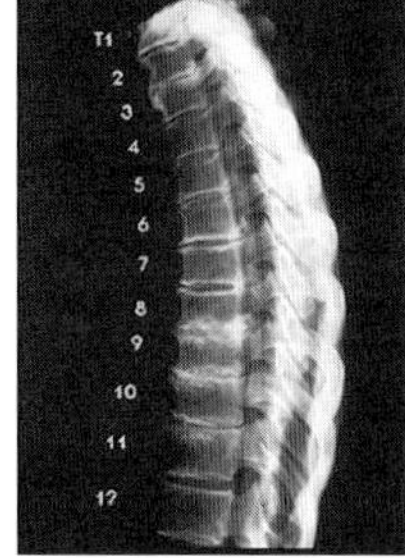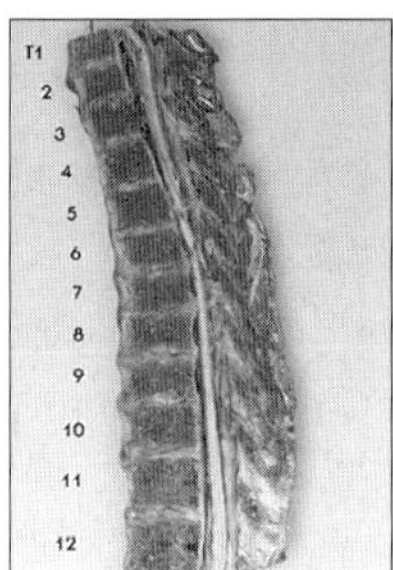

Plates 4-2 A & B	Plates 4-3 A & B	Plates 4-4 A & B
UPPER THORACIC CURVE REVERSAL	Thoracic Anterolesthesis: Upper Thoracic II	Thoracic Spine: Antrolesthesis: Upper thoracic II
Anterolisthesis Upper Thoracics I		
Pg. 88-89	Pg. 90-91	Pg. 92-93

SECTION III:
Subluxations with a reversal of the lower curve (3 pairs)

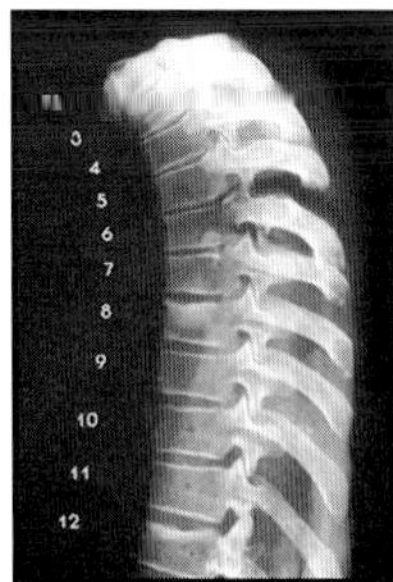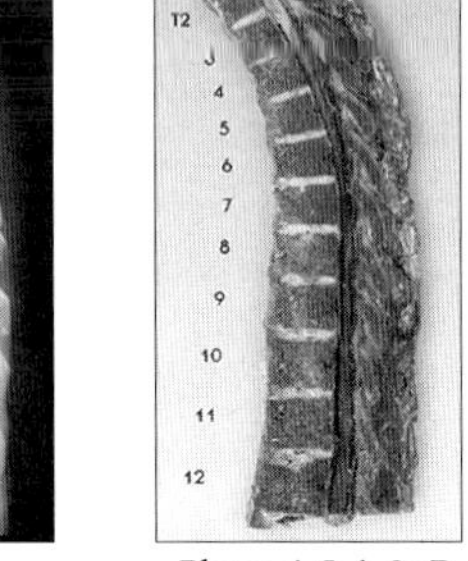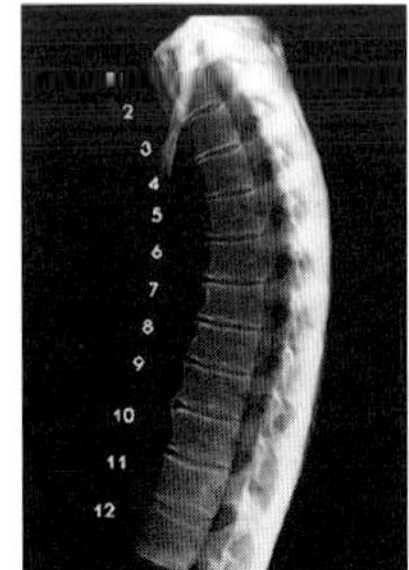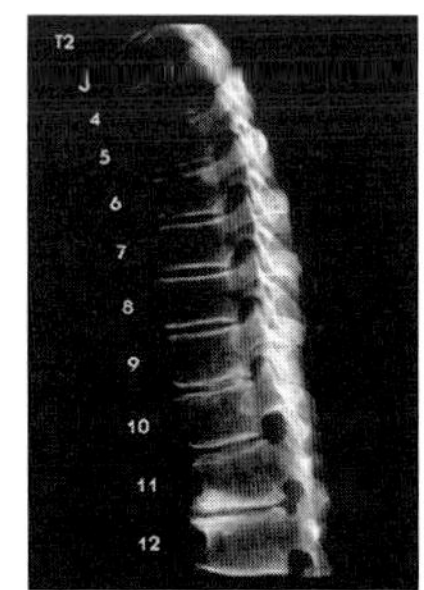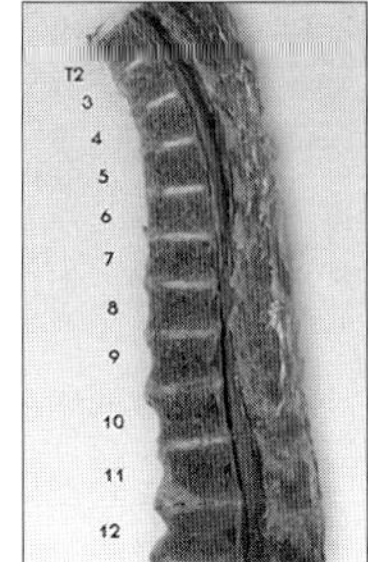

Plates 4-5 A & B	Plates 4-6 A & B	Plates 4-7 A & B
LOWER THORACIC CURVE REVERSAL	LOWER THORACIC CURVE REVERSAL	LOWER THORACIC CURVE REVERSAL
(T7-11)	Thoracic Spine: Anterolisthesis of lower	
Thoracic Spine : Anterolisthesis lower thoracics	thoracics	
Pg. 94-95	Pg. 96-97	Pg. 98-99

CHAPTER FOUR — EXPANDED TABLE OF CONTENTS
Atlas of Subluxations of the Thoracic Spine

SECTION IV:
Subluxations with anterolisthesis of the upper and lower thoracic vertebrae (3 pairs)

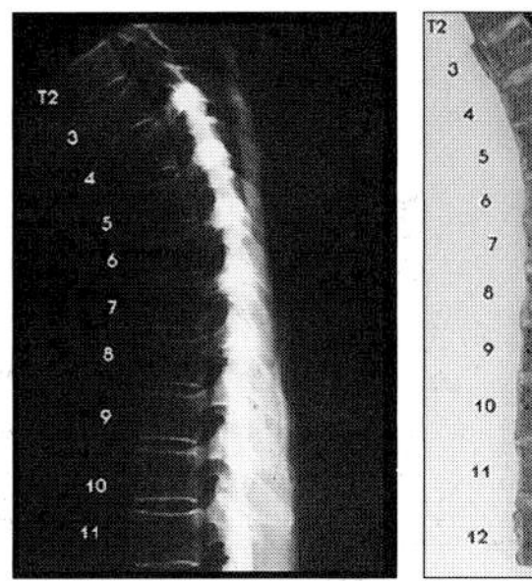
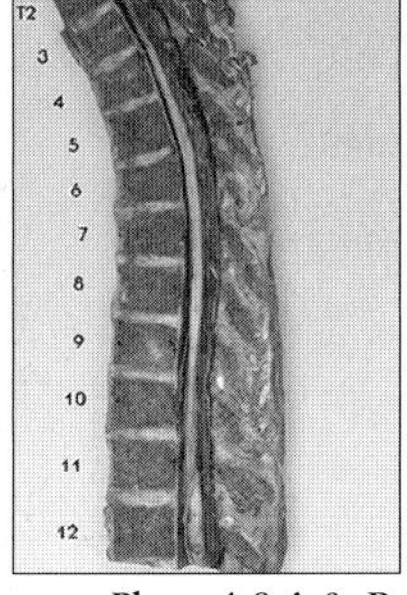

Plates 4-8 A & B
THORACIC UPPER POSTERIOR AND
LOWER ANTEROLISTHESIS

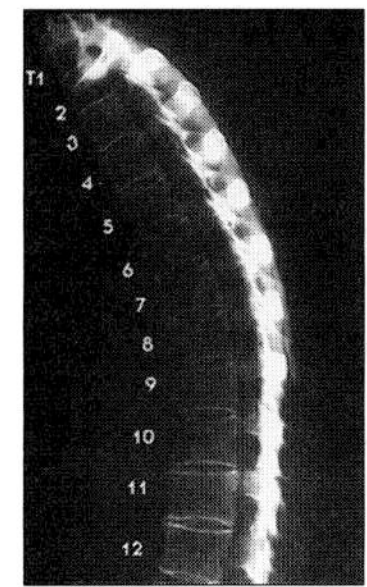
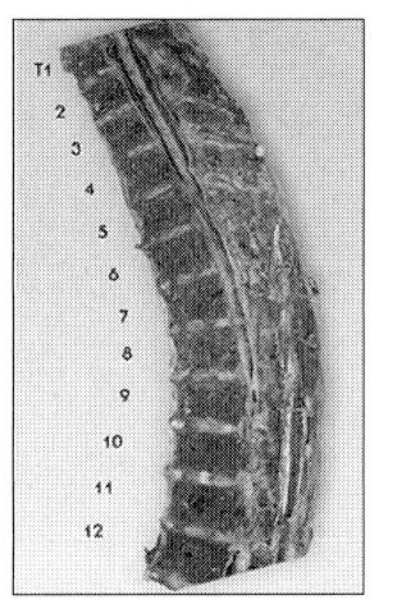

Plates 4-9 A & B
Thoracic Spine - antrolesthesis upper and lower
vertebrae

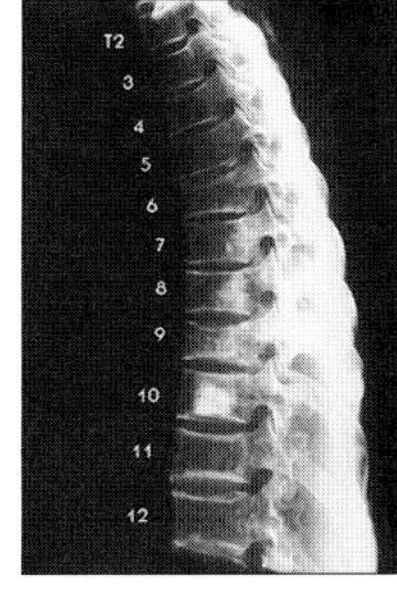
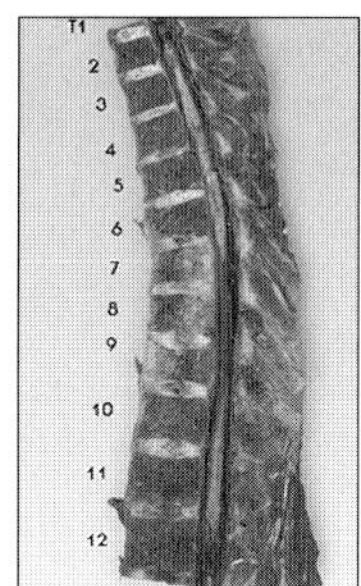

Plates 4-10 A & B
Thoracic Spine: Upper and lower antrolesthesis

Pg. 100-101

Pg. 102-103

Pg. 104-105

SECTION V:
Hyperkyphosis of the thoracic curve (3 pairs)

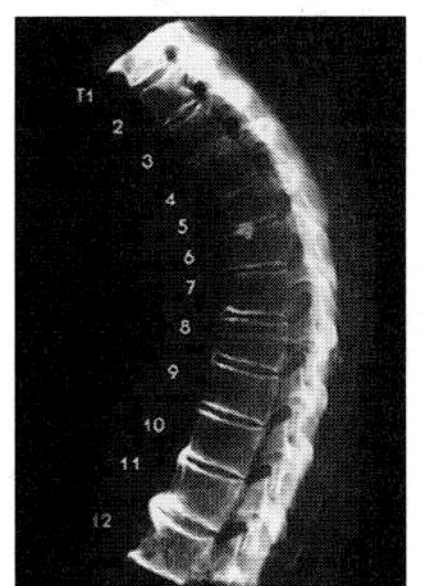
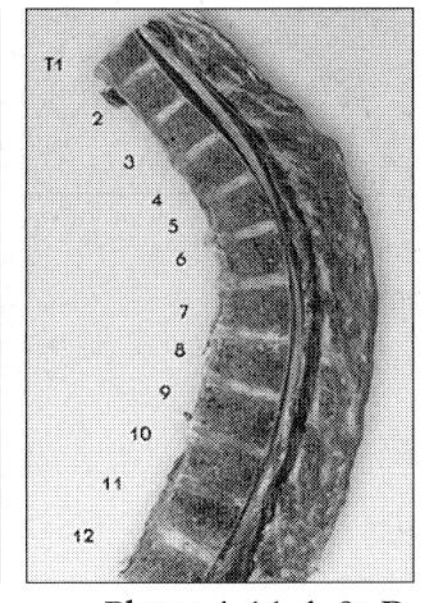

Plates 4-11 A & B
HYPERKYPHOSIS
Thoracic Spine: Progressive Spurring with
Osteoporosis and Hyperkyphosis

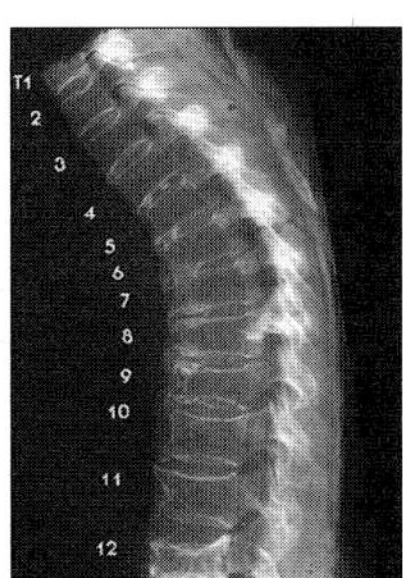
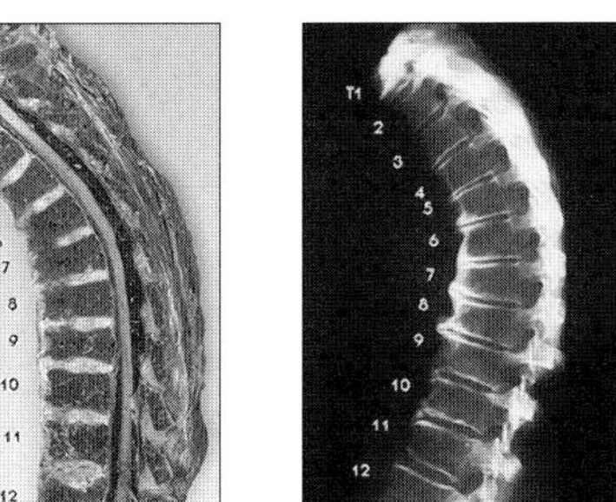

Plates 4-12 A & B
Progressive Spurring with Hyperkyphosis
caused by Osteoporosis

Plates 4-13 A & B
Progressive Spurring and Hyperkyphosis.

Pg. 106-107

Pg. 108-109

Pg. 110-111

Additional X-rays and MRIs

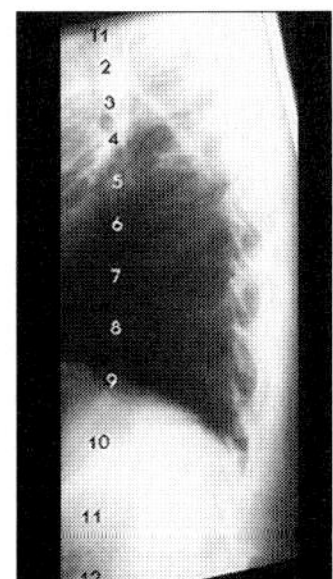
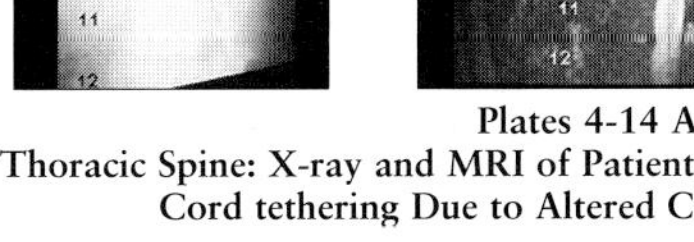
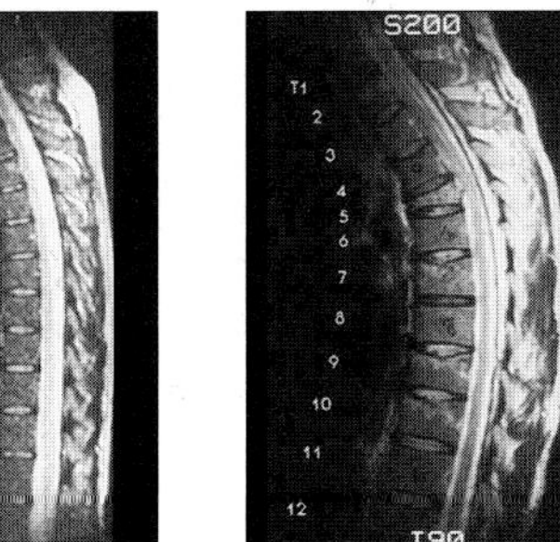
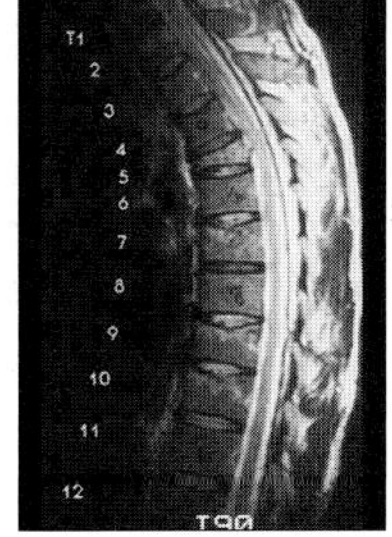

Plates 4-14 A & B
Thoracic Spine: X-ray and MRI of Patient with
Cord tethering Due to Altered Curves

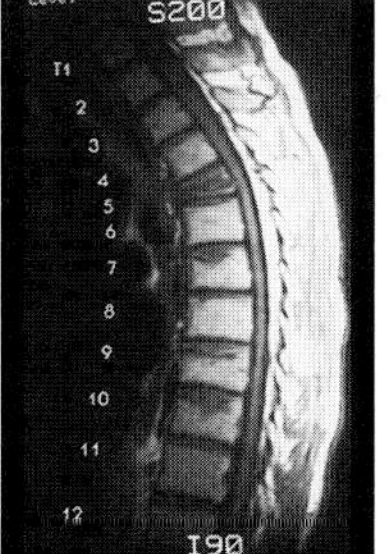

Plates 4-15 A & B
Hyperkyphosis due to Compression Fracture

Pg. 112-113

Pg. 114-115

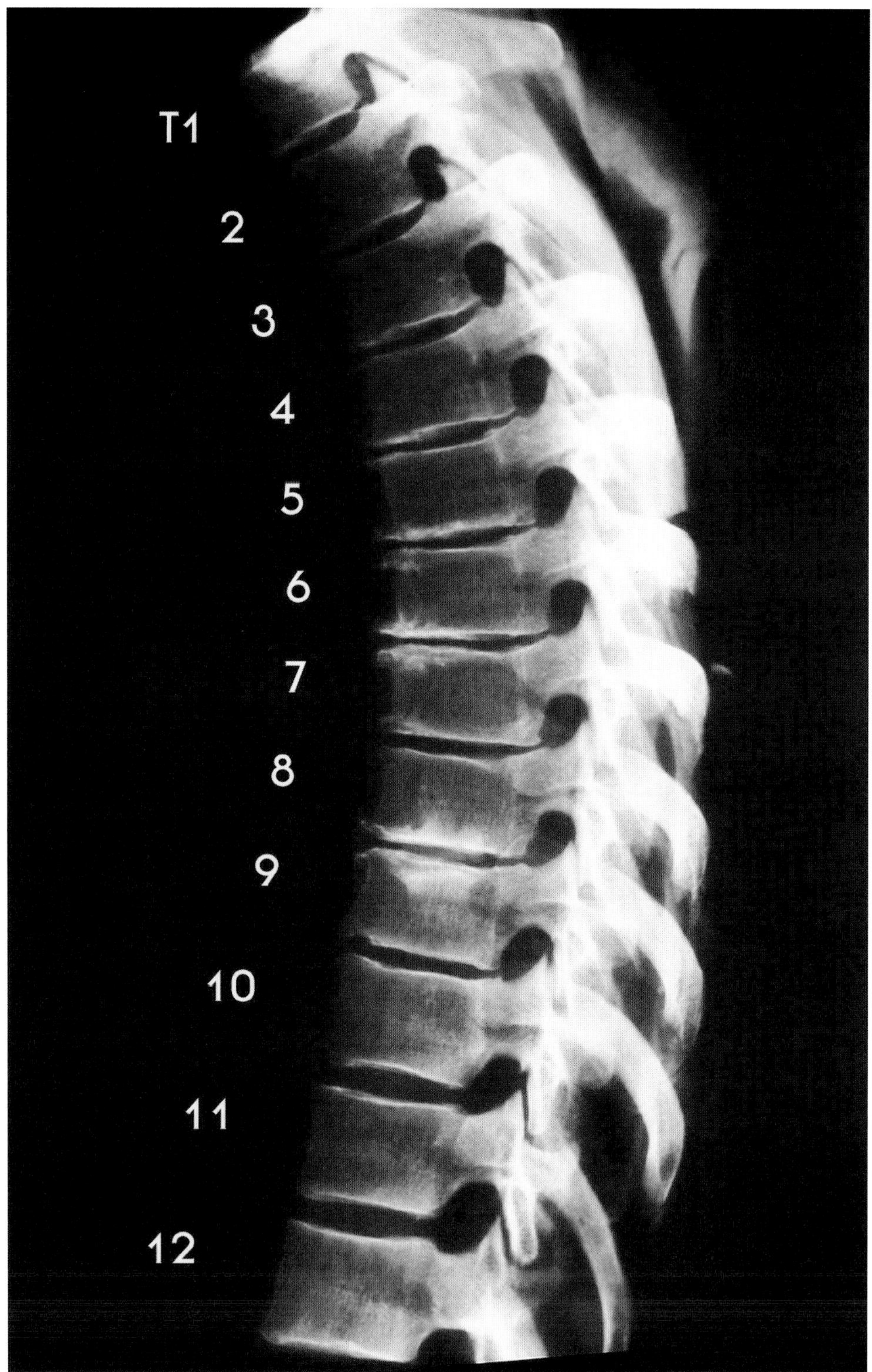

Plates 4-1 A & B
SUBLUXATIONS WITH A NORMAL KYPHOTIC CURVE
This shows the thoracic spine with minor compression fractures and multiple disc herniation.

All the discs in this specimen show anterior brown degeneration indicating poor imbibition (fluid exchange) and chronically low hydration of that part of the disc. Signs of trauma are seen in the end plate disturbances of the inferior body of T3 down to the superior endplate of the body of T10. This is a result of the subluxations of T1 to T10

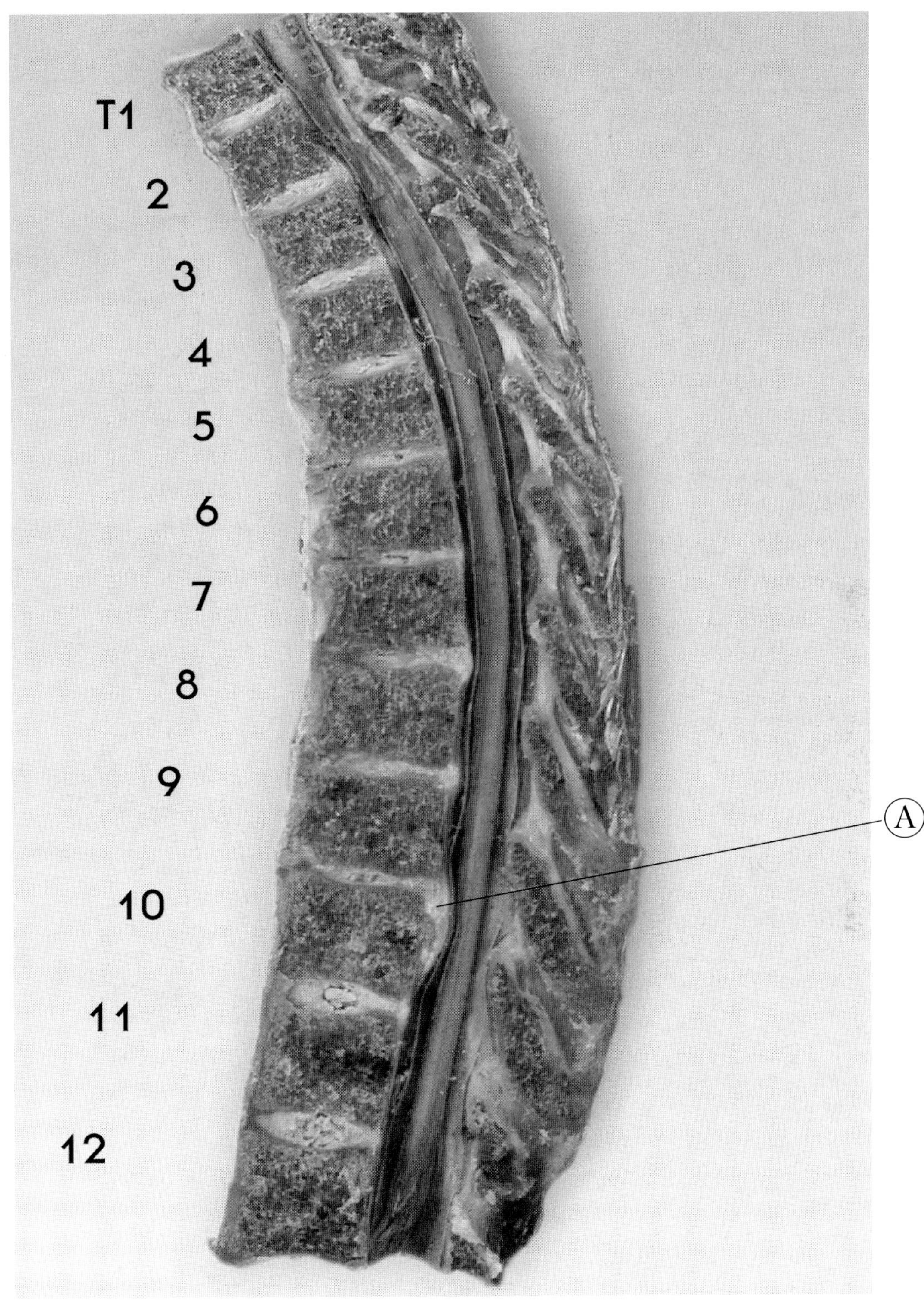

and the resulting osteophyte development of the affected segments.
T2 is retro to T1 with disc bulging slightly; T3 is retro to T2 with disc herniation and cord contact; T3 and T4 have signs of compression and there are misalignments of T5 to T9. T8 anterior to T7 with disc herniating and mild cord contact;T9 -10 disc herniating with cord contact; note normal alignment and appearance of T11 and T12.

(A) Disc herniation

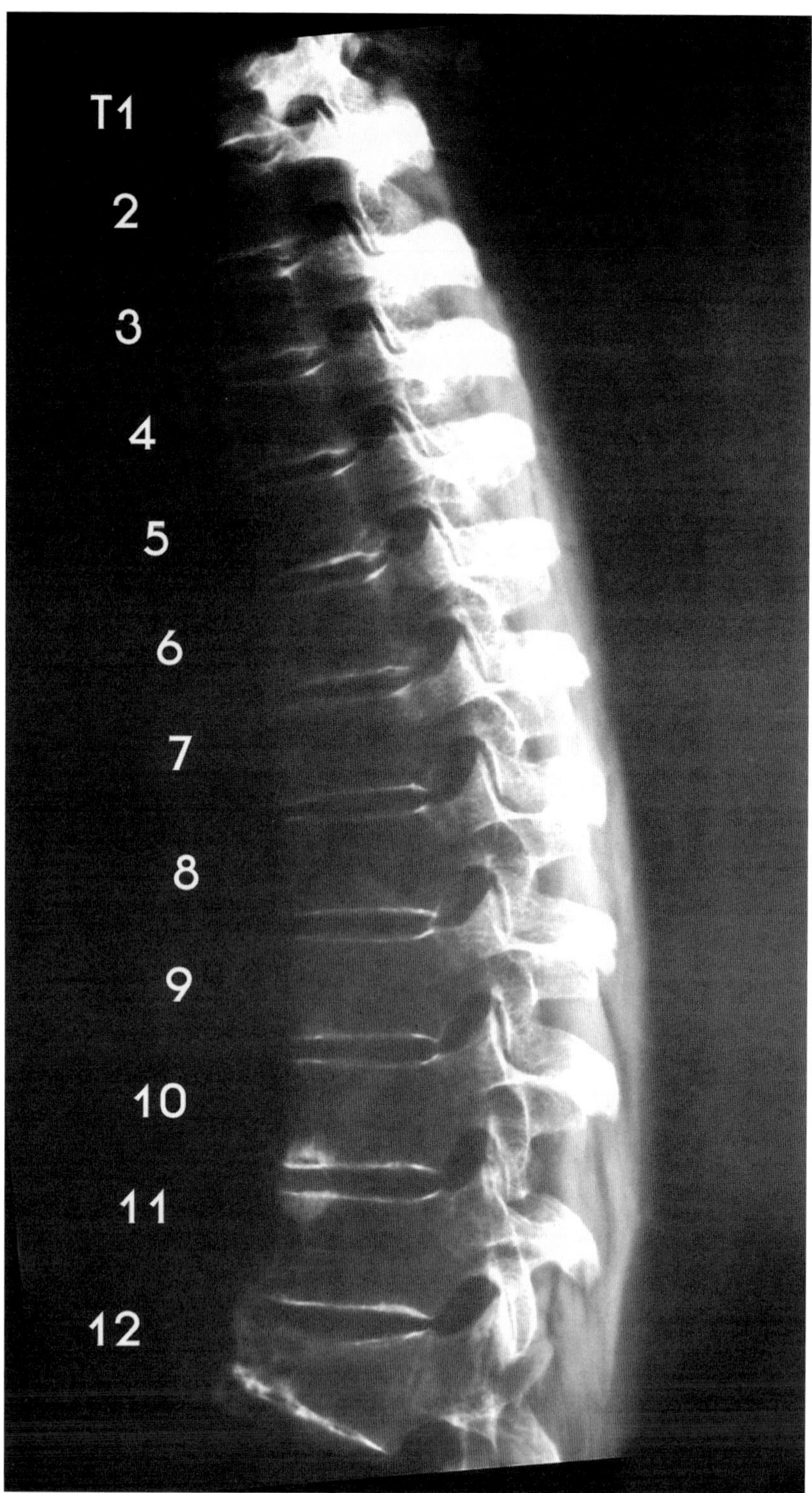

Plates 4-2 A & B
UPPER THORACIC CURVE REVERSAL
Anterolisthesis Upper Thoracics I

The compression fracture of T12 has created a wedge shaped vertebral body. The reversal of the normal kyphotic curve between T2 and T5 could be an adaptive response to this trauma or a posterior to anterior force occurring in this area. This has resulted in a "dishing" or indentation of

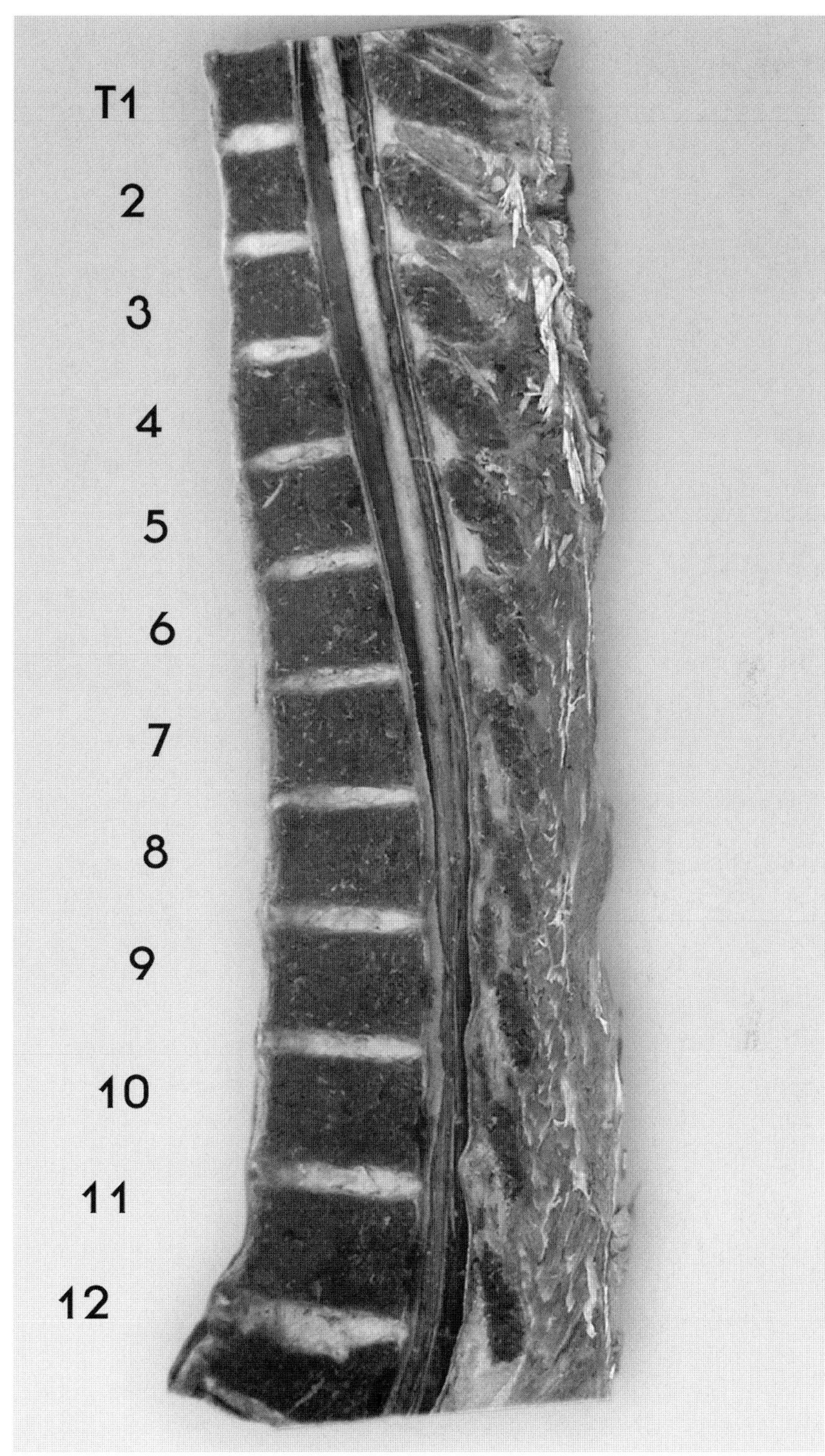

this portion of the thoracic spine. T4 is a complete anterolesthesis and the apex of this curve reversal. From the T4-5 disc and below, there is anterior brown degeneration that indicates poor hydration in this portion of the discs. T6 - T11 looks aligned except for T10-T11 with slight anterior spurring. The T6-11 area is slightly off the sagital plane.

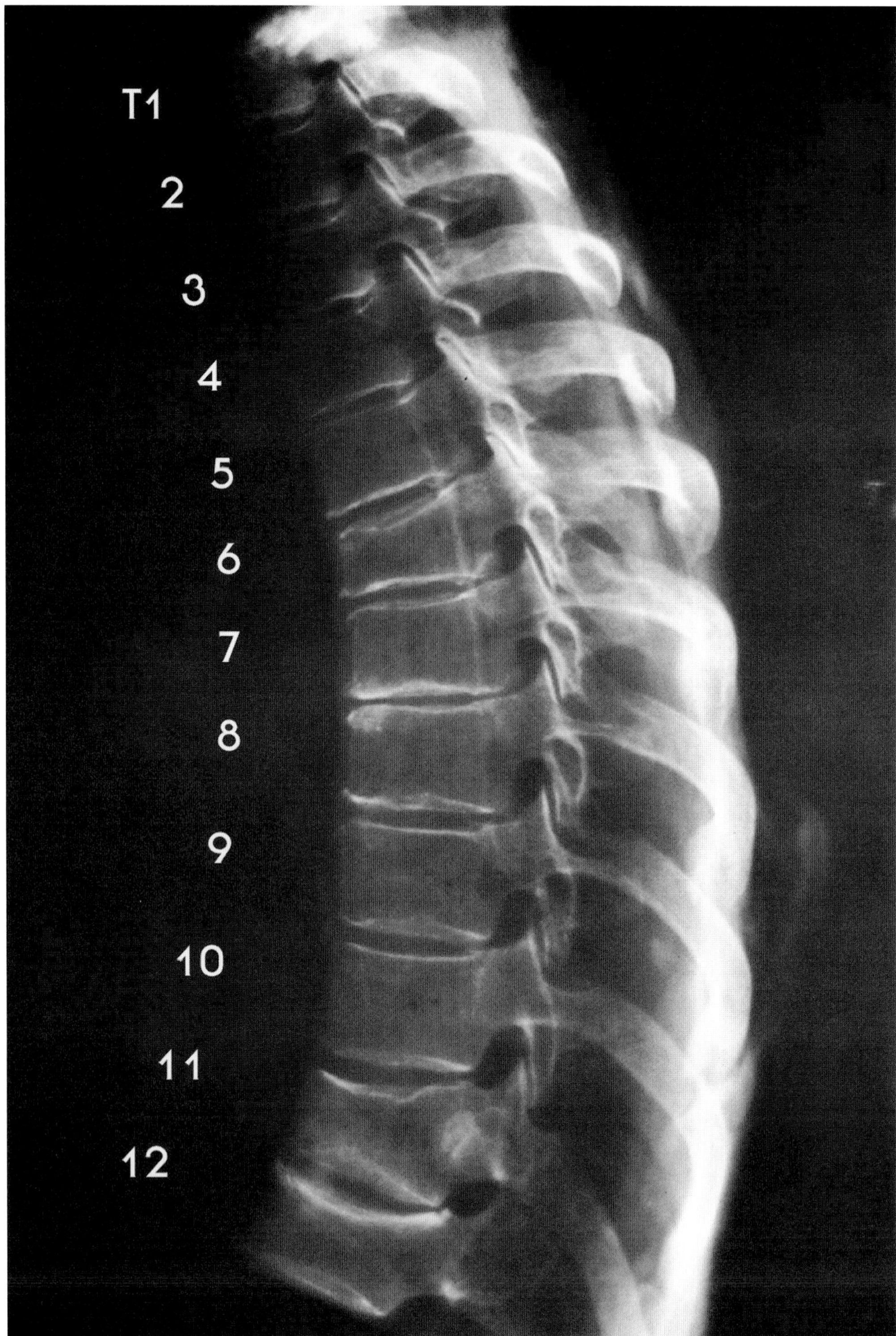

Plates 4-3 A & B
Thoracic Anterolesthesis: Upper Thoracic II

This specimen has definite signs of trauma with compression fractures from T6 through T12. There is a disc herniation at T11-12 with cord contact. The upper thoracic curve reversal could be an adaptive response to the lower thoracic trauma and resulting deformity or to a direct posterior to anterior event.

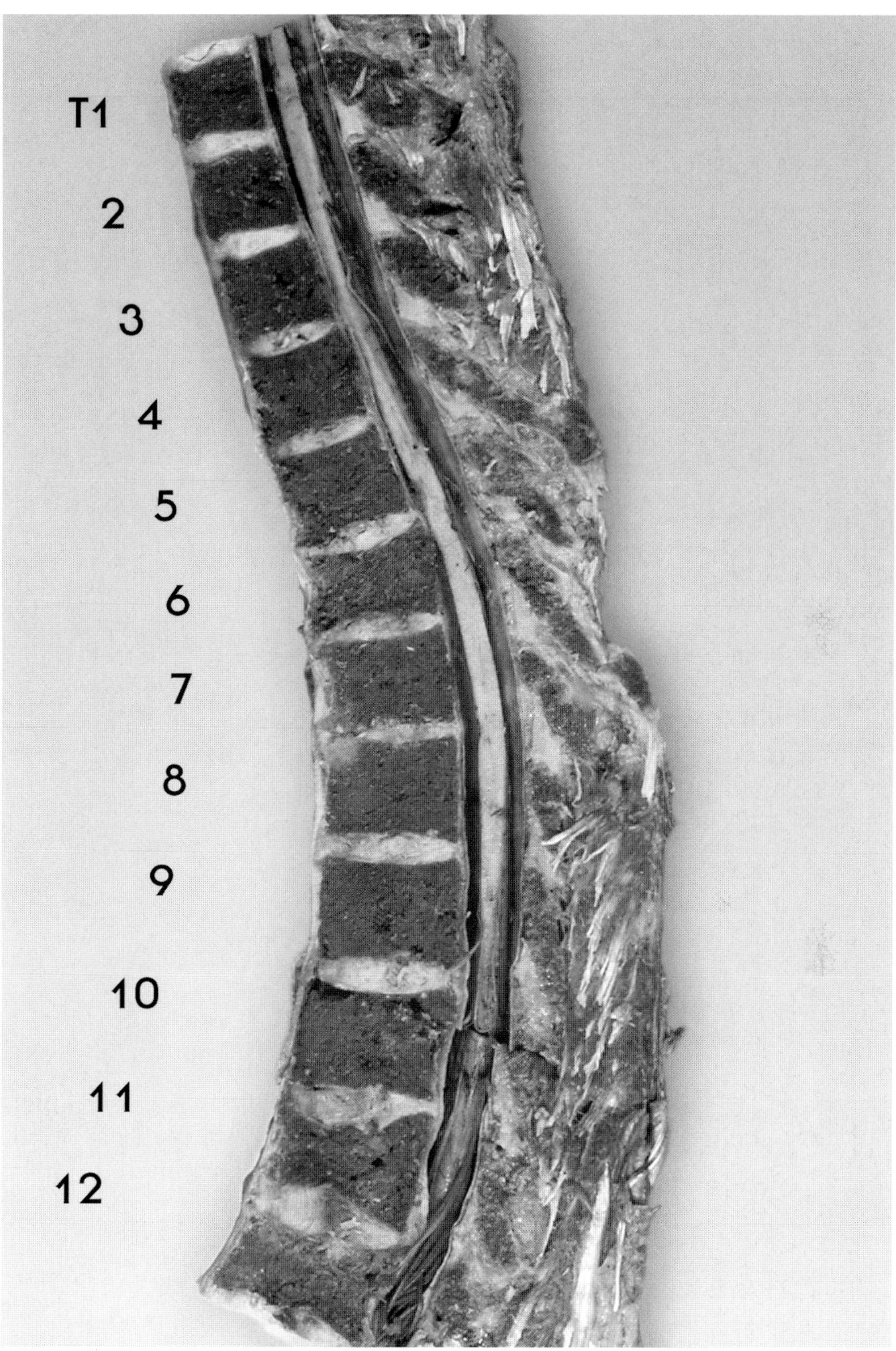

The anterior reverse apex is at T4-5 with a complete antrolesthesis of T5. Despite the compression fractures, a kyphotic curve returns to the lower thoracic spine.

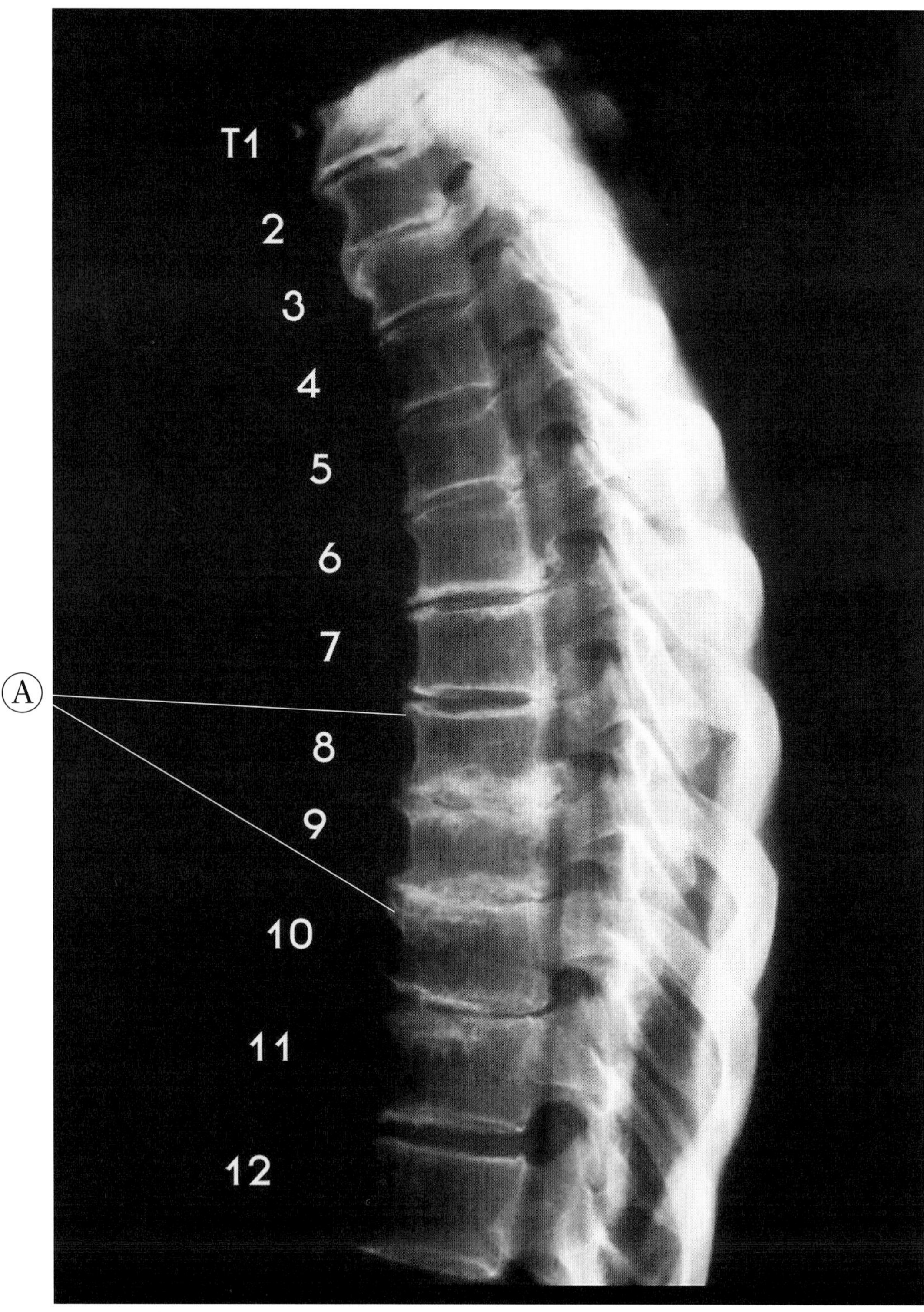

Plates 4-4 A & B
Thoracic Spine: Antrolesthesis: Upper thoracic II

This specimen has signs of old trauma with multiple segments compressed and sclerotic. There is loss of normal disc height and spurring anteriorly and posteriorly. The curve reversal has an anterior apex of T3-4 with stairstepping subluxations of T4 to T12. Disc degeneration has advanced to near fusion of T8-9 and T9-10 with posterior bulging and near cord contact in the neutral position. (This means that flexion of any part of the vertebral column could make those posterior disc protrusions clinically significant.)

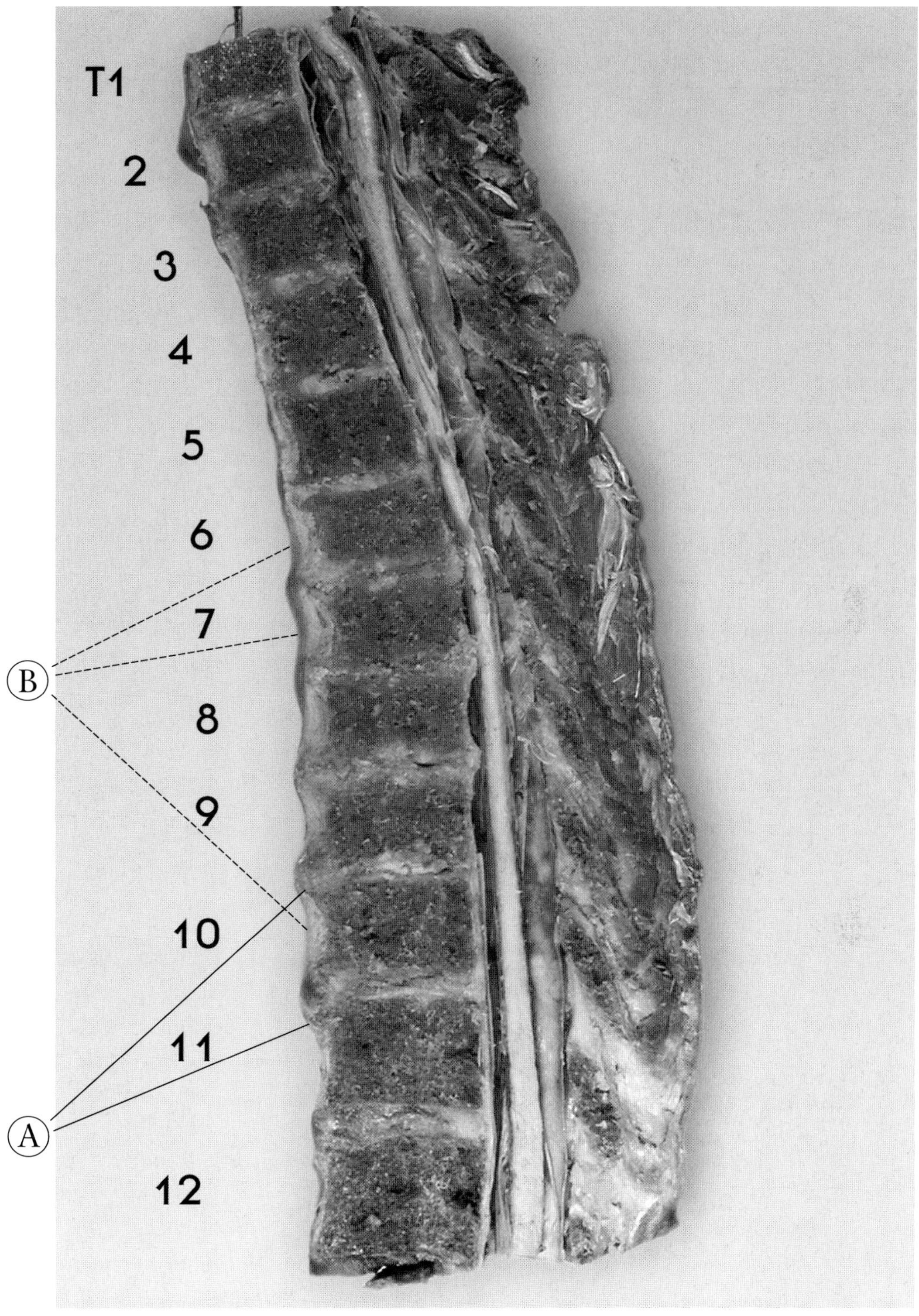

The anterior endplate spurring and disc bulging is associated with anterior longitudinal ligament thickening from T5 to T11.
(A) Anterior spurs and endplate changes
(B) Hypertrophy of A.L.L.

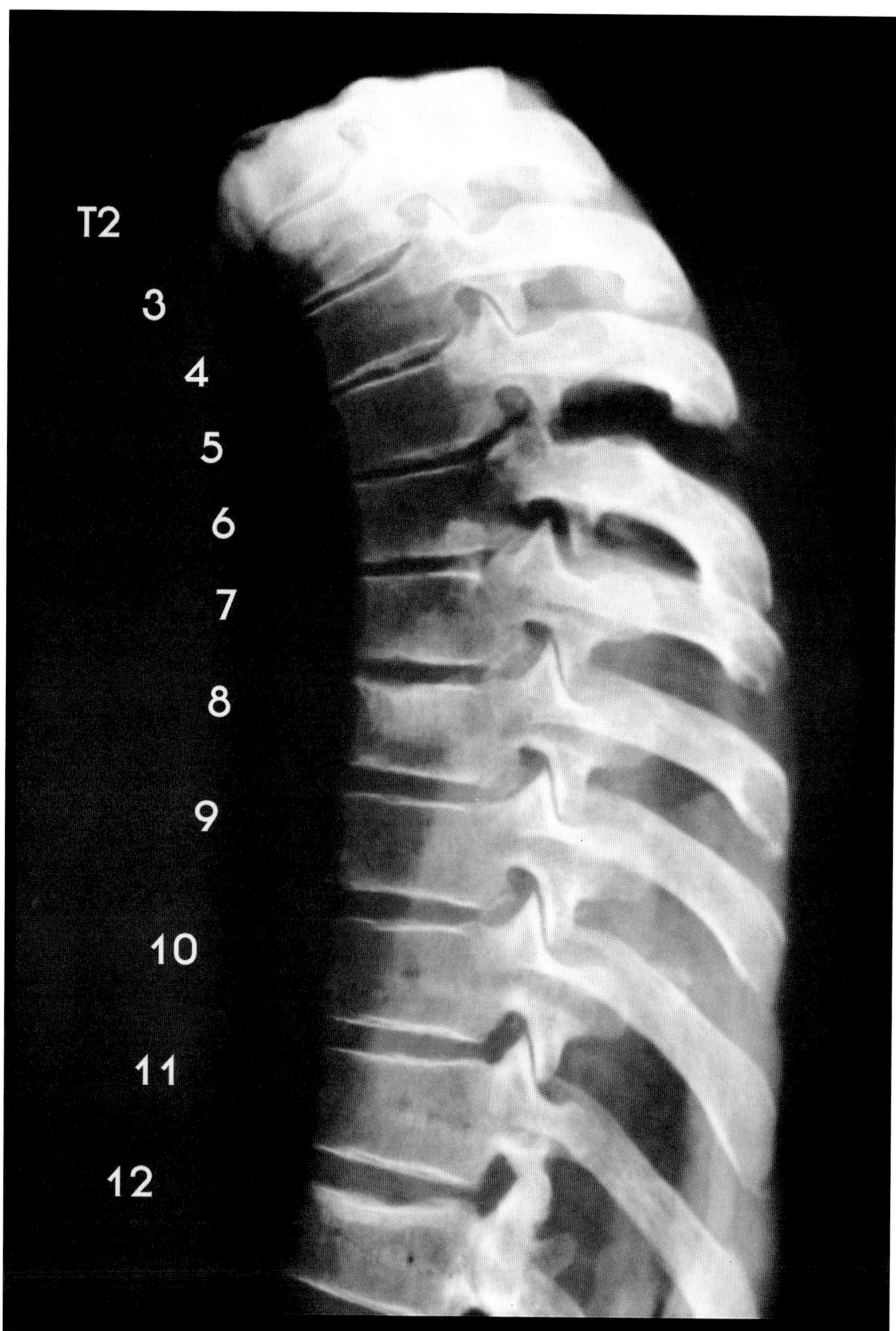

Plates 4-5 A & B
LOWER THORACIC CURVE REVERSAL (T7-11)
Thoracic Spine: Anterolisthesis lower thoracics

T2-6 appear normal except for endplate damage with slight spurring anteriorly with all segments, indicating an anterior weight bearing in this person's posture. There is a mild reversal of the thoracic curve with an anterior apex at T10. Compression damage from T7 to

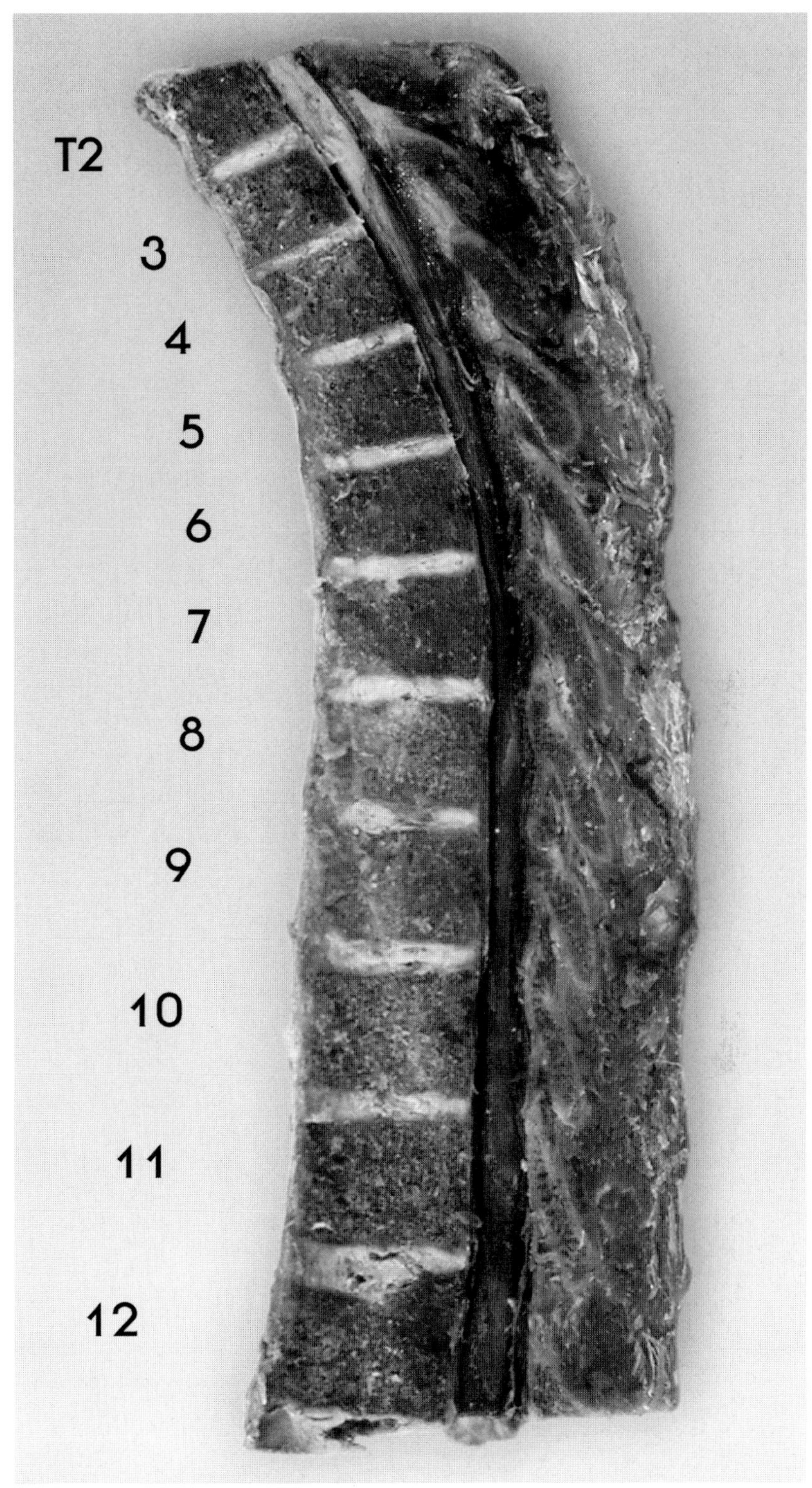

T12 and all endplates have signs of repair. All discs have anterior brown degeneration with a Schmoral's node in the superior T8 endplate; T12 vertebral body has suffered a compression fracture. Near normal alignment was maintained and disc pathology is only moderate to absent.

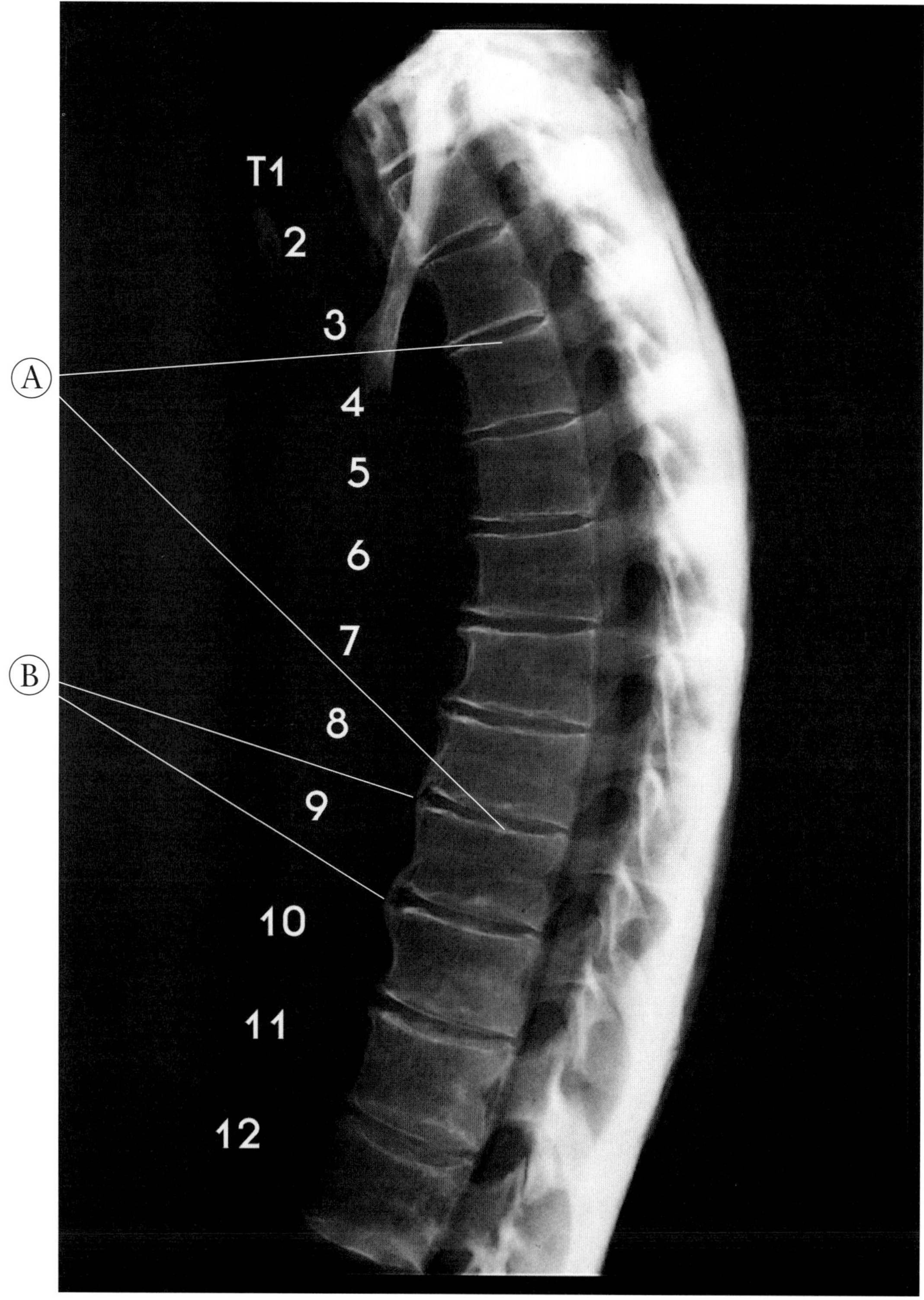

Plates 4-6 A & B
LOWER THORACIC CURVE REVERSAL
Thoracic Spine: Anterolisthesis of lower thoracics

This specimen has a moderate reversal of the kyphotic curve from T8 to T11 with an anterior apex at T9. T1-2 disc looks OK with slight brown degeneration of disc; T3 retro to T2 with anterior spurring of T2-T3 with slight disc tearing Hand bulging. From T3 to T12 there is anterior spurring, loss of disc height anteriorly with brown degeneration; T6 retro to T7 with compression of T6 or Schmoral's node on the inferior end-plate of T6; T7-8 tearing

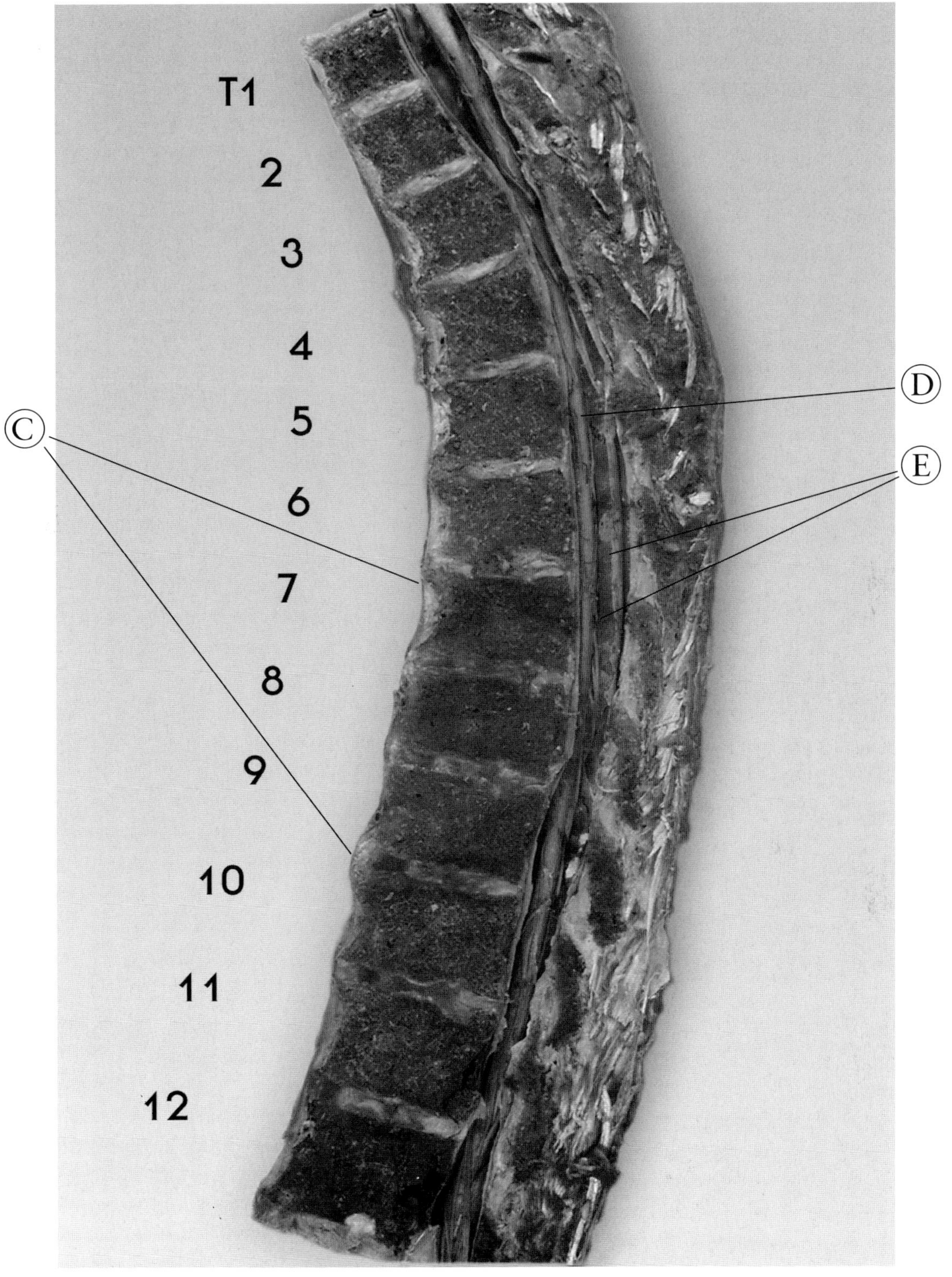

with degeneration; T7-11 are aligned with marginal and non-marginal phytes. All endplates appear to have repaired from significant axial loading.

(A) All endplates appear disrupted in various degrees
(B) Para-spinal phytes, T8-9, T9-10; ossification of A.L.L.
(C) Appearance of hypertrophy of A.L.L. T3-T7
(D) Spinal cord. Note anterior position in canal
(E) There are intrathecal or subarachnoid adhesions on the dorsal aspect of the cord with nerve and vascular entrapment

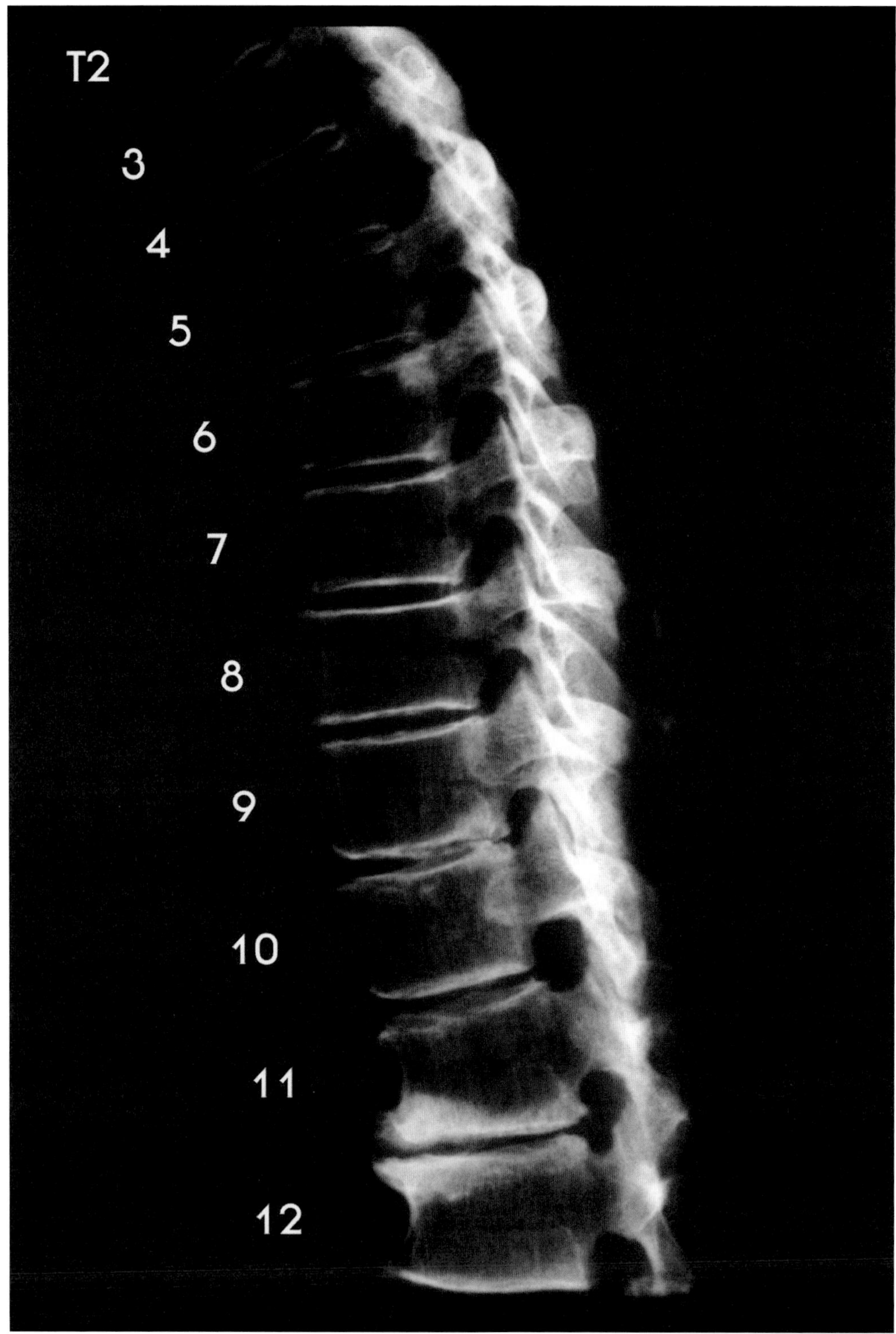

Plates 4-7 A & B
LOWER THORACIC CURVE REVERSAL
This specimen has a reversal of the kyphotic curve from T7 to T11 with an anterior apex at T9. T2-6 look normal except for the anterior disc degeneration. There are subluxations of T7 to T12 with varying degrees of degeneration, anterior spurring, endplate sclerosis, and

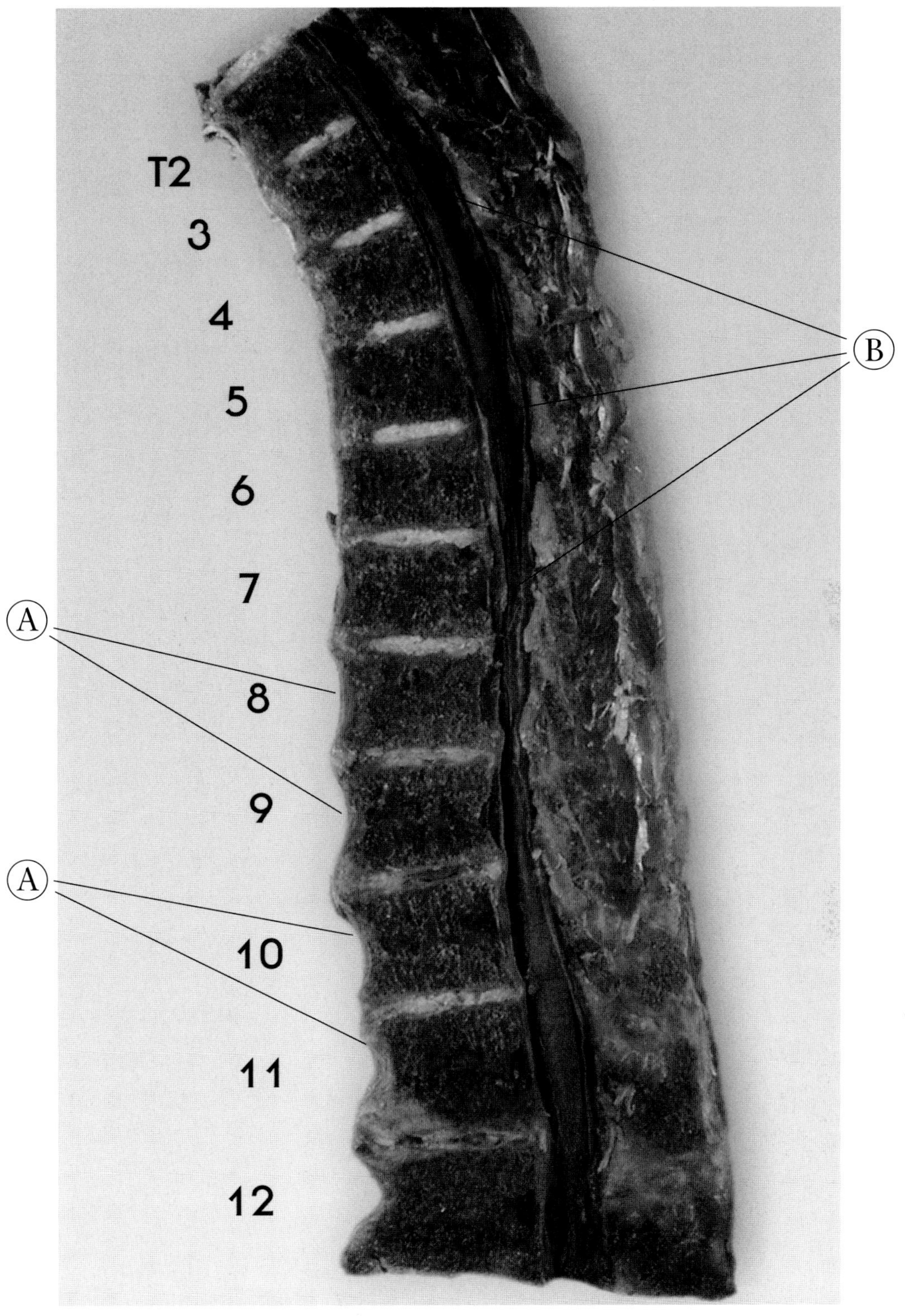

anteriorly bulging discs. T11 is a complete retrolisthesis with T12 having signs of compression repair, anterior spurring, and slight posterior spurring. There is severe DJD with cavitation of the disc.

(A) Hypertrophy of the A.L.L. from T8 to T11

(B) The spinal cord is anteriorly displaced from T2-T7

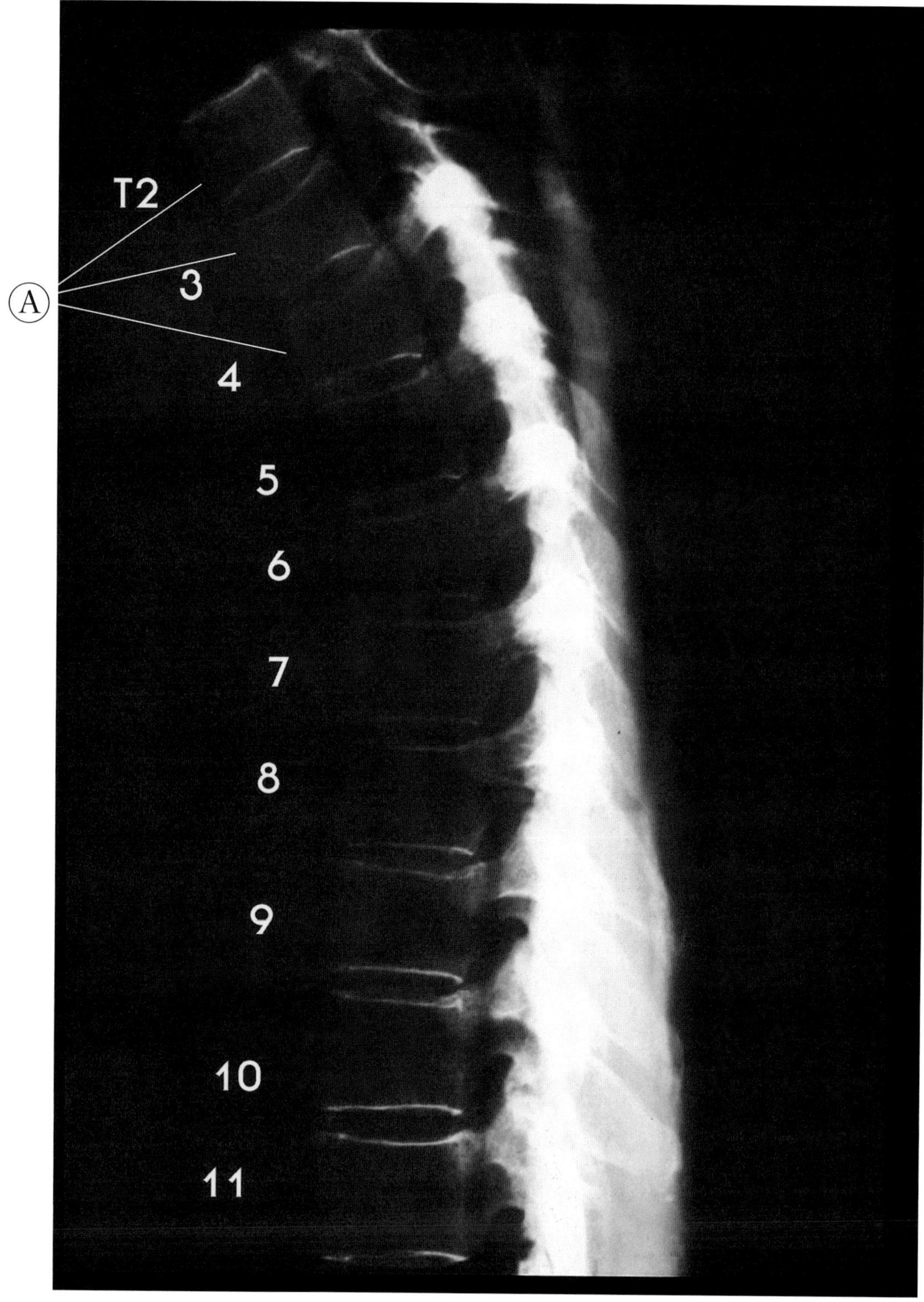

Plates 4-8 A & B

THORACIC UPPER POSTERIOR AND LOWER ANTEROLISTHESIS

T3 is retro to T2 with compression of T3 anteriorly, loss of the vertebral body height anteriorly and degeneration of the anterior disc T2-3. Note cord in anterior canal to T7; T4 antro to T5; compression fracture of T5 anteriorly in loss of vertebral bodies height with disc degeneration in anterior; T6 is retro to T5 with anterior disc bulge and degeneration; T7 is anterior to T8

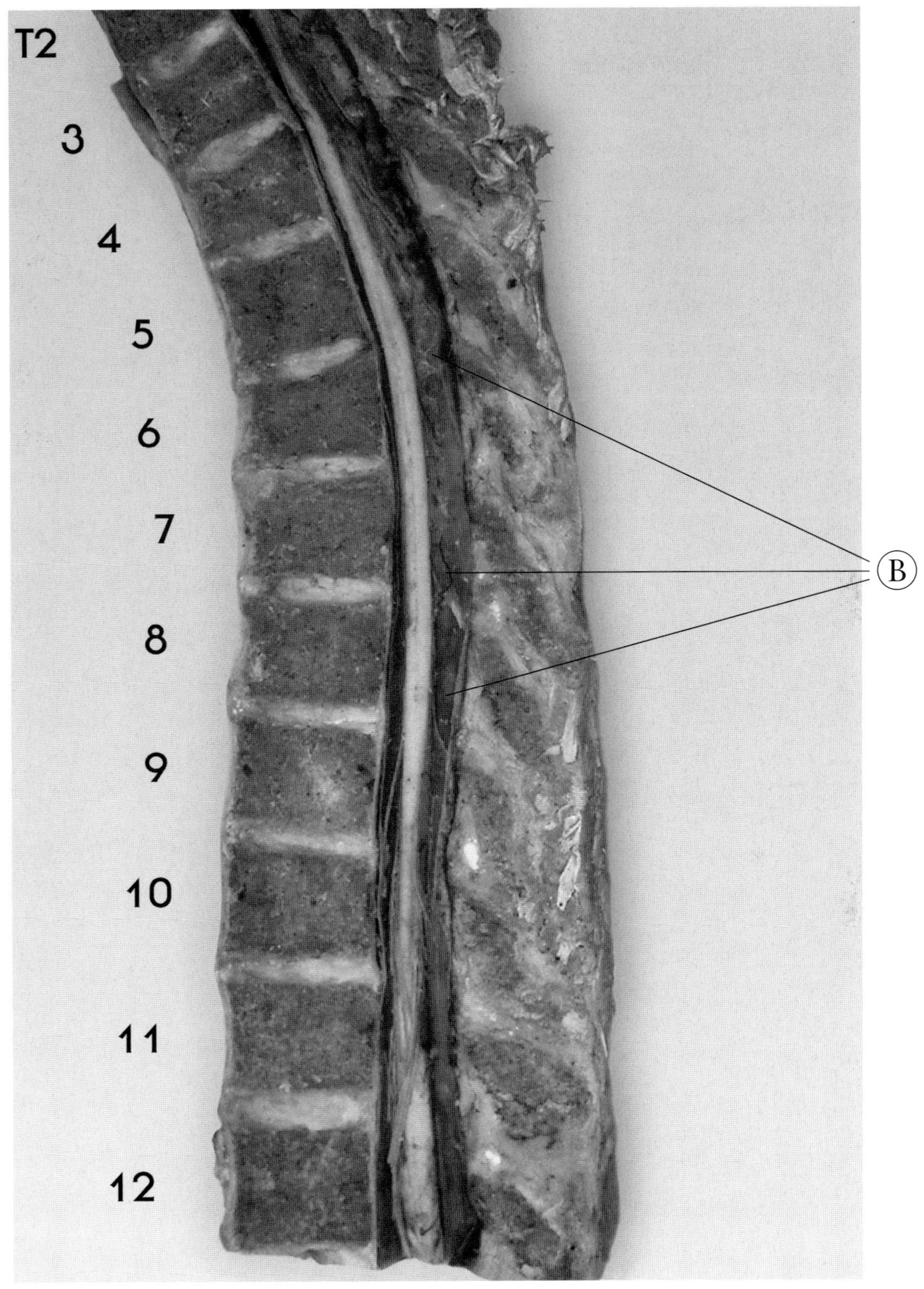

with anterior disc degeneration; T8 retro to T9 anterior disc degeneration with very slight posterior disc bulge; T9 is retro to T10 with anterior disc degeneration and very slight posterior disc bulge; T10-T11 is normal except for slight dehydration and degeneration.

(A) T2-4 appear to have slight nuclear compressions
(B) The intrathecal adhesions entrapping nerve roots and blood vessels

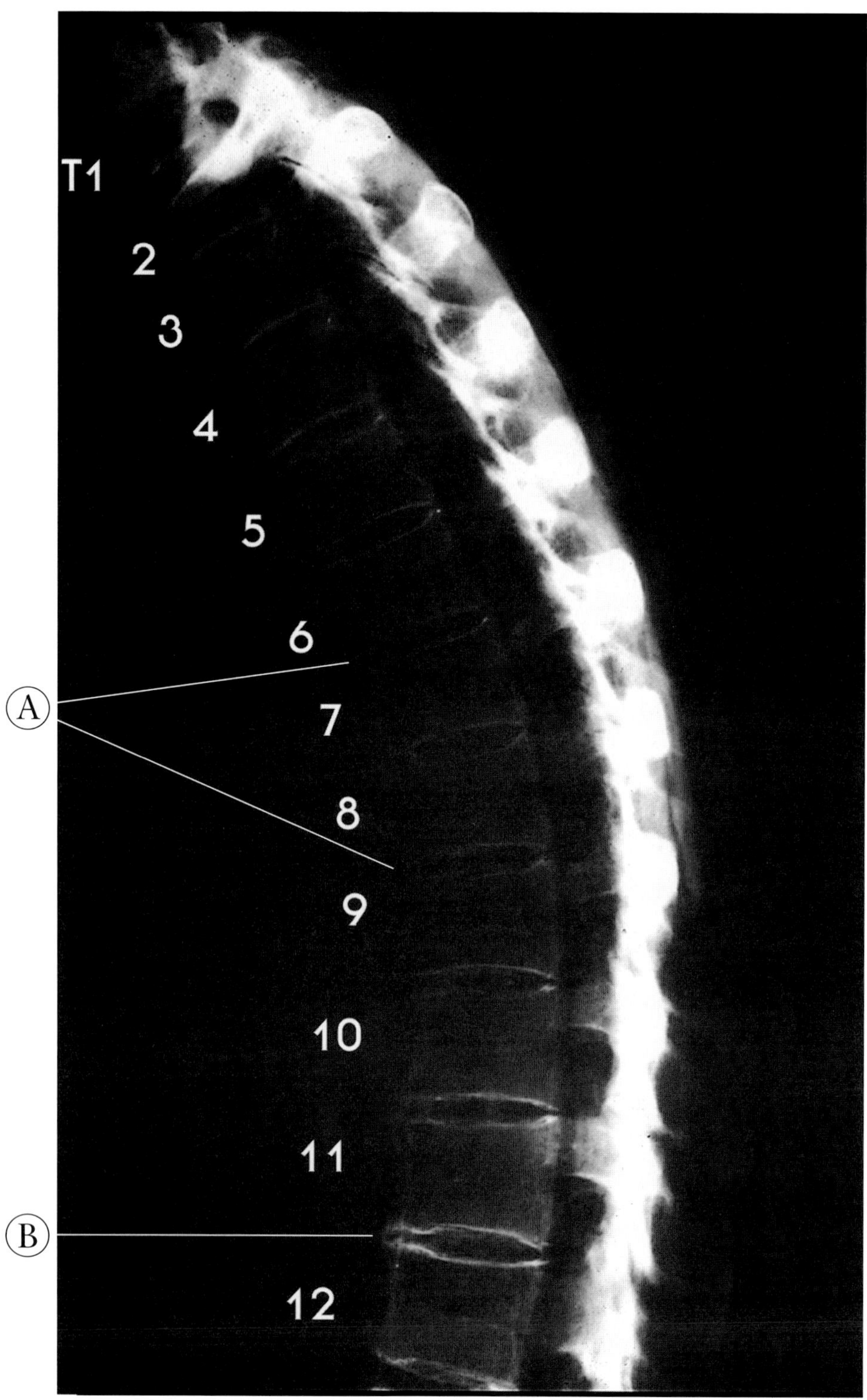

Plates 4-9 A & B
Thoracic Spine - antrolesthesis upper and lower vertebrae
T1-2 look normal with slight brown degeneration; T3 is retro to T2 showing disc tearing with anterior and posterior bulging; T4 is retro to T3, with slight anterior spurring (marginal osteophyte); T5 is retro to T4. There is slight brown degeneration on all discs.

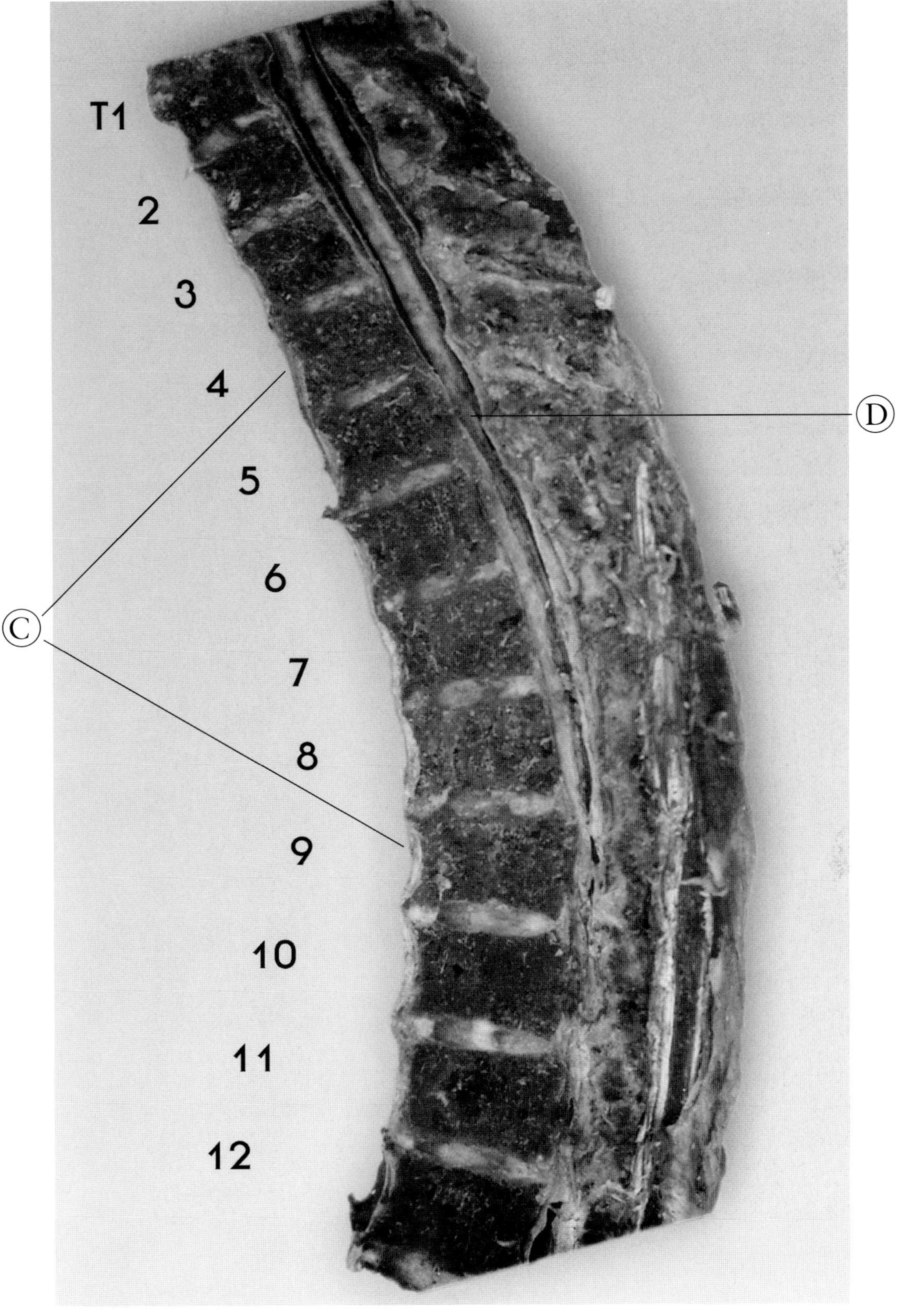

There is loss of the mid sagittal plane at T3 and below exposing part of the outside and inside edge of the thecal sac.

(A) Beginning of calcification of discs T6-7 to T11-12
(B) Para-spinal phytes of T10-T12
(C) Hypertrophy of anterior longitudinal ligament from T3 to Tll
(D) Spinal cord on anterior wall of canal

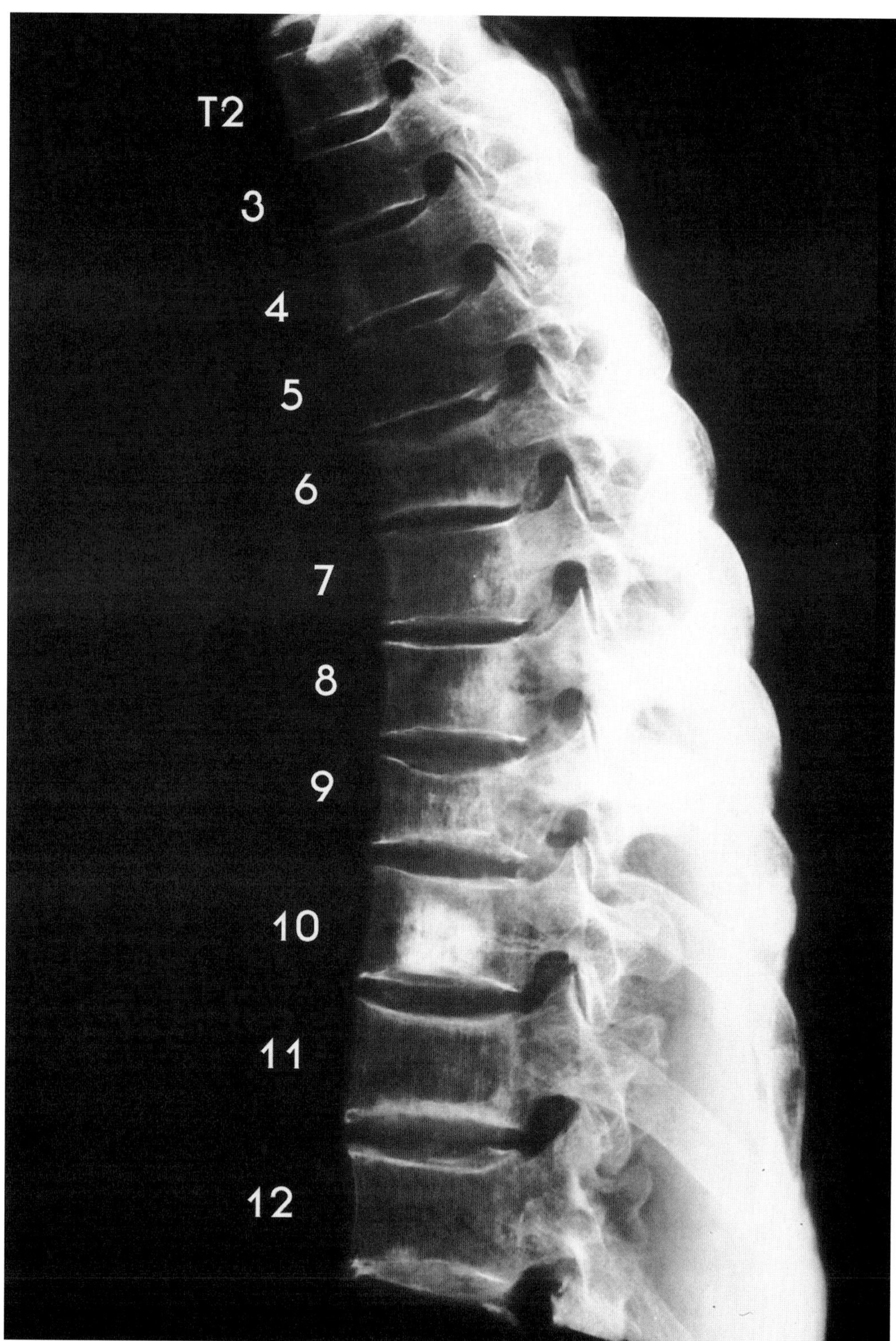

Plates 4-10 A & B
Thoracic Spine: Upper and lower antrolesthesis
There are compression fractures with loss of height of T6 and T9.
Alignment looks OK throughout. All discs have slight to moderate DJD.

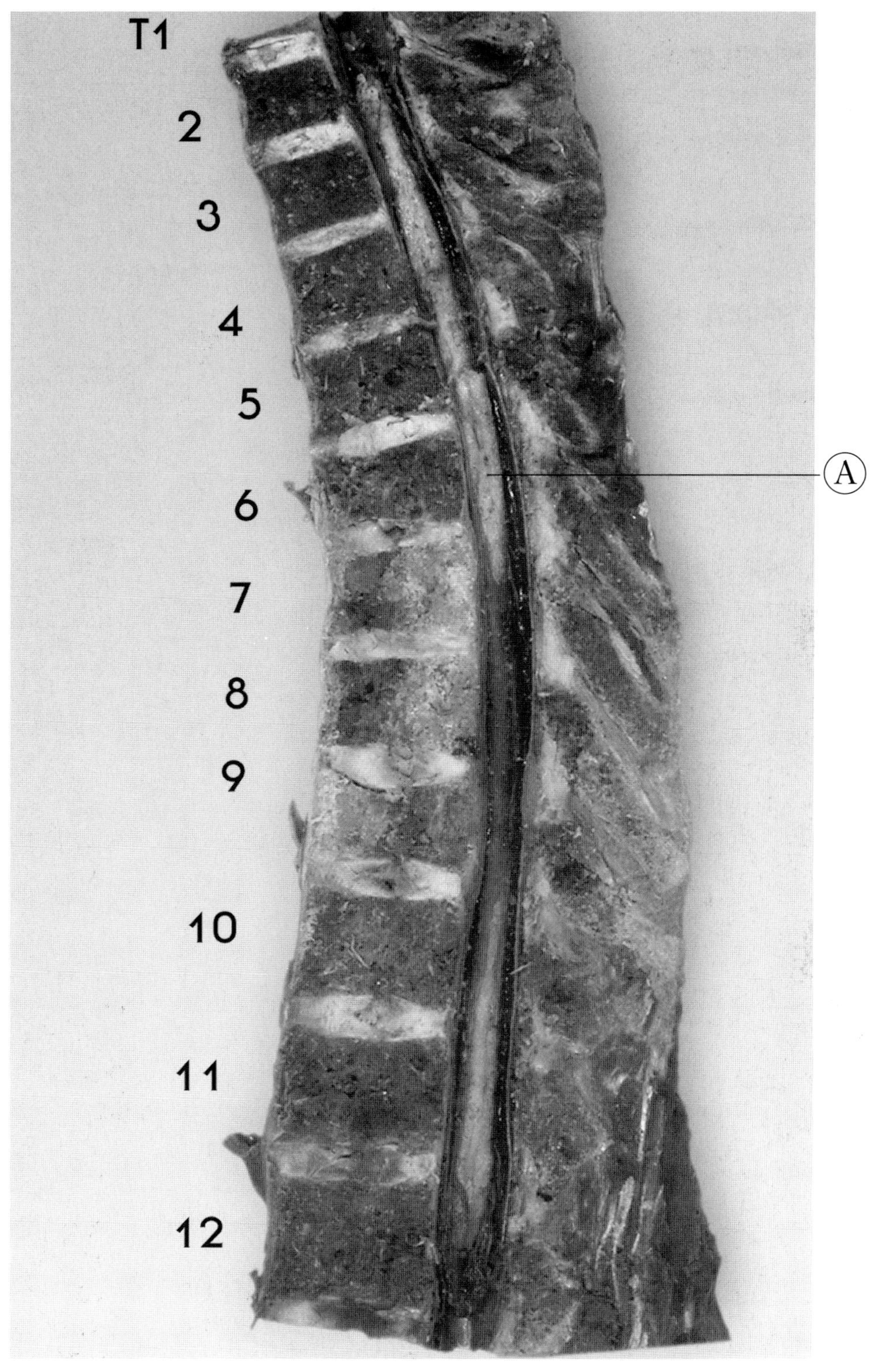

Compression Fracture T9, not a Schmoral's node; T9-10 cavitation; T10-11 tearing; T11 is a slight but complete anterolisthesis; T12 is retro to T11 with disc tearing, slight cavitation, and DJD.
  (A) Spinal cord

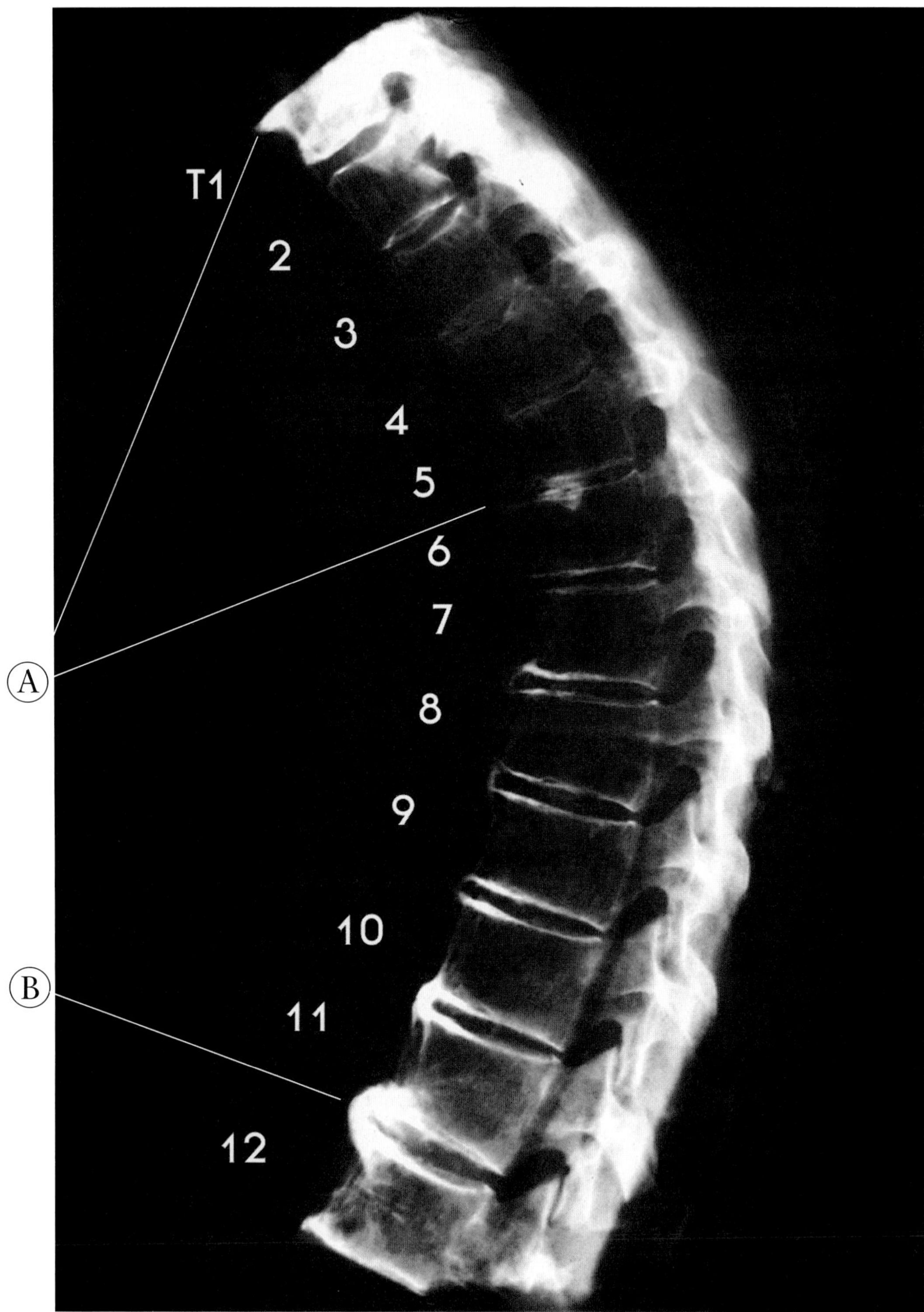

Plates 4-11 A & B
HYPERKYPHOSIS
Thoracic Spine: Progressive Spurring with Osteoporosis and Hyperkyphosis
This specimen has an increase in the kyphotic curvature with signs of trauma and calcification of a part of the anterior longitudinal ligament. Almost all of the endplates are disrupted with anterior disc narrowing from T2 to T7 and brown degeneration throughout. T3-T11 look aligned.

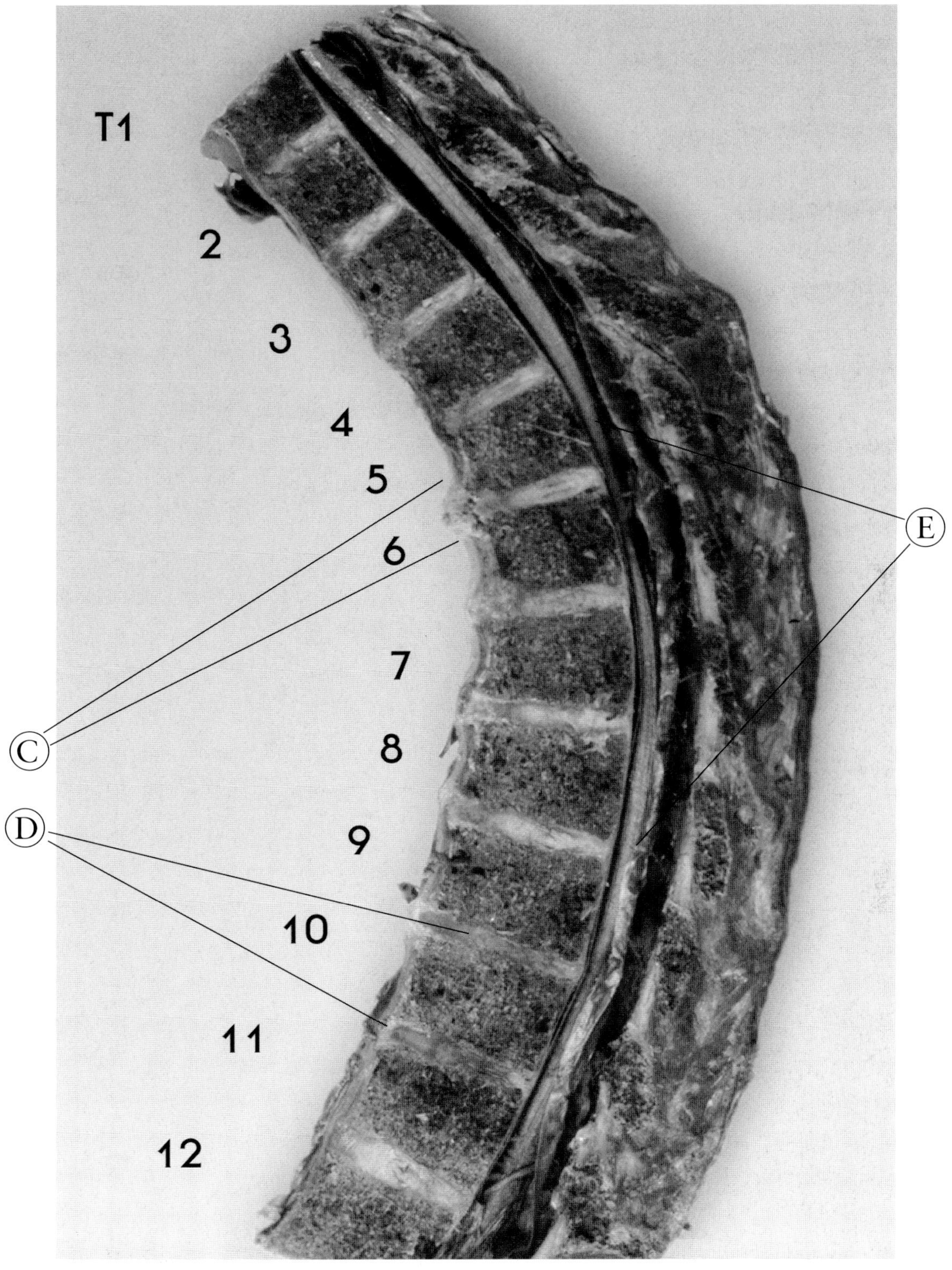

(A) Major marginal osteophytes at T5-T6
(B) T11-T12 has significant calcification of anterior disc and A.L.L.
(C) The hypertrophy of the A.L.L. from T4-T8, only part is calcified. T3-4 and inferior
     segments have hypertrophy of the A.L.L. as a result of compression and stress
(D) T9-10 and T10-11 have significant disc dehydration and calcification
(E) Note anterior placement of cord T5-9. This condition of the A.L.L. hypertrophy from
     T3-T12 could qualify as "DISH" because more than three consecutive segments
     are involved. (An early stage?)

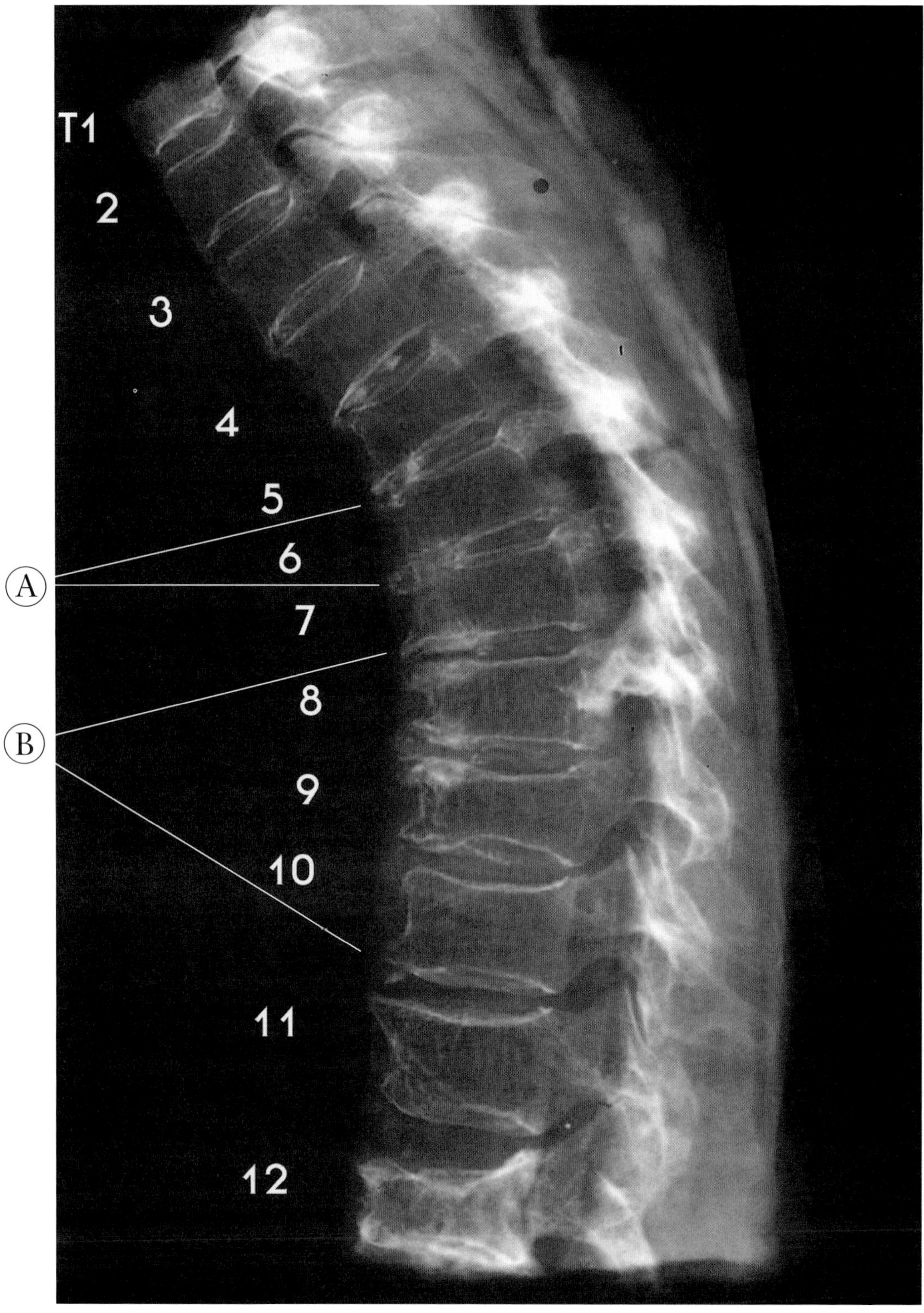

Plates 4-12 A & B
Progressive Spurring with Hyperkyphosis caused by Osteoporosis
This specimen has an increase in the kyphotic curvature as a result of subluxations, compression fractures, and loss of anterior disc height between T4 and T9. There is a very slight compression fracture of T4. T5 is retro to T4 with very slight compression fracture of T5 with calcification of the disc. T6-T12 have normal alignment but changes due to compression fractures of T6-T12.

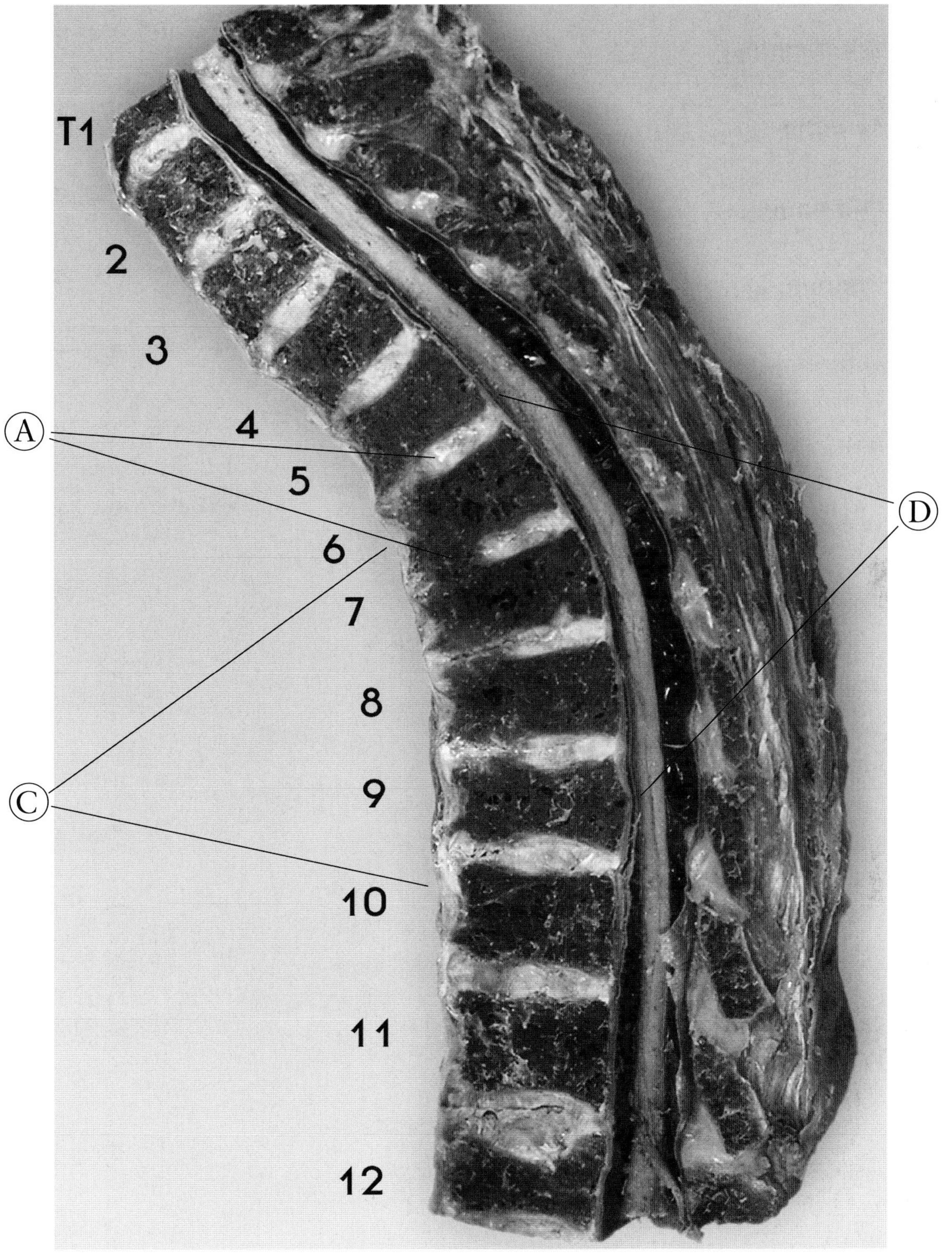

(A) Some discs have dark brown areas that correspond to calcified appearance on X-ray
(B) There is anterior vertebral body spurring from T3 to T12
(C) Hypertrophy of A.L.L. from T5-T12
(D) There is spinal cord/canal contact from T5 to T9

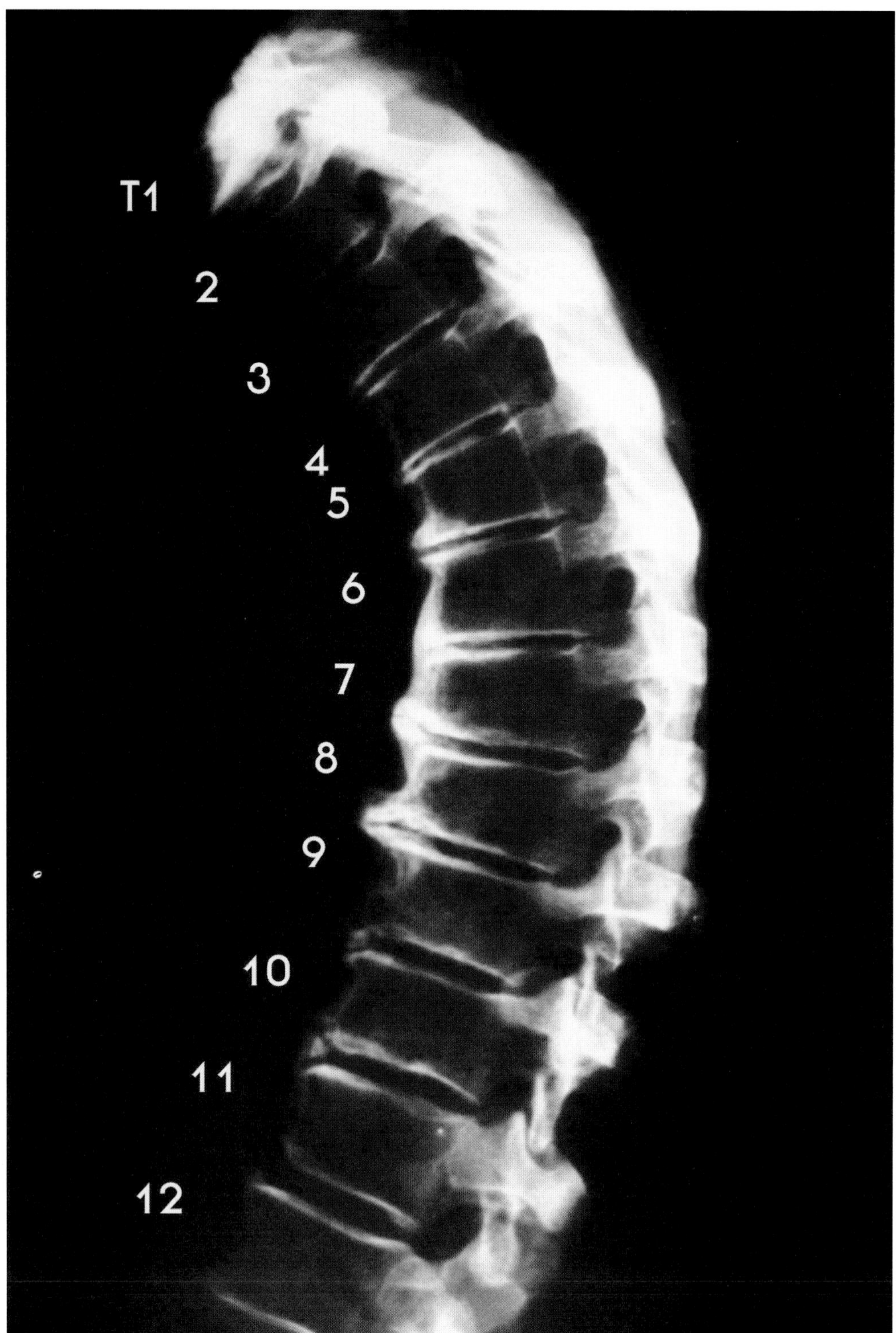

Plates 4-13 A & B
Progressive Spurring and Hyperkyphosis.
There appear to be no anterior/posterior subluxations. The hyperkyphosis is due to compression fractures of T5 to T11 with some loss of disc height. T6 to T9 has an anterior fusion with para-spinal phytes of four segments [DISH].

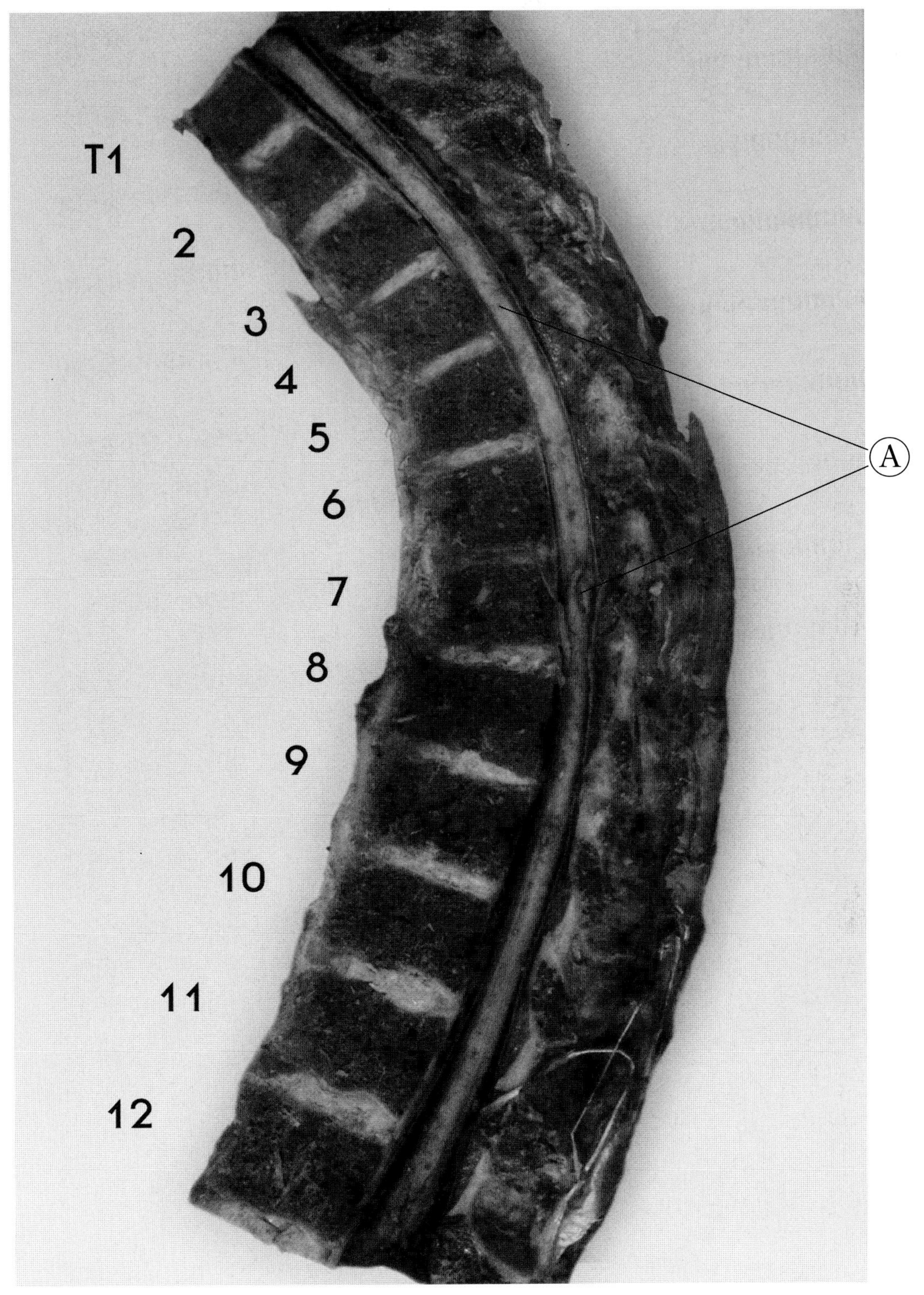

(A) Cord and canal contact. Note: This individual had a near normal cervical curve and lumbar curve

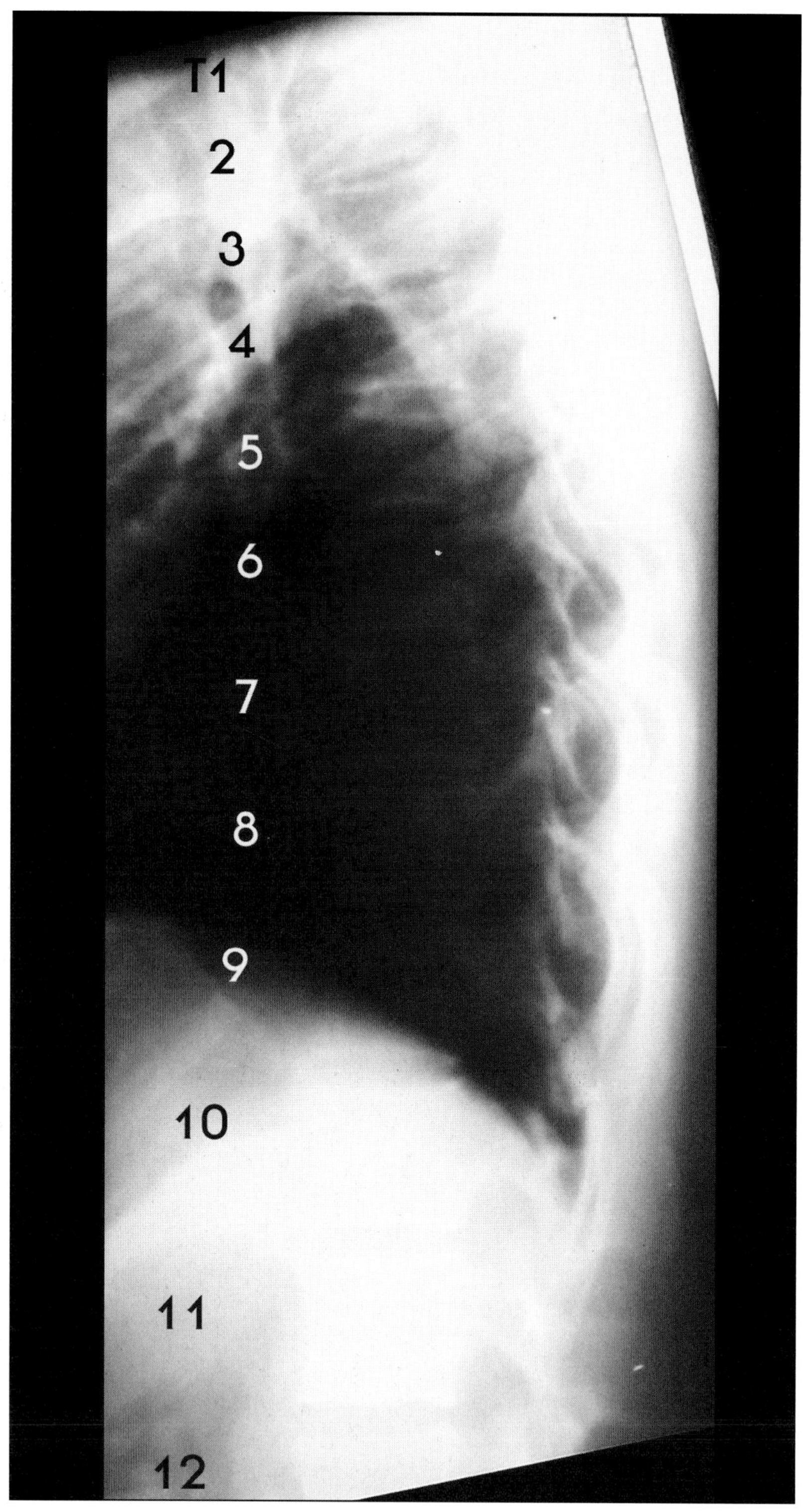

Plates 4-14 A & B
Thoracic Spine: X-ray and MRI of Patient with Cord tethering Due to Altered Curves
Note the hypokyphosis and cord- canal contact from T3 to T9.

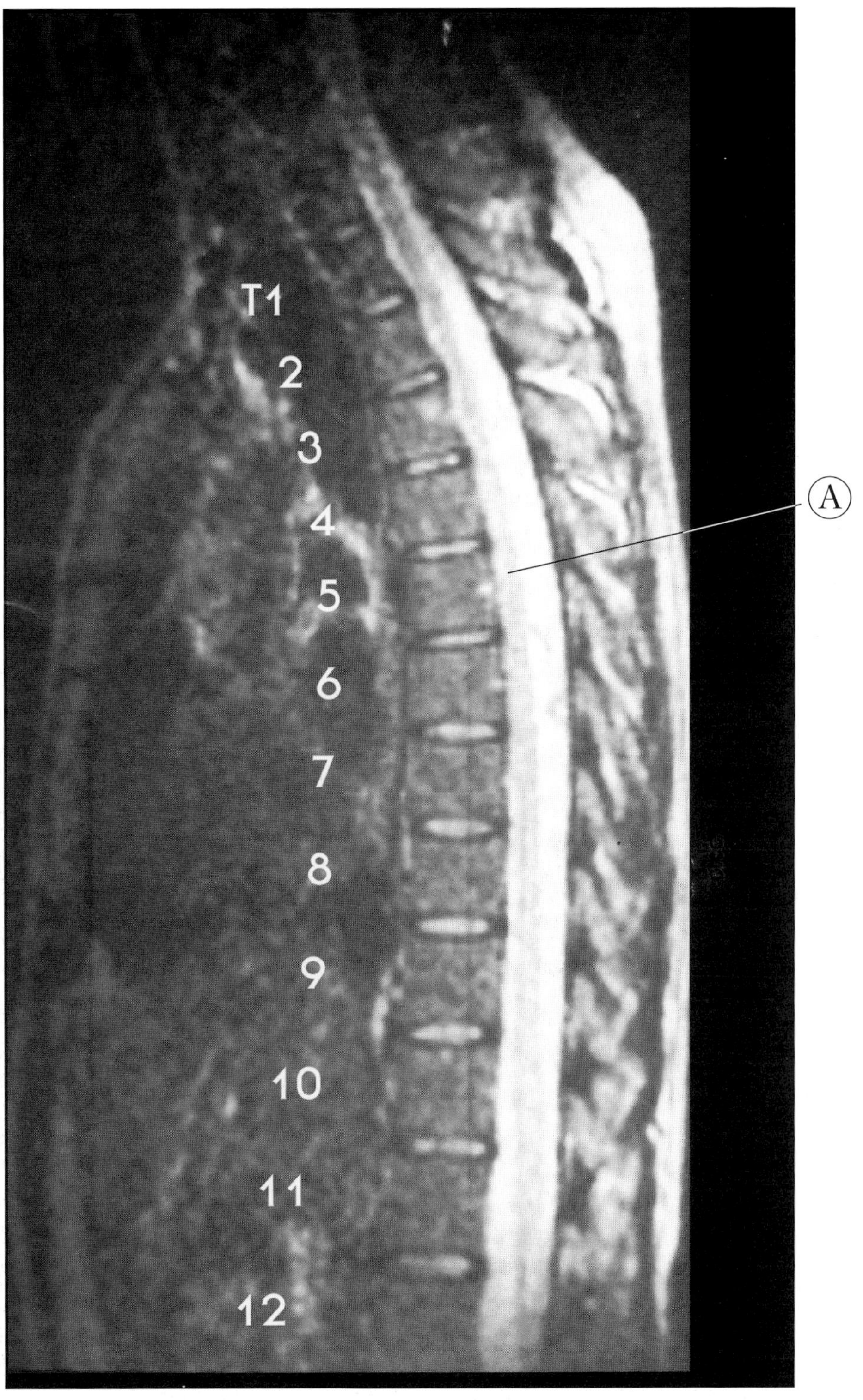

This patient has many internal organ symptoms that are worsened by sitting at her desk. When she is away from work her digestion, ulcer, bowel and bladder complaints "mysteriously" go away.

(A) Spinal cord

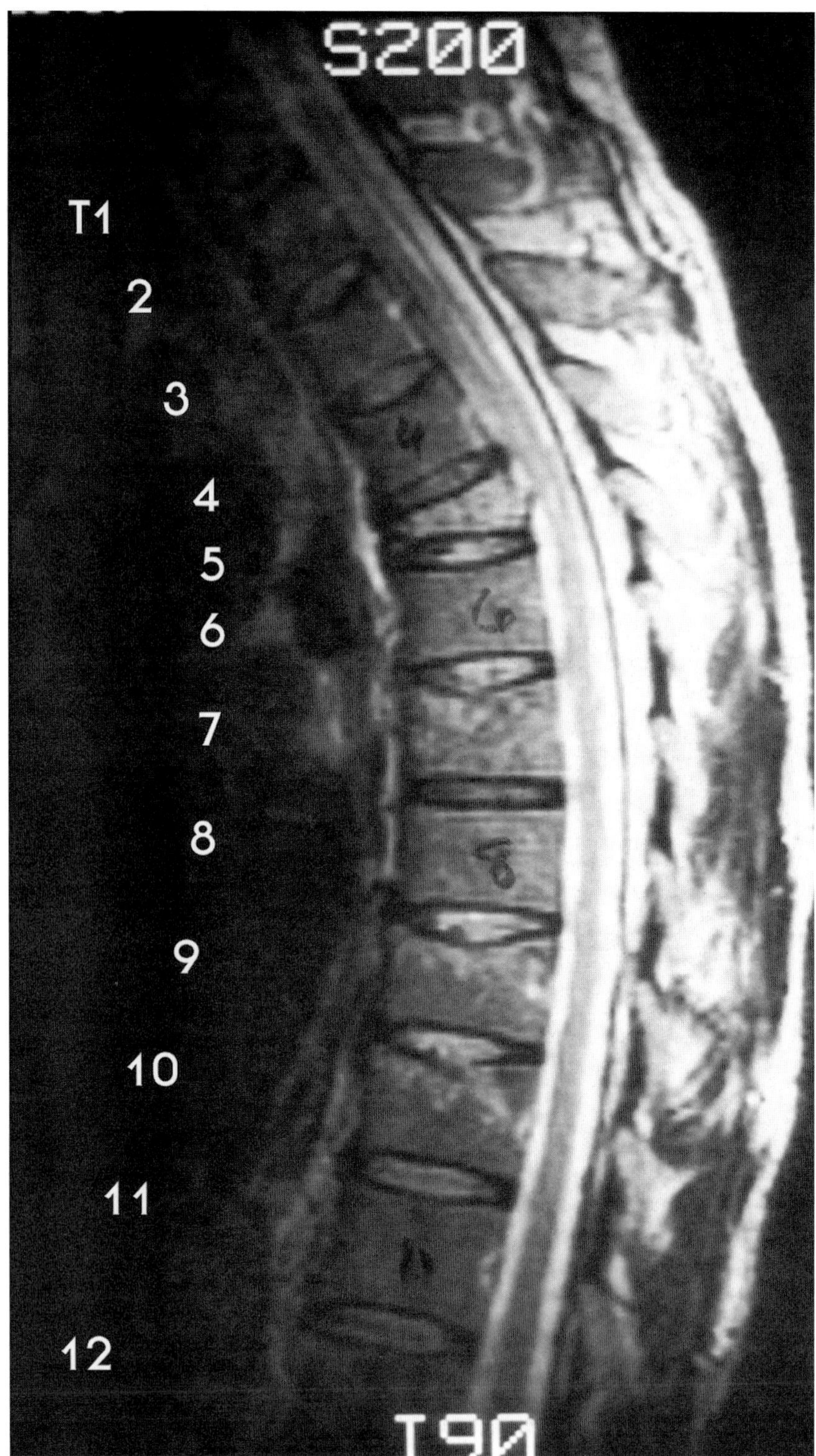

Plates 4-15 A & B
Hyperkyphosis due to Compression Fracture
Here are two MRIs of the same individual with different contrasts or
"signals." There are compression fractures of T5, T7, T9, and T10, with only
T5 suffering a major change of shape. There is a moderate retropulsion of
T5 into the canal, with spinal cord contact in the supine positition.

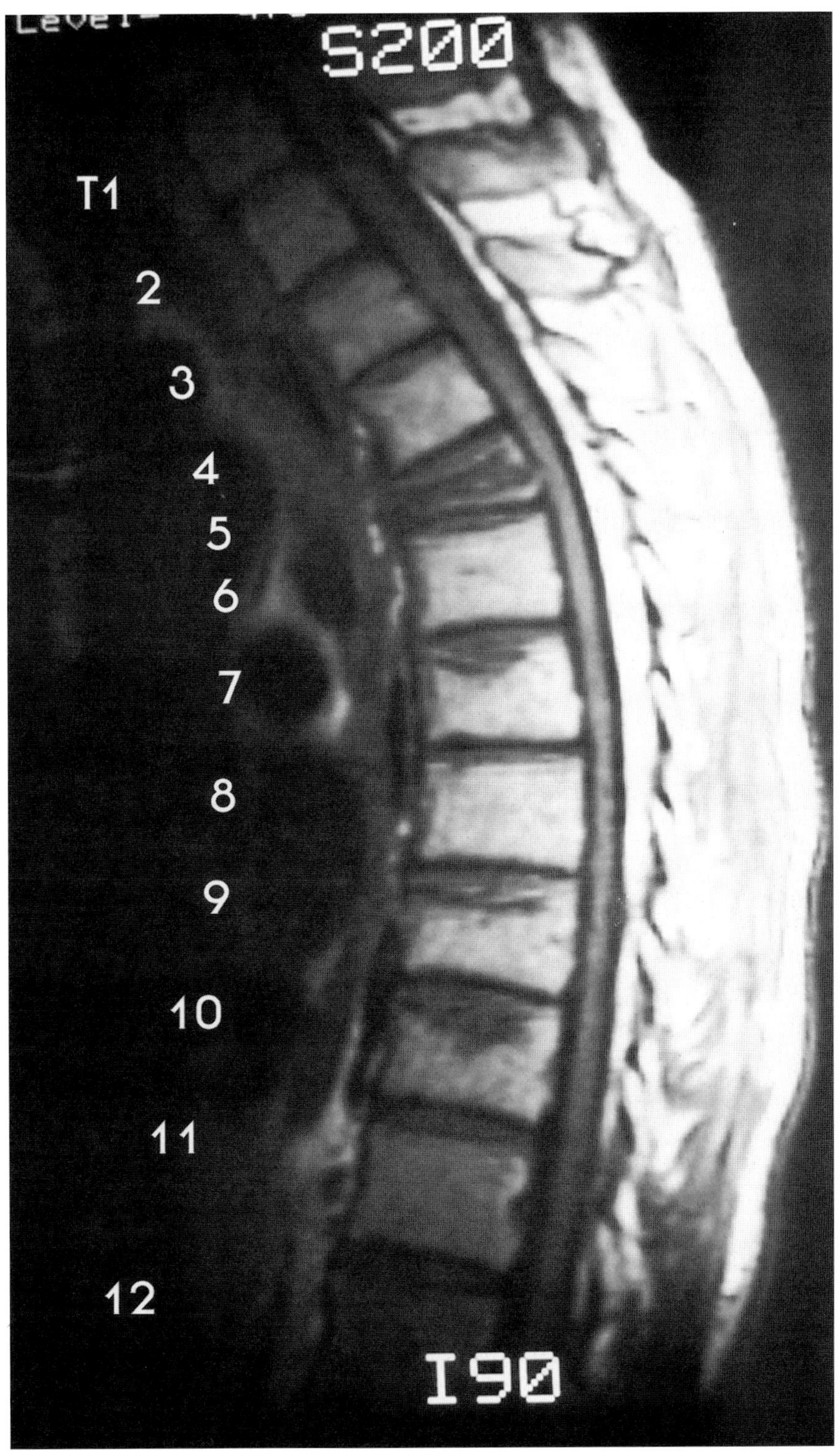

Certain flexed positions caused moderate to severe radiating rib and chest pain in the T5-6 area. Cervical hypolordosis adversely affects the spinal cord after an injury to the thoracic spine. There is tractioning of the cord from T3-T9 caused by cervical hypolordosis and hyperkyphosis of the thoracic spine. This image is taken in the recumbent position which gives the patient relief. The symptoms appear while sitting and worsen with neck flexion.

CHAPTER FIVE
Subluxations Of The Lumbar Spine

Discussion

The lumbar spine bears more of the body's weight than any other part of the vertebral column, as its massive body and robust facets indicate. Normally, a lordotic curve is present or should be present in the lumbar spine. Both the angles of the facets and the angle between the pedicles and vertebral bodies necessitate this curvature. Separations of the spinous processes and facets (flexion) increase the length of the posterior wall of the spinal canal and put all the weight bearing on the discs. A three point weight bearing system exists with the two pairs of facets and vertebral bodies each bearing roughly a third of the gravitational load. Anatomical studies of trabecular patterns of the bone clearly indicate that the facets are weight-bearing joints. In **Figure 5-1** a CT Scan of L4 shows hypertrophy of the left articular facets and loss of joint space, common features of subluxation.

Alteration of the curve of the lumbar spine can cause these articular facets to separate or hyper load. Shifting of most of the gravitational load to the discs and vertebral bodies can occur with an unequal loading of the articular facets. Note the osteophytes and altered joint space is on the left in **Figure 5-1**. Chronic subluxation of the lumbar spine stops normal motion of the discs and interrupts their hydraulic function (**See Figure 5-2**). This specimen has three levels of disc degeneration. Notice the alignment of L1 and L2 and the condition of the disc. There is misalignment of L3 posteriorly to L2, with wedging, tearing, and bulging of the disc. This condition is caused by subluxation and the resulting loss of normal motion and hyper loading. The L3-4 disc is even more distressed, which is caused by the retrolisthesis of L4. There is significant dehydration, tearing, cavitation, and loss of disc height.

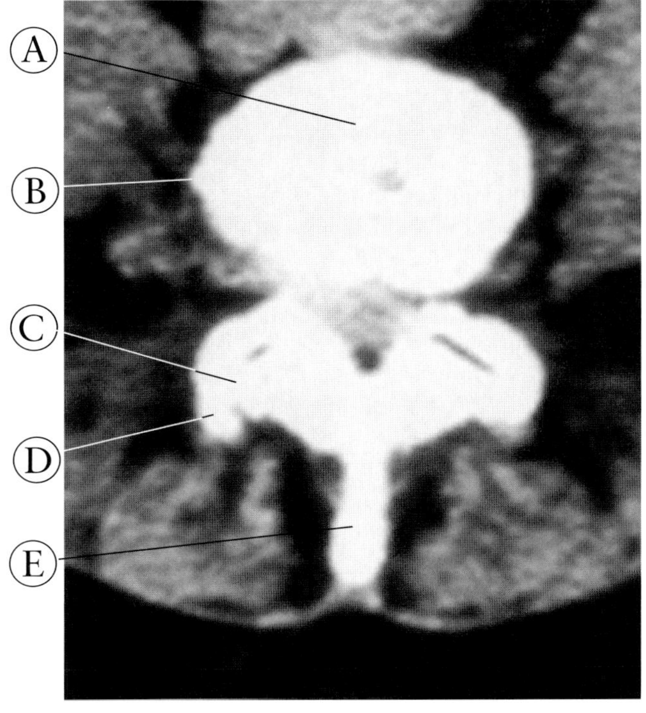

Figure 5-1
CT SCAN OF L4 IN AN INDIVIDUAL WITH CHRONIC LUMBAR SUBLUXATIONS AND OSTEOARTHRITIS.
The altered weight bearing has affected the facets and body of the vertebrae. Note that the hypertrophy of the vertebrae in the body and articular facet is on the left.
  (A) Body of vertebrae
  (B) Osteophytes or "spurs"
  (C) Diminished joint space
  (D) Altered facet
  (E) Spinous process

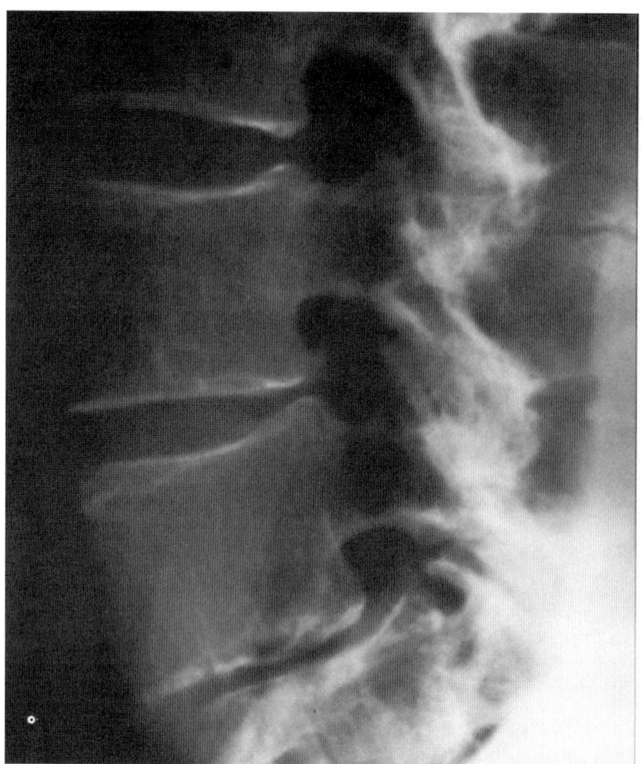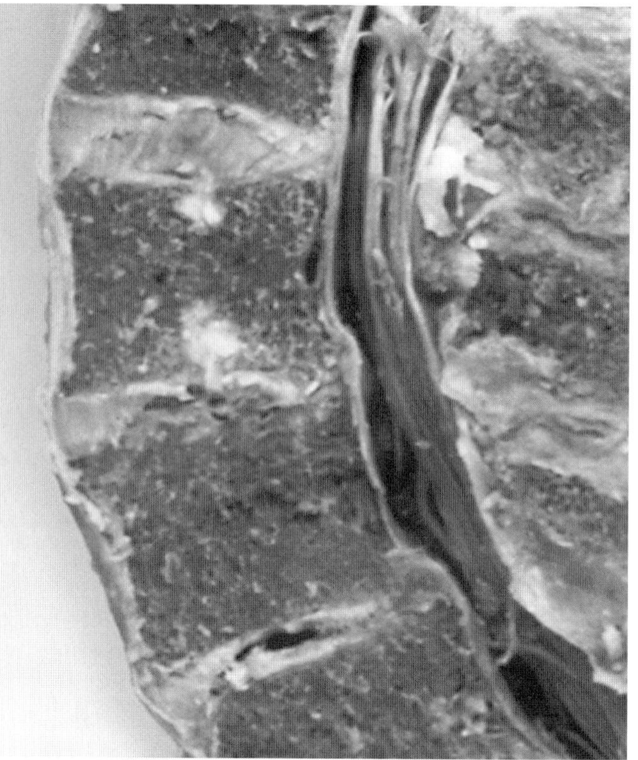

Figure 5-2

A VIEW OF VARYING DEGREES OF DISC HEALTH.

Note the different conditions of the discs in the same individual. The subluxations and disc degeneration are intimately related. When normal alignment is maintained the disc can be in good health regardless of age. All the discs in this specimen are the same age but only the subluxated motor units degenerate.

Figure 5-3

THE HYDROPHILIC DISC.

The L2-3 and L3-4 discs have been exposed to tap water after the lumbar spine was cut in a sagittal plane. The nucleus pulposus in this cadaver have absorbed the water and have bulged. This is an expected phenomenon. The annular walls and end plates normally contain this water absorbing glycoprotein matrix. These discs convey motion between and transmit the load to the vertebrae.

(A) Nucleus pulposus

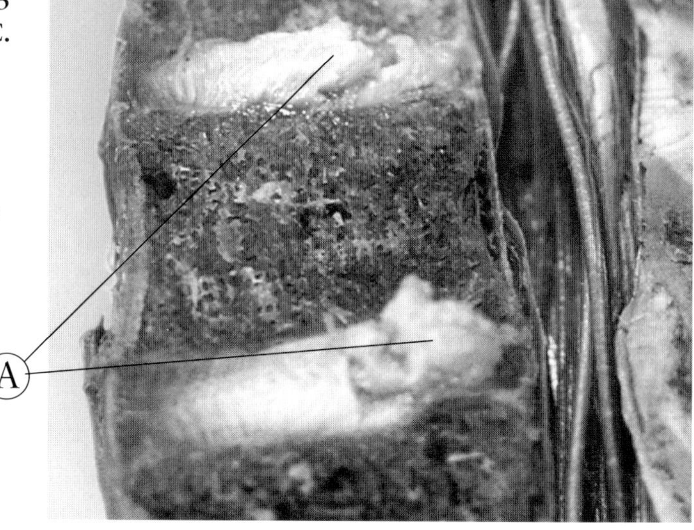

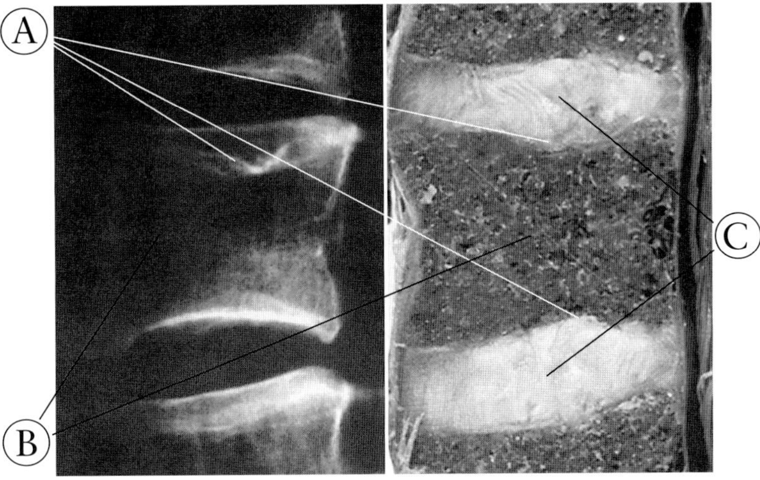

Figure 5-4
**THE SHOCK ABSORBING
VERTEBRAL BODY.**
The superior and inferior end plates have
been damaged and repaired with the
deforming force being absorbed by the
L2 vertebral body. Under the load the
endplates deflect more than the annular
walls. Notice the discs have remained
relatively healthy and that the alignment
was not disturbed by the trauma.
  (A) Damaged end plates
  (B) Vertebral body
  (C) Discs

Discs are not Shock-Absorbers.

The intervertebral disc is the largest avascular structure in the body. To remain healthy, it is dependent upon the constant, slow influx of fluid. In **Figure 5-3** the hydrophilic nature of the nucleus pulposus is demonstrated in near normal discs. After exposure to water the newly cut edge of the nucleus pulposus bulged out with the absorbed water. The normal disc has between 76 to 89% volume of water. Many studies have been conducted on the subject, but the latest research indicates that loading and unloading during normal spinal motion is the primary mechanism for disc nutrition and fluid exchange. This exchange primarily takes place through the top and bottom end plates and not, as previously thought, through the annular walls.

Additional studies indicate that the disc, contrary to popular belief, is not primarily a shock absorber. To demonstrate this point, **Figure 5-4** shows an anatomical specimen and its lateral X-ray. The vertebral bodies, the end plates, and the medullary bone in particular, deflect more during loading than the annular rings. In other words, the bulging of the annular rings is less than the bowing and bending of the end plates into the medullary bone of the vertebral bodies during loading. The nucleus pulposus is not spherical in shape, contrary to the impression created by illustrators (**See Figure 5-5**). In the lumbar spine it has a kidney bean shape in cross section, and in coronal section, is uniform in height, and resembles a column. The whole nucleus pulposus is wider than it is high.

Figure 5-5
**CROSS SECTION OF A NORMAL
LUMBAR DISC**
The lumbar discs and vertebrae have a kidney
bean shape, with a slight impression at the
posterior side. The nucleus pulposus is in the
posterior portion of the disc.
  (A) Annulus fibrosus (annular rings)
  (B) Nucleus pulposus
  (C) Posterior impression

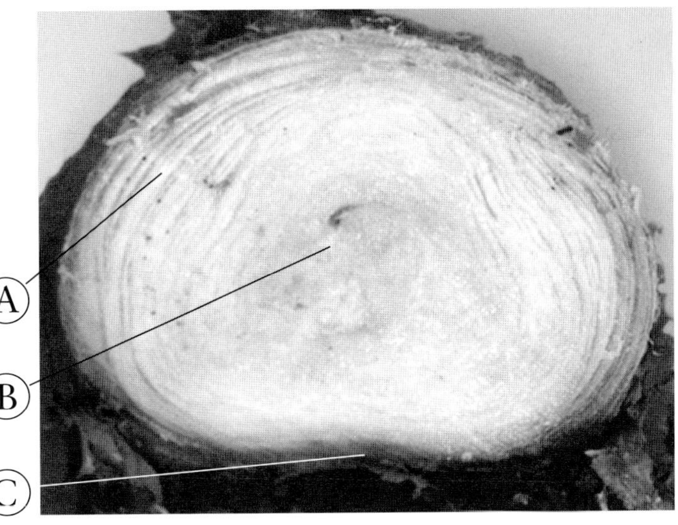

The lumbar spine in **Figure 5-6** shows that although the L2 vertebra has sustained a compression fracture, the adjacent discs have remained intact, with the alignment near normal. The L2 vertebral body and end plates have taken the brunt of the force, deforming to the point of crushing. The disc is, for mechanical purposes, a closed hydraulic system, as only a small amount of fluid (about 11%) is lost during normal compression. The remaining disc fluid is not deformable, since the annular rings are normally inelastic. The end plates do deform, compressing the trabeculae of the medullary bone. This is the mechanism for the vertebrae to absorb force. The science of hydraulics shows that force introduced at one

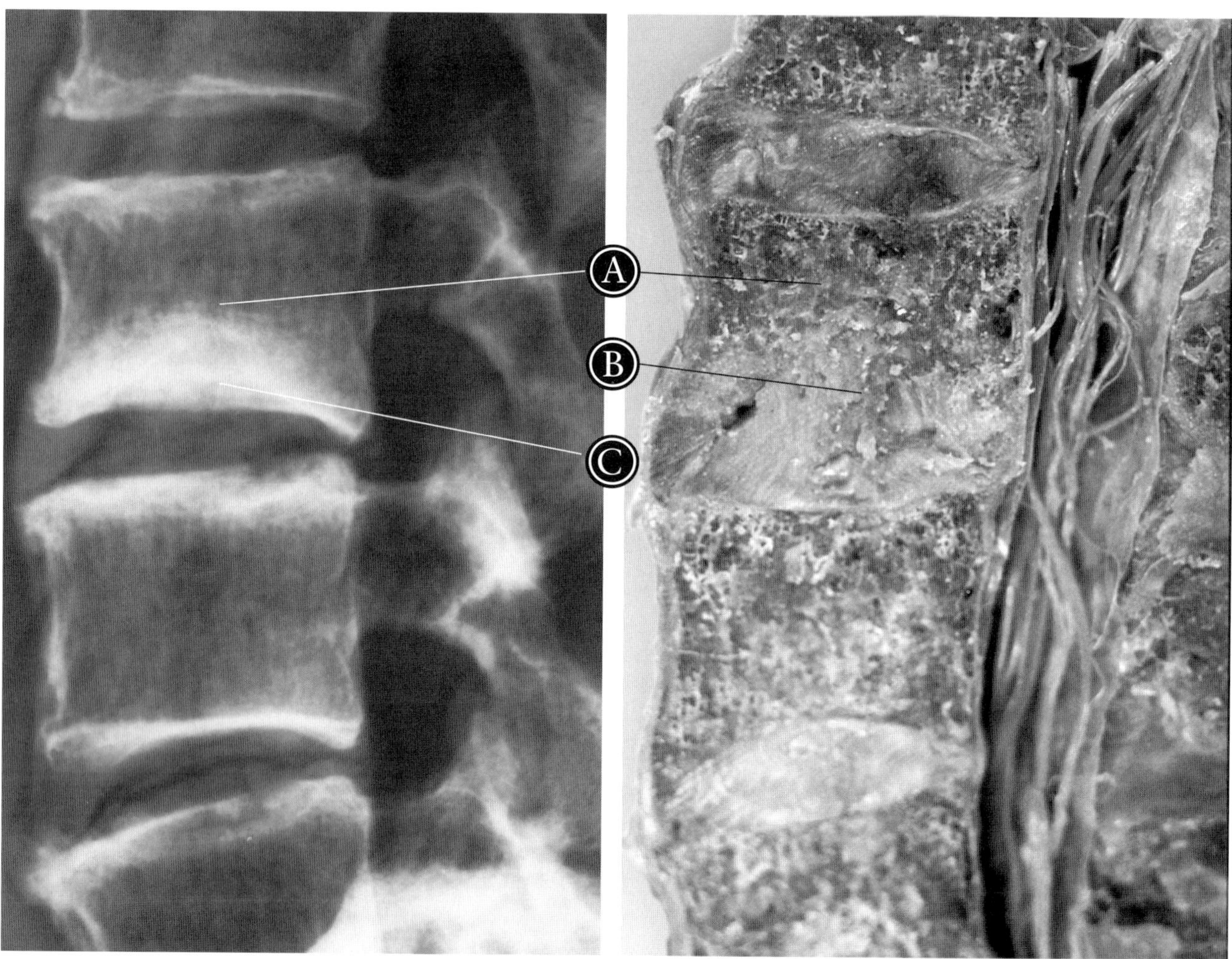

(A) L2 vertebral body
(B) Nucleus pulposus
(C) Repaired compression injury to L2

Figure 5-6

A LARGE NUCLEUS PULPOSUS PROTRUSION INTO L2.
The L2-3 disc has protruded up into L2. Note on the X-ray a bone repair has taken place that happened some time ago. This is another example of the vertebral body absorbing the deforming force of trauma with the nucleus pulposus expanding into the vertebral body of L2.

end of a fluid filled system is automatically transferred to the other end of that system; that is, the force is transmitted, not absorbed. Thus, when the lumbar spine is compressed, the force is transmitted to the vertebral bodies so that they absorb the load (or shock). As **Figure 5-7** demonstrates, when the force is too great, the vertebral bodies can actually collapse. The ver-

tebral bodies of L2 through L5 have all suffered compression fractures but the A to P alignment was not significantly altered and the discs have remained relatively healthy. The discs, being hydrophilic, create an osmotic pressure that will cause the disc to expand to fill the available space.

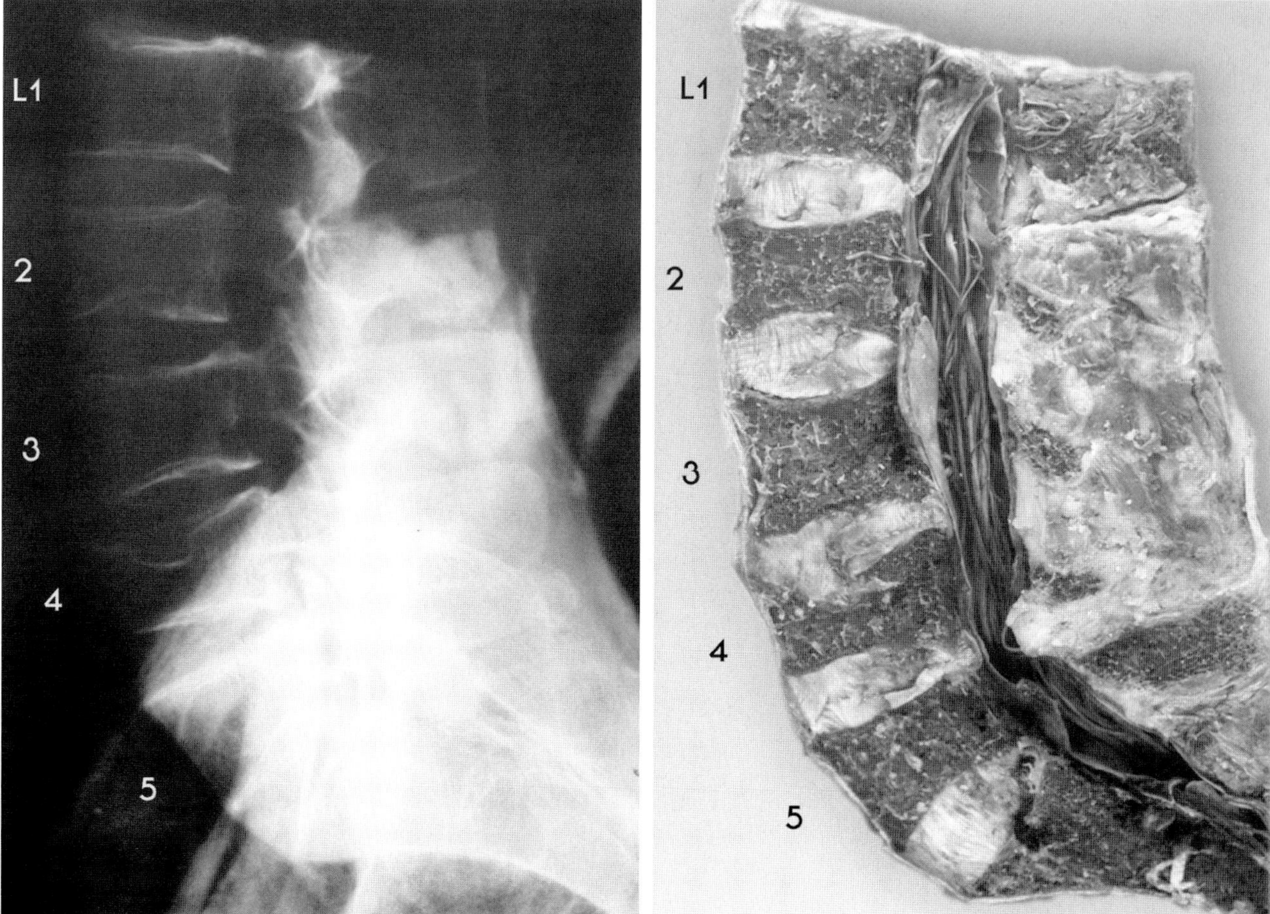

Figure 5-7
COMPRESSION FRACTURES OF THE LUMBAR SPINE WITH NEAR NORMAL ALIGNMENT
This specimen has compression fractures of L2, 3, 4, and 5. The lordotic curve and the A to P alignment have been maintained despite the trauma. Notice that the disc height has actually increased in certain areas.

Types of Lumbar Subluxations

The Subluxations of the lumbar spine are classified according to the changes in architecture. The lordotic curve of the lumbar spine is an essential architectural feature. Subluxations generally cause less neural involvement if the lordotic curve is maintained. **Figure 5-8** is a comparison of lumbar spines. In **Figure 5-8a**, L5 is anterior to L4 with disc tearing and other signs of degeneration. The sacrum has moved anteriorly to L5 and the disc has totally desiccated, indicating an old, long standing condition. Note the lack of osteophytic spurs and canal stenosis. The lordotic curve preserved normal weight bearing of most of the joints and major bony changes did not occur.

In **Figure 5-8b** the lordosis is lost with the subluxation of L3 and L4 and widening of the vertebral bodies has taken place. This occurs at the site of the subluxation only. Note the change in spinal canal width at the subluxation and overall canal length.

Figure 5-8c shows a lumbar spine with the characteristic "stair-stepping" of vertebral bodies that have buckled under deforming stress. There clearly is a loss of normal alignment between L3-L4 and L4-L5 resulting in a reversal of the lordotic curve. The vertebral segments have undergone chronic degeneration as a result of the altered weight bearing. Displacement of opposing end plates causes a shearing of the annulus and nucleus. The uncoupling of facets, stress on facetal capsules, or hyper-loading, and stress on the disc annulus, cause a proprioceptive guarding by the paraspinal muscles and the intrinsic muscles of the vertebral column. This locks the vertebrae into the buckled position, and thus interrupts the pumping motion that is necessary for normal flow of fluid in and out of the discs. The discs, of course, begin a slow process of dehydration and degeneration.

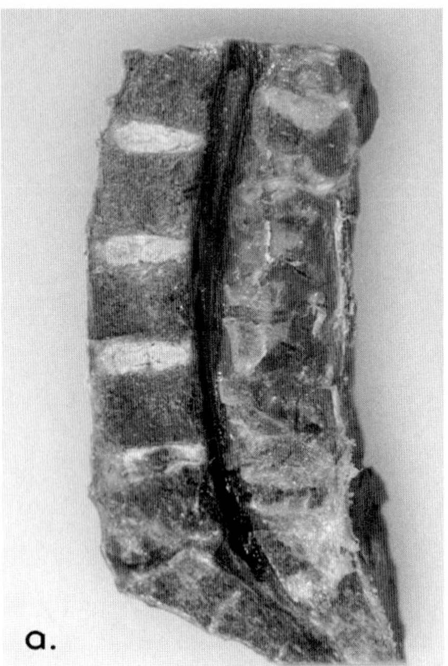
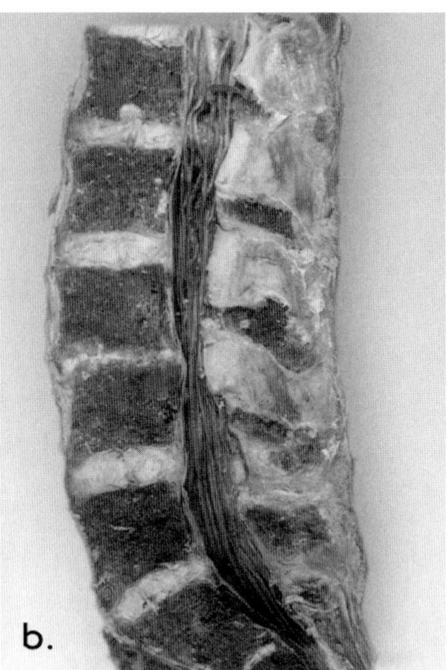
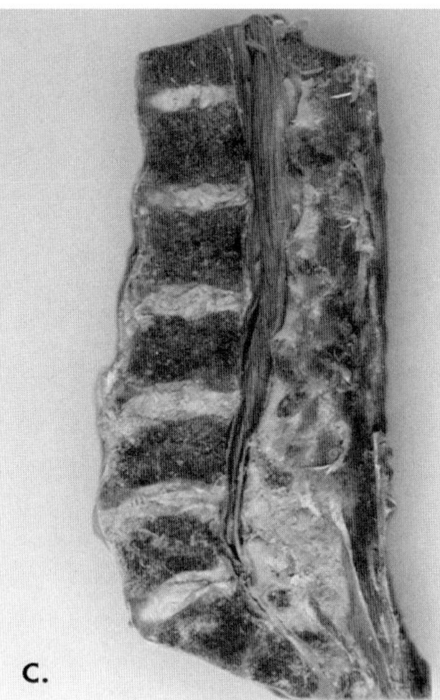

Fig. 5-8

A COMPARISON OF SUBLUXATIONS WITH A LORDOTIC CURVE, WITHOUT A CURVE AND A REVERSED CURVE.

In this small set of lumbar spines the curve and the shape of the canal are intimately involved. In comparing (a) to (b), the difference in the spinal canal length can be noted, no longer being in (b). The spine in (c) has an even longer spinal canal than (a) or (b). Also the patterns of degeneration are different. Subluxations occurring with the curve intact have milder degenerative changes. In (b) the canal stenosis is apparent and in (c) the vertebral body widening and spurring are obvious.

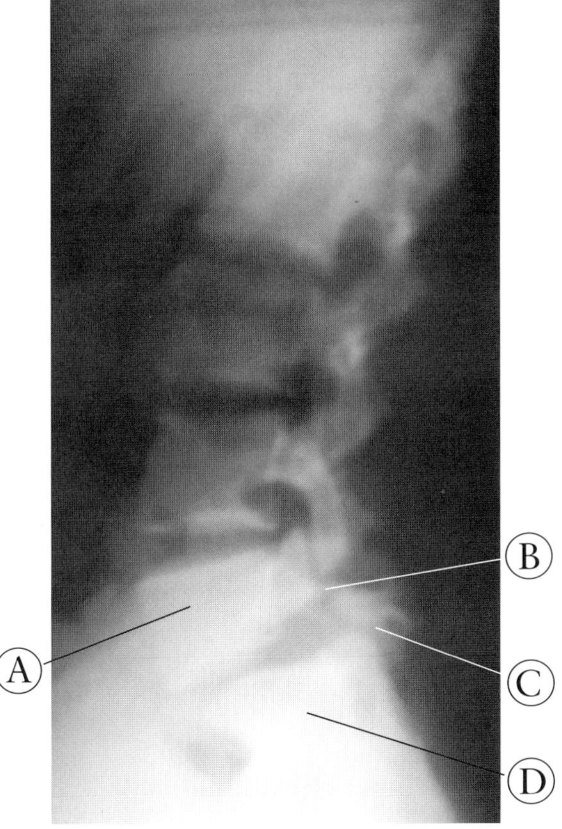

Figure 5-9

Lateral Lumbar X-ray of a 20 year old with L5 spondylolisthesis. The fifth lumbar vertebra is broken and separated. The entire spine including the L5 vertebral body and superior articular joint have subluxated anteriorly.

(A) Body of L5 vertebra
(B) Break in articular arch of L5
(C) Inferior articulations of L5
(D) Sacrum

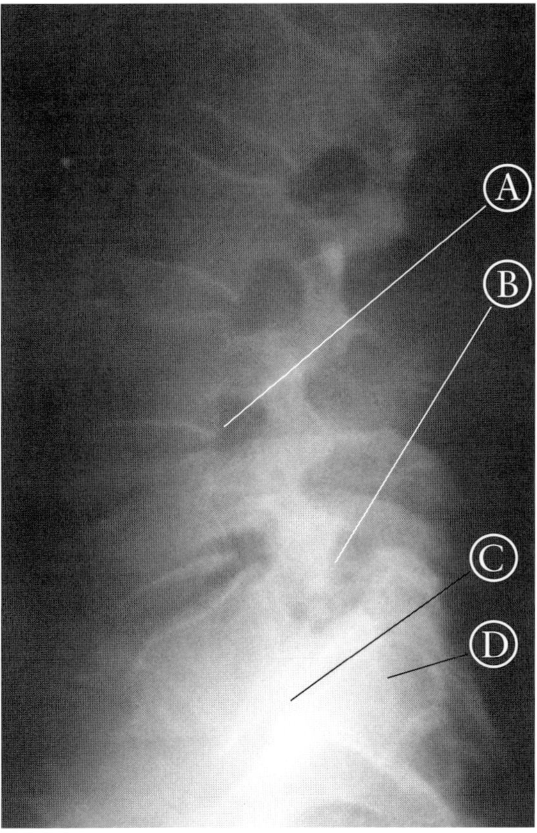

Figure 5-10

Lateral lumbar X-ray of 75 year old with spondylolisthesis. The fifth lumbar vertebra is broken and separated. The fifth lumbar vertebral body is fused to the sacrum. Patient denies chronic pain. Note maintenance of Lumbar curve.

(A) L3-4 subluxation
(B) Break in L5 vertebra
(C) Fused L5-S1 joint
(D) Sacrum

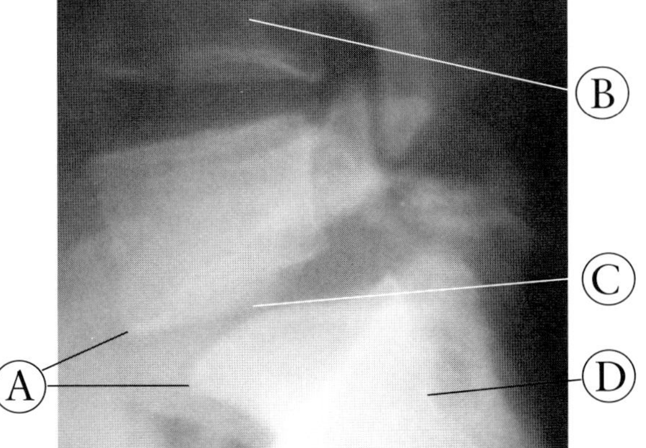

Figure 5-11

Closeup of L5 spondylolisthesis in 20 year old. This injury occurred at age 6. The fifth lumbar disc is sheared by the shifted end plates and signs of anterior spurring are present. The loss of disc height adds to the picture of a chronic injury in a young person.

(A) Anterior spurs
(B) L4 subluxated posteriorly to L5
(C) Narrowed L5-S1 disc
(D) Sacrum

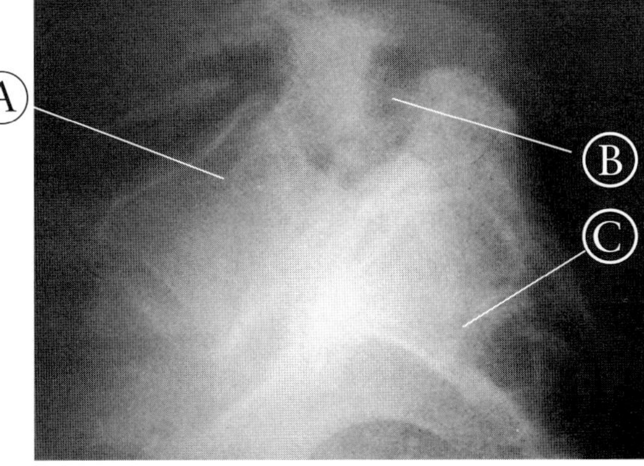

Figure 5-12

Closeup of spondylolisthesis in a 75 year old. Note the L5 vertebra has fused in the anterior position relative to the sacrum. The gap between the anterior part of L5 and the posterior part is still visible.

(A) L5
(B) Gap in L5
(C) Sacrum

The etiology of osteoarthritis of the spine is subluxation. Loss of the normal curves increases the forces that change the vertebrae. Subluxation increases the weight-bearing on the vertebral body, which then increases the vertebral body loading. This will cause an increase in the cross-sectional area of the vertebral bodies (See **Figure 5-8c**). This enlargement of the vertebral bodies and endplates manifests as spurs, osteophytes, encroachment into the spinal canal (stenosis), and encroachment of the intervertebral foremen, often leading to damage and stress in the nervous system. The degenerative changes of subluxations cause less stenotic changes to the intervertebral foramen and spinal canal if the normal lordotic curve is maintained.

Lumbar and sacral subluxations can be fixed with contracture of the lumbo-sacral aponeurosis or thoraco-lumbar fascia. (**See Figures 5-9 - 5-12.**)

Soft tissue adaptation to a subluxation complex can restrict motion of nearby joints. For example, the superior displacement of the apex of the sacrum can become permanent with a shortening of the 5 to 7 mm. thick anchoring of the lumbo-sacral fascia and tendinous attachments of the erector spinae musculature to the lower sacrum. This is the normal motion of the facets of at least the lower lumbar spine.

The condition created by subluxations results in what is commonly referred to as degenerative arthritis, degenerative disc disease, or spondylosis. In osteoarthritis of the spine, the etiologic agent is the subluxation which causes altered weight bearing. Many studies demonstrate that the subluxation occurs traumatically, either instantly or repetitively, and that increased degeneration takes place over time at those levels.

CHAPTER FIVE — EXPANDED TABLE OF CONTENTS
Atlas of Subluxations of the Lumbar Spine
SECTION I
Subluxations of the lumbar spine with a lordotic curve (15 pairs)

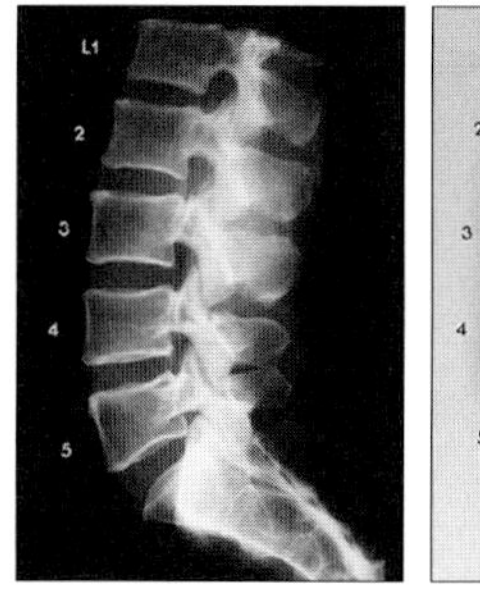 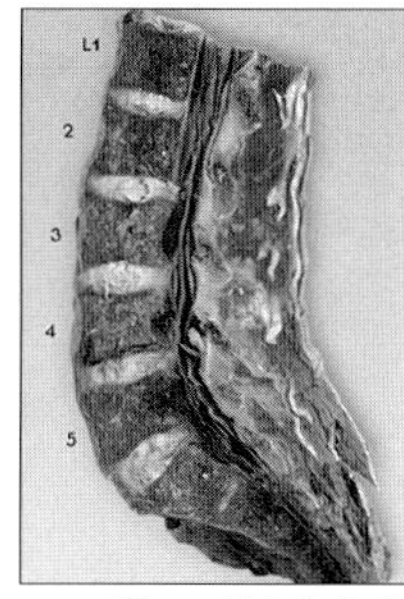

Plates 5-1 A & B
LUMBAR SPINE - near normal,
slight subluxations

Pg. 128-129

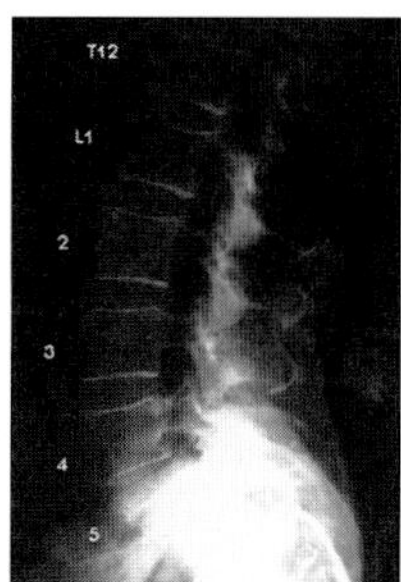 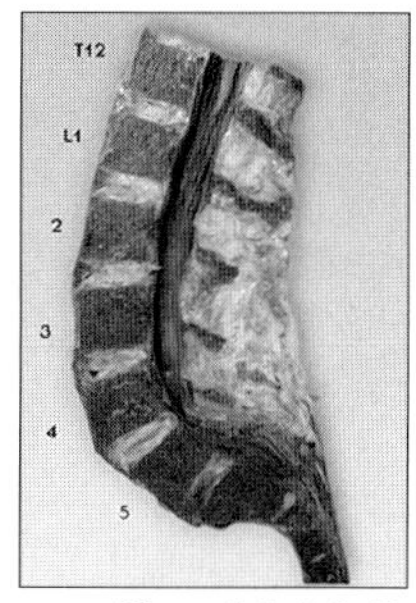

Plates 5-2 A & B
LUMBAR SPINE variations in
"normal" lumbar curve

Pg. 130-131

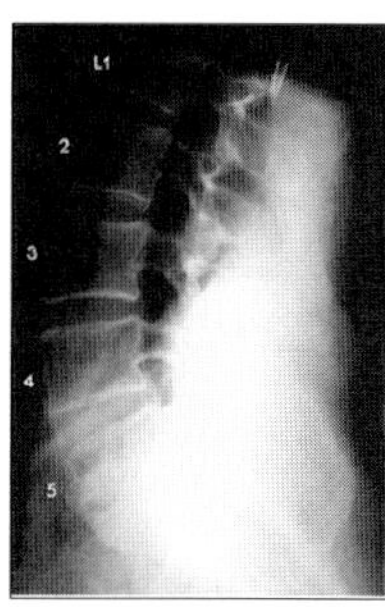 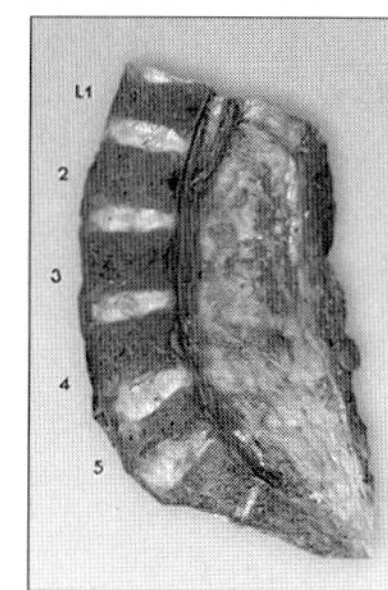

Plates 5-3 A & B
LUMBAR SPINE - L5 has a compression
fracture with sclerosis and healthy discs.

Pg. 132-133

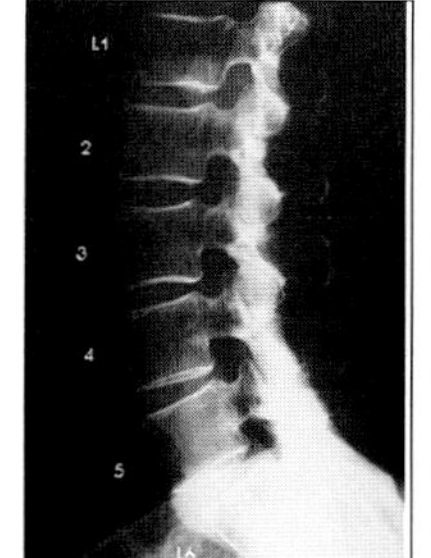 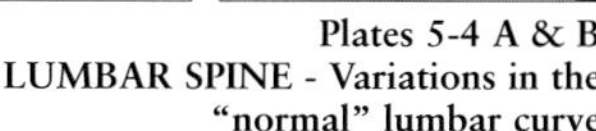 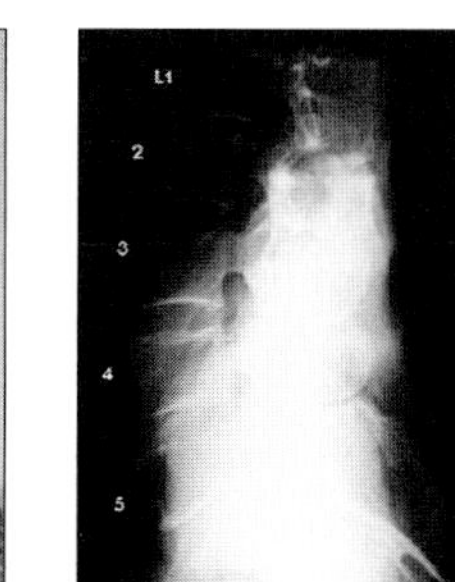

Plates 5-4 A & B
LUMBAR SPINE - Variations in the
"normal" lumbar curve

Pg. 134-135

Plates 5-5 A & B
LUMBAR SPINE - A near normal lordotic
curve with L5-sacral wedging

Pg. 136-137

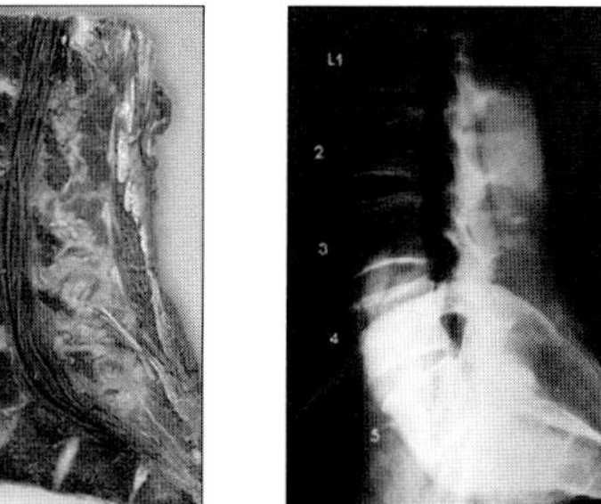 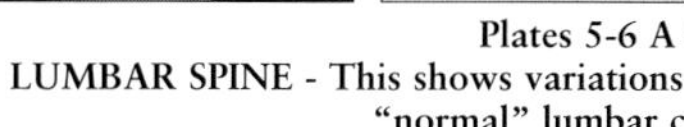

Plates 5-6 A & B
LUMBAR SPINE - This shows variations in a
"normal" lumbar curve

Pg. 138-139

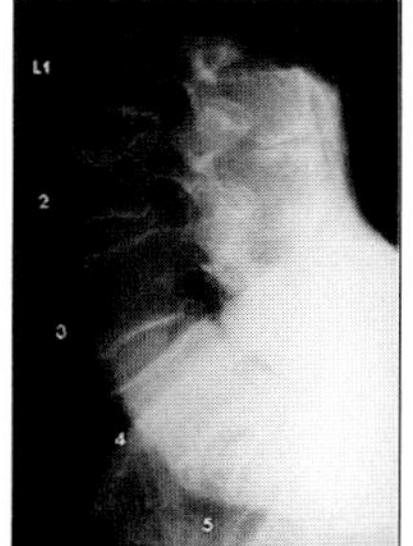 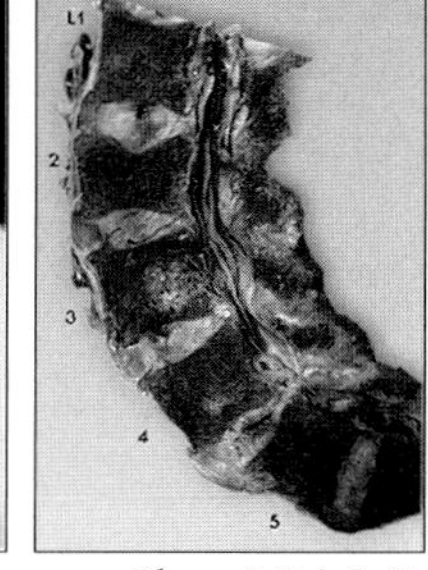

Plates 5-7 A & B
LUMBAR SPINE - This specimen has
subluxated segments with the curve maintained

Pg. 140-141

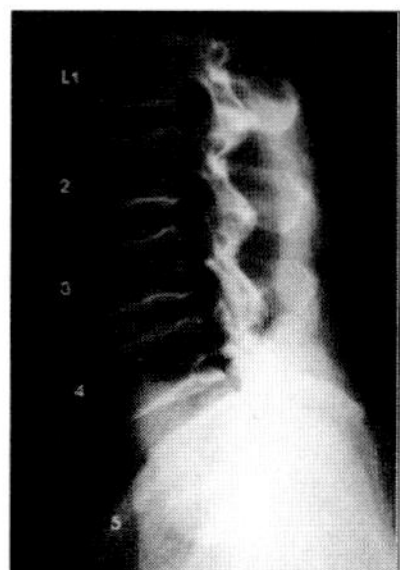

Plates 5-8 A & B
LUMBAR SPINE - variations in
"normal" lumbar curve - I

Pg. 142-143

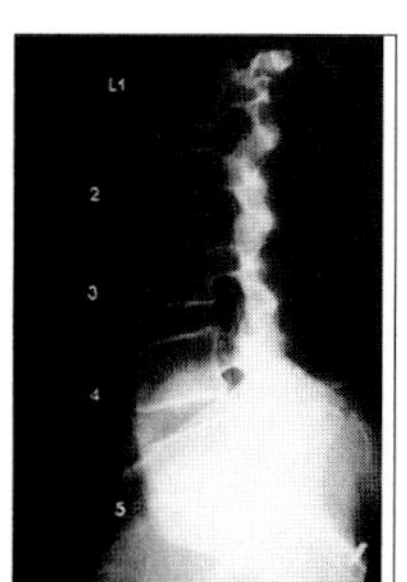 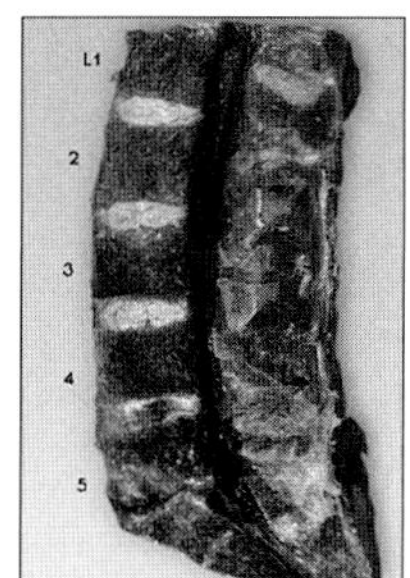

Plates 5-9 A & B
LUMBAR SPINE - Normal discs above a major
subluxation with damaged discs

Pg. 144-145

CHAPTER FIVE — EXPANDED TABLE OF CONTENTS
Atlas of Subluxations of the Lumbar Spine

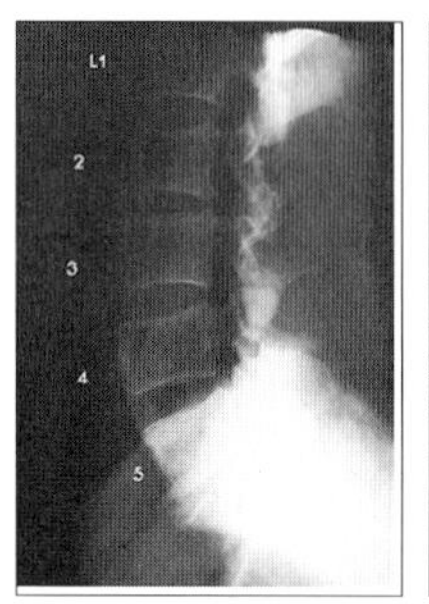 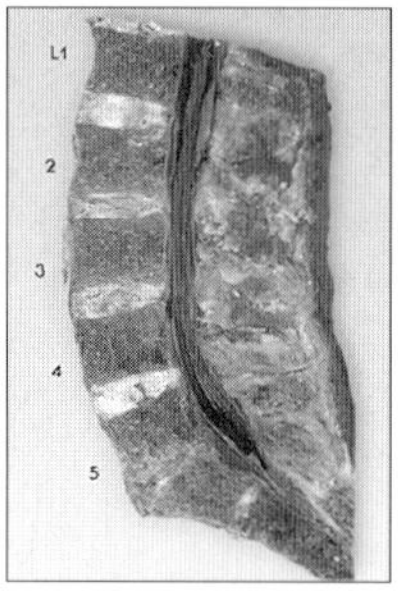

Plates 5-10 A & B
LUMBAR SPINE - This demonstrates
L5-sacrum wedging with anterior
displacement of the sacrum

Pg. 146-147

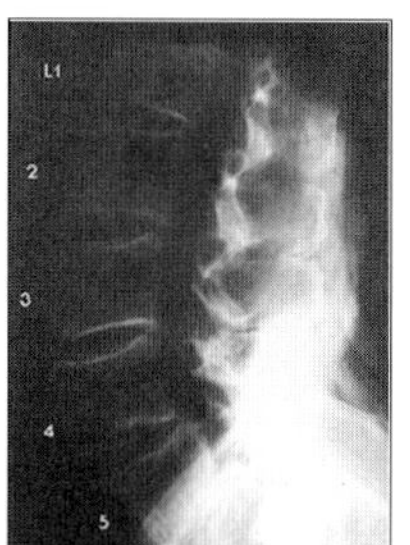 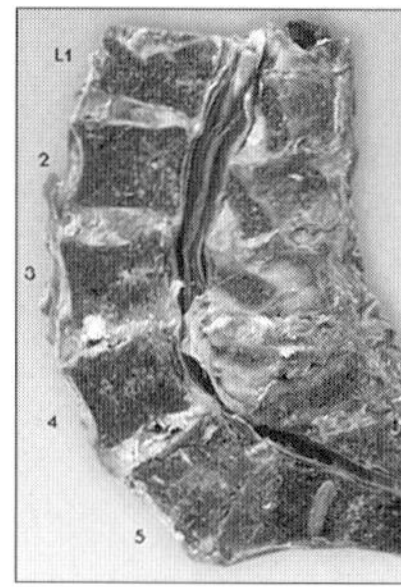

Plates 5-11 A & B
LUMBAR SPINE - This shows complete
anterolisthesis of L4 and partially of
L5 and S1 with end stage fusion

Pg. 148-149

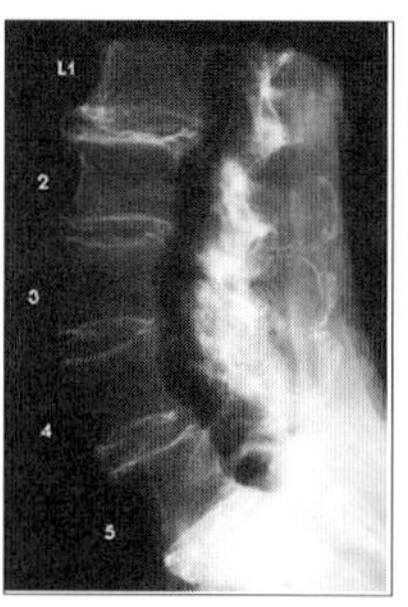 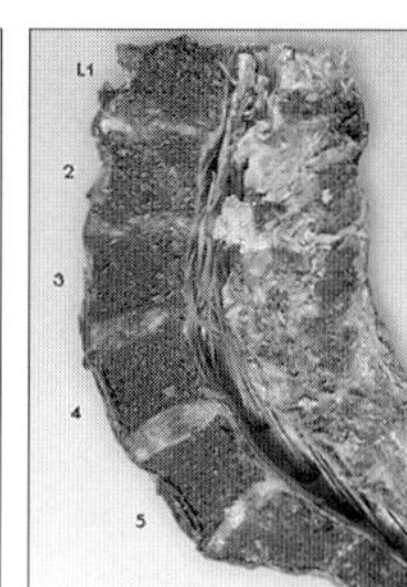

Plates 5-12 A & B
LUMBAR SPINE - This illustrates normal discs
below damaged discs with lordosis maintained

Pg. 150-151

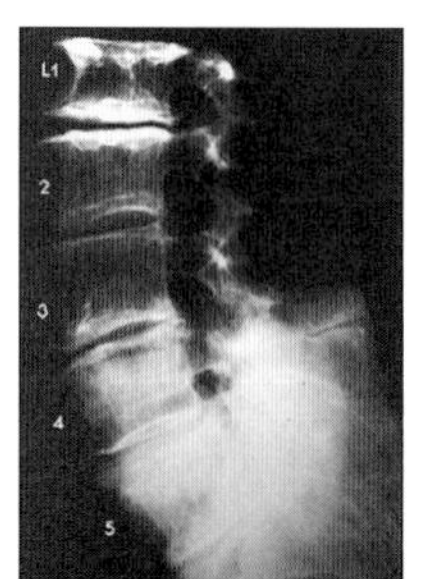 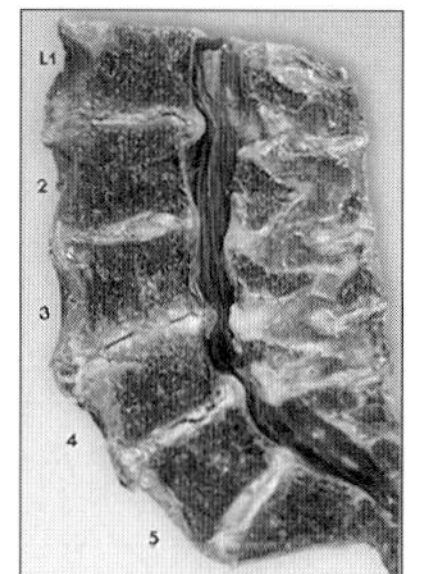

Plates 5-13 A & B
LUMBAR SPINE - The end-stages of
degeneration, post trauma

Pg. 152-153

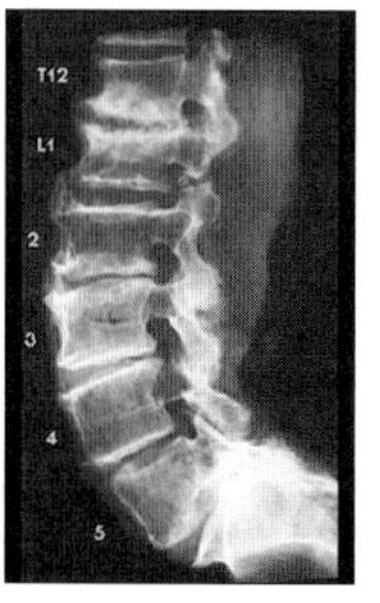

Plates 5-14 A & B
LUMBAR SPINE - This has subluxated segments
with the curve maintained, sequential retrolisthesis
to the segment below, or stairstepping

Pg. 154-155

SECTION II:
Subluxations of the lumbar spine with a loss of lordotic curve (6 pairs)

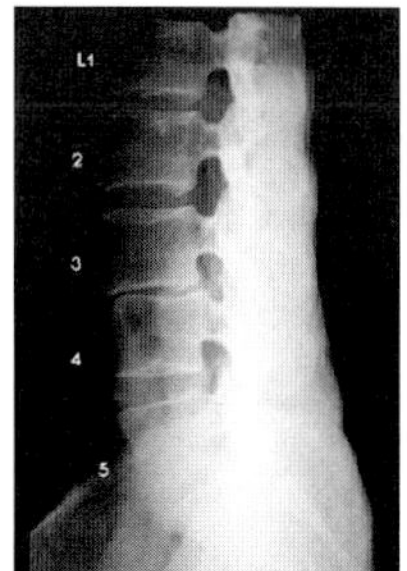 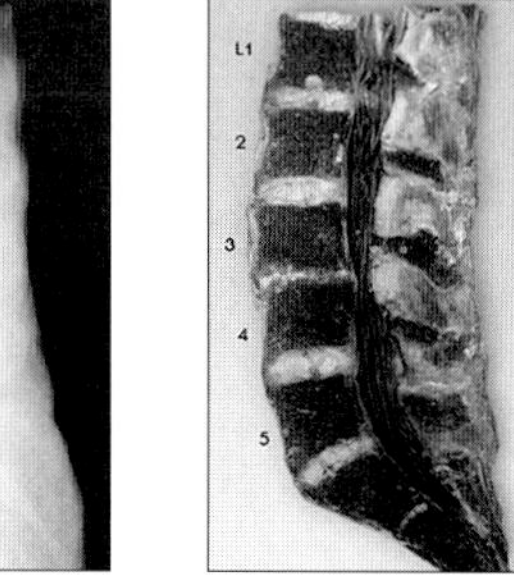

Plates 5-15 A & B
LUMBAR SPINE - This shows hypolordosis
with one significant subluxation

Pg. 156-157

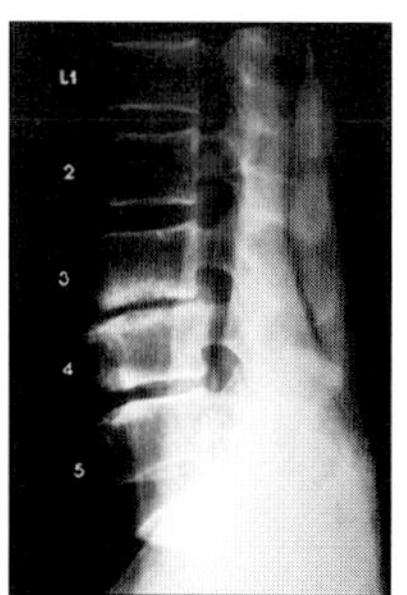 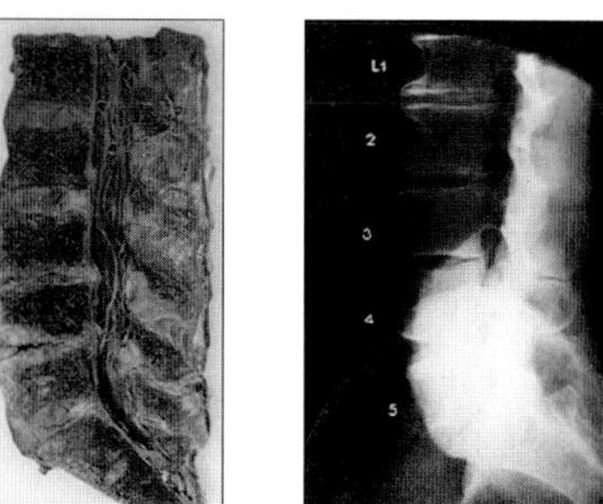

Plates 5-16 A & B
LUMBAR SPINE - This illustrates
subluxations with a loss of lordotic curve
and various stages of disc degeneration

Pg. 158-159

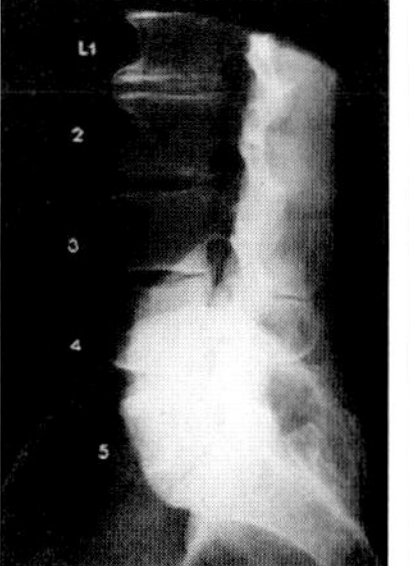 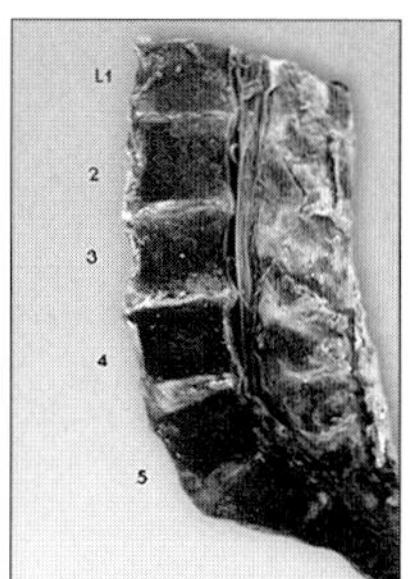

Plates 5-17 A & B
LUMBAR SPINE - The subluxation complex of
this specimen involves the entire lumbar spine

Pg. 160-161

CHAPTER FIVE — EXPANDED TABLE OF CONTENTS
Atlas of Subluxations of the Lumbar Spine

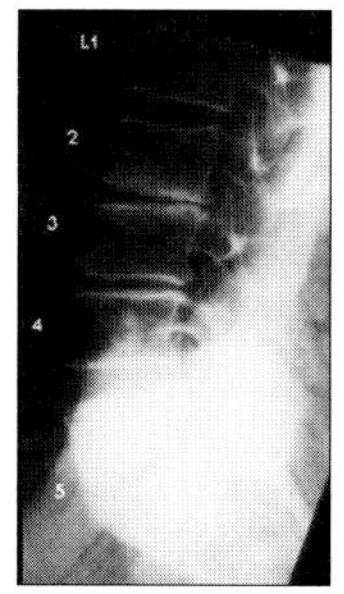

Plates 5-18 A & B
LUMBAR SPINE - This shows multiple
subluxations with loss of curve

Pg. 162-163

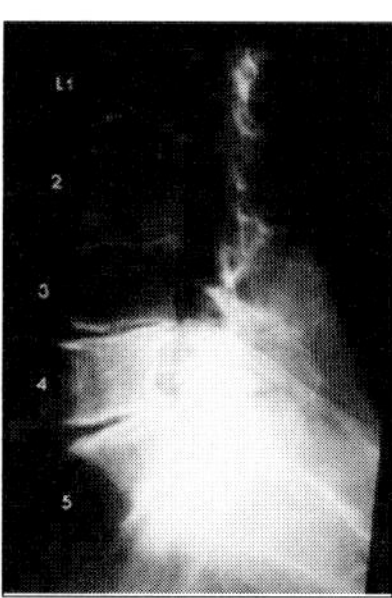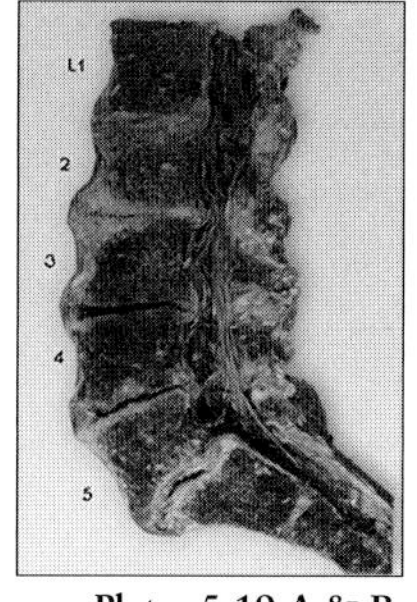

Plates 5-19 A & B
LUMBAR SPINE - This illustrates subluxations
in end-stages of degeneration with a loss of
lordotic curve

Pg. 164-165

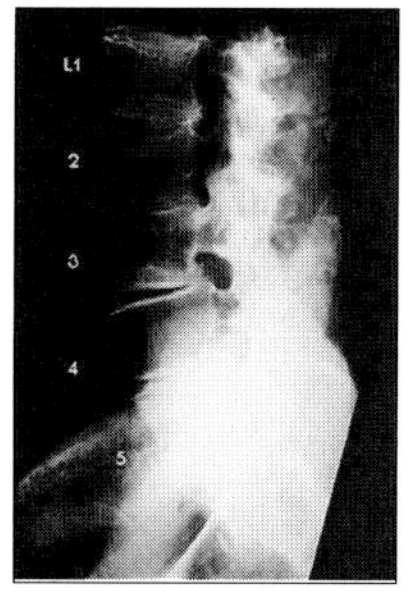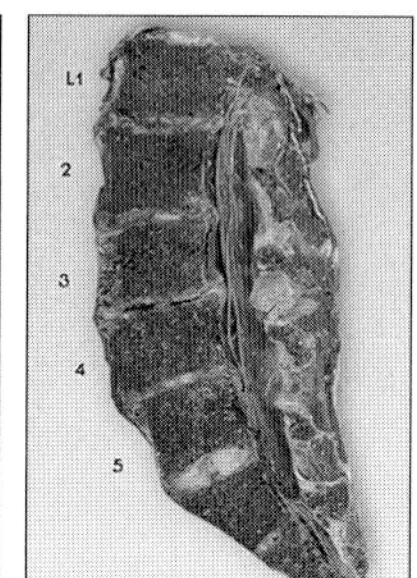

Plates 5-20 A & B
LUMBAR SPINE - This specimen has multiple
subluxations and the end-stages of degeneration

Pg. 166-167

SECTION III:
Subluxations of the lumbar spine with a reversal of the lordotic curve (4 pairs)

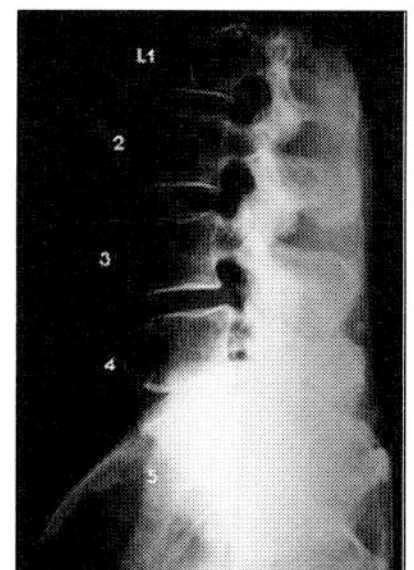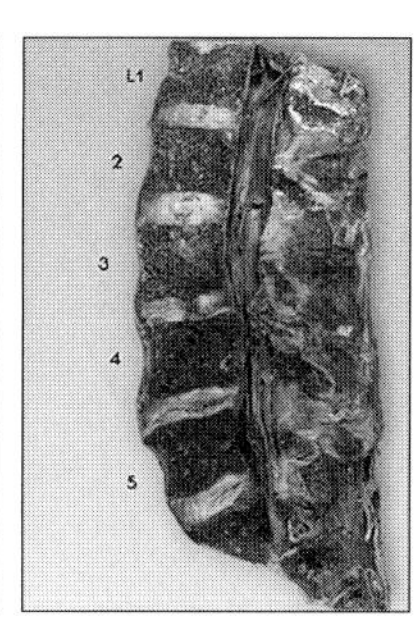

Plates 5-21 A & B
LUMBAR SPINE - This individual has a
reversal of lumbar lordotic curve
with complete retrolisthesis of L4

Pg. 168-169

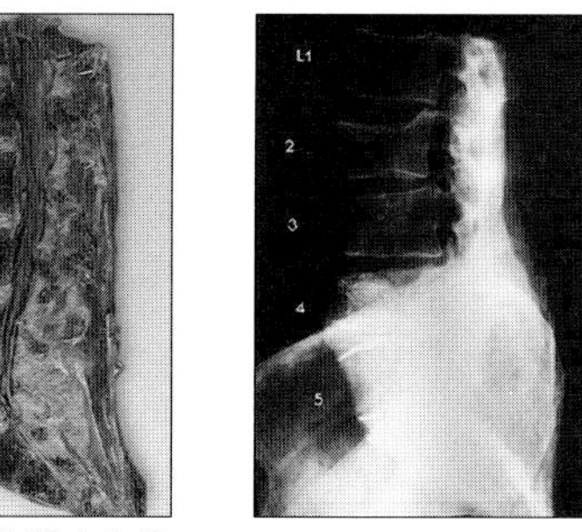

Plates 5-22 A & B
LUMBAR SPINE - Sequential retrolisthesis
forming a "stairstepping" of L1-L5 into a
reversal of the lordotic curve

Pg. 170-171

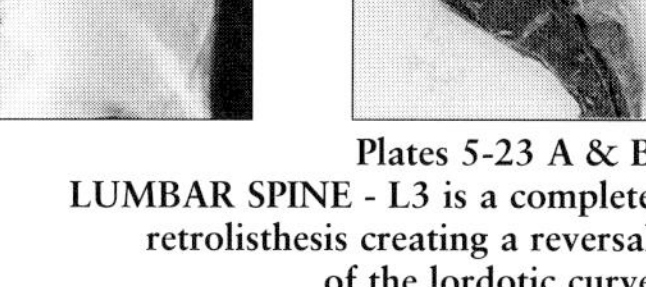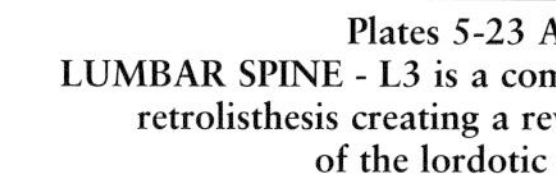

Plates 5-23 A & B
LUMBAR SPINE - L3 is a complete
retrolisthesis creating a reversal
of the lordotic curve

Pg. 172-173

Additional X-ray/MRI Comparison

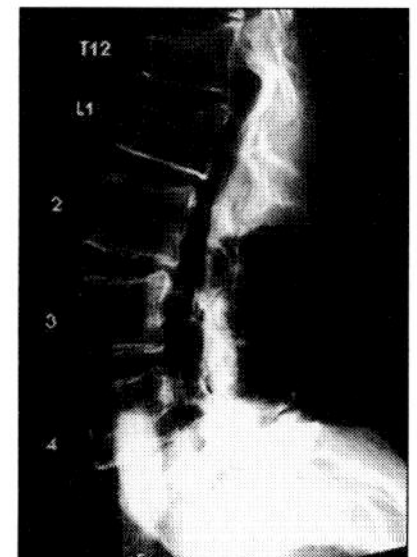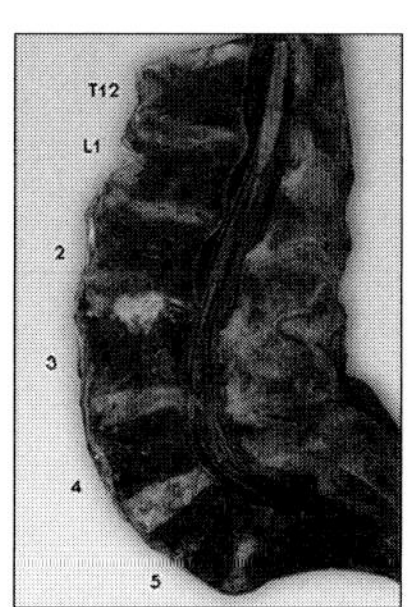

Plates 5-24 A & B
LUMBAR SPINE - This shows a reversal of the
lordotic curve in the upper lumbar spine

Pg. 174-175

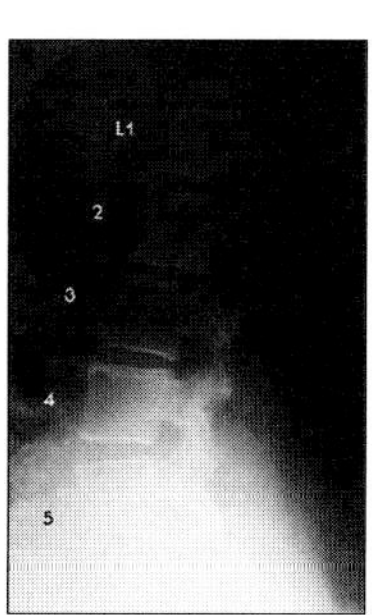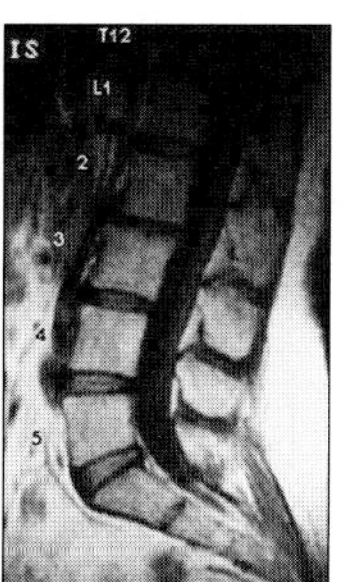

Plates 5-25 A & B
SUBLUXATIONS WITH A LOSS OF LORDOSIS
An X-ray and MRI comparison

Pg. 176-177

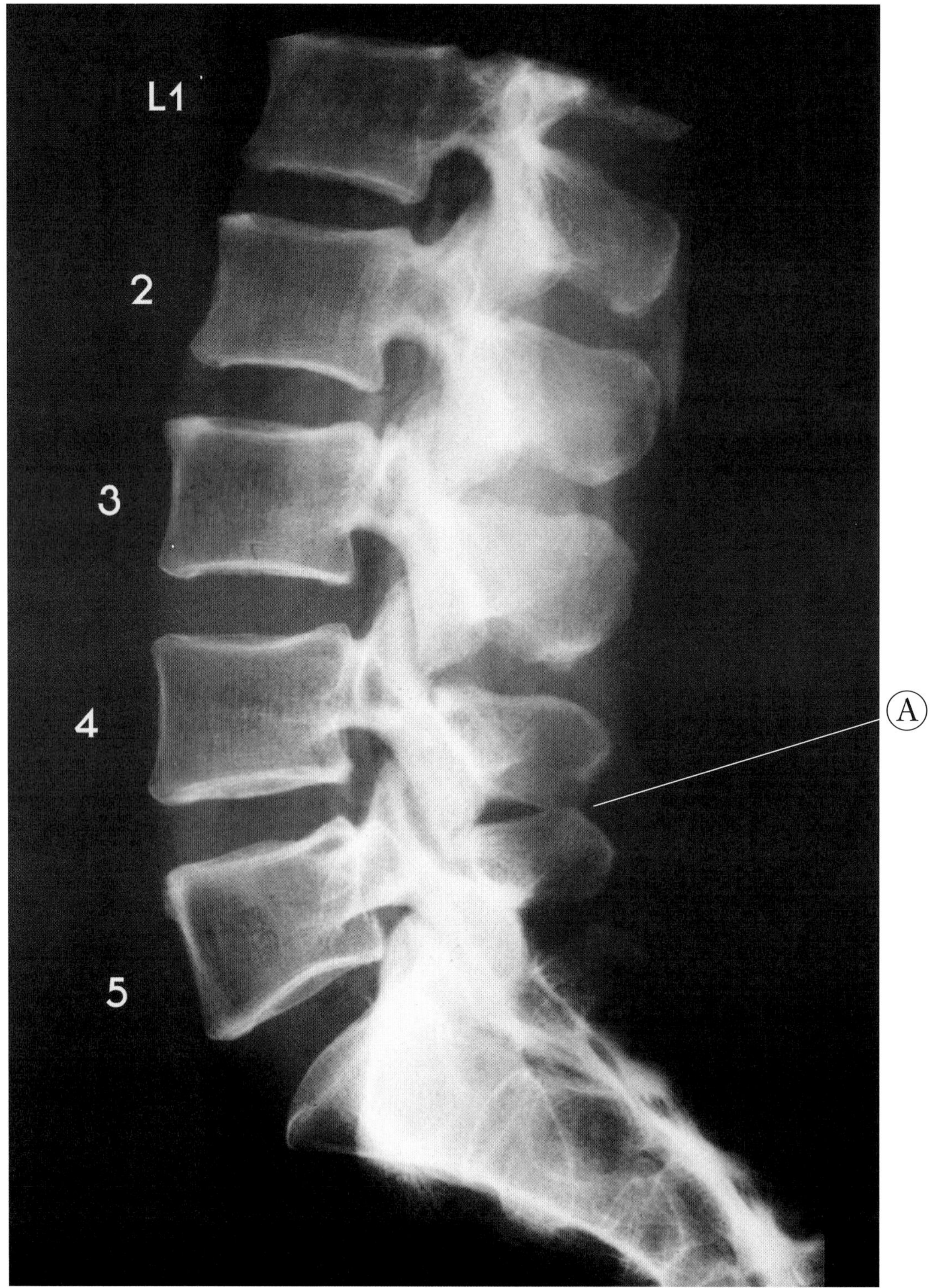

Plates 5-1 A & B
LUMBAR SPINE - near normal, slight subluxations

Some of the lordotic curve in this specimen has been maintained.
L1 and L2 look aligned. The rest of the spine is a reversed stairstepping with each vertebrae being posterior to the next inferior vertebrae. L2 is slightly retro to L3 with slight disc bulging.

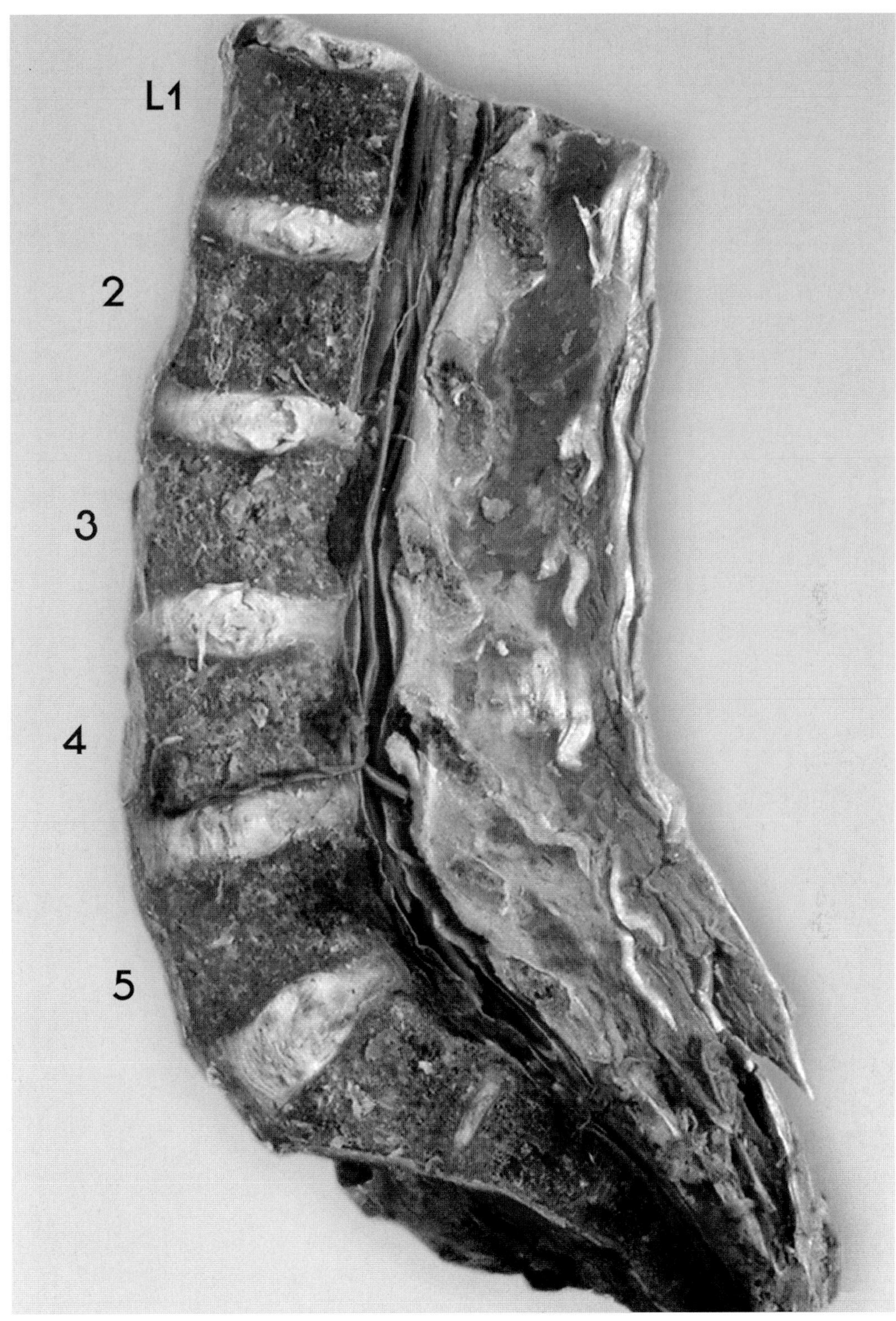

L3 slightly retro to L4 with disc bulge; L4 retro to L5 with disc wedging; L5 is slightly retro to the sacrum with disc wedging and bulging.
  (A) L4-L5 have spinous process contact

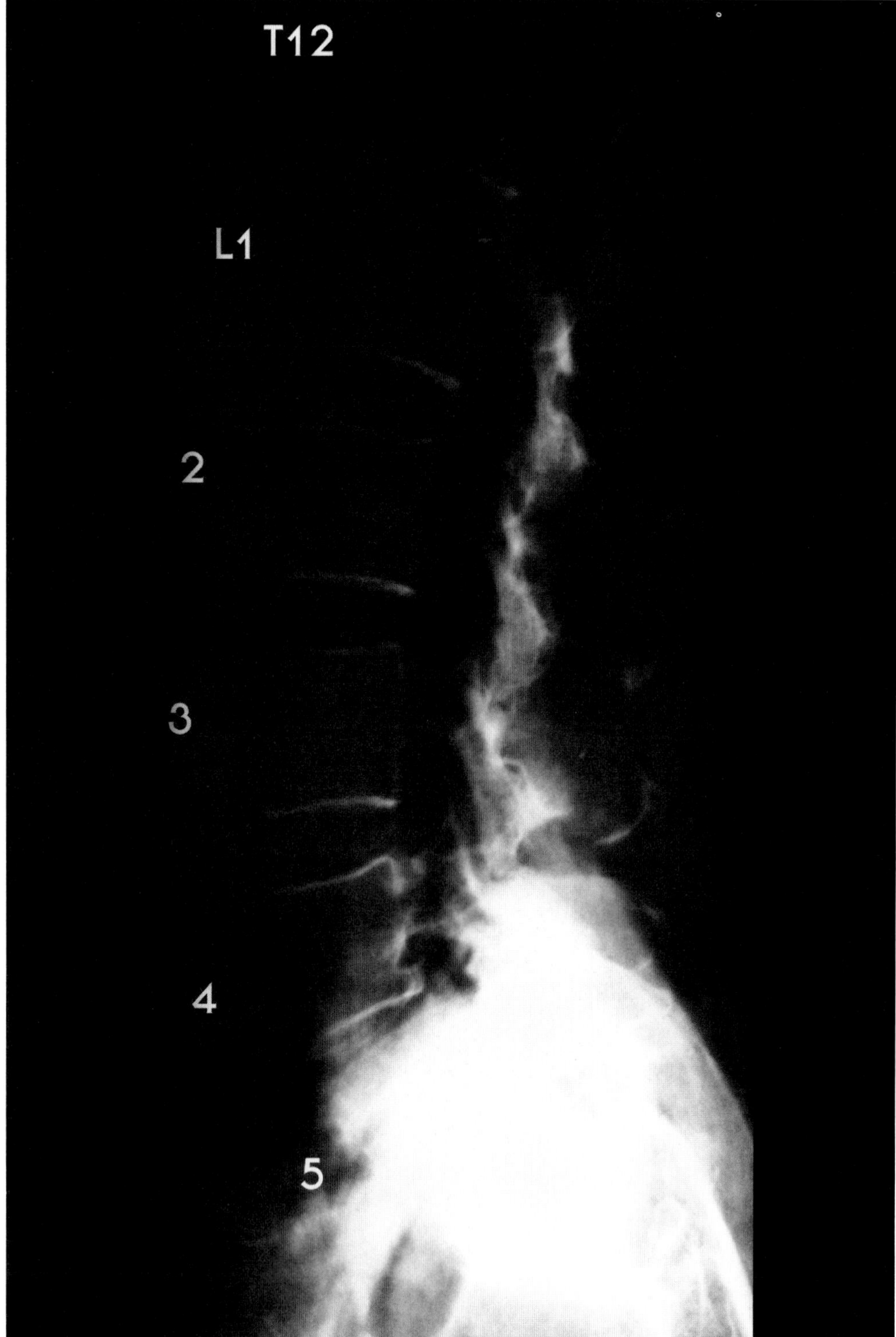

Plates 5-2 A & B

LUMBAR SPINE variations in "normal" lumbar curve

This is a good example of slight degeneration processes in the discs with minor antro and retro displacement.

L1 is slightly antro to T12 with a small posterior bulge, slight tearing, and the beginnings of brown degeneration anteriorly. L2 is slightly antro to L1 with slight tearing and anterior

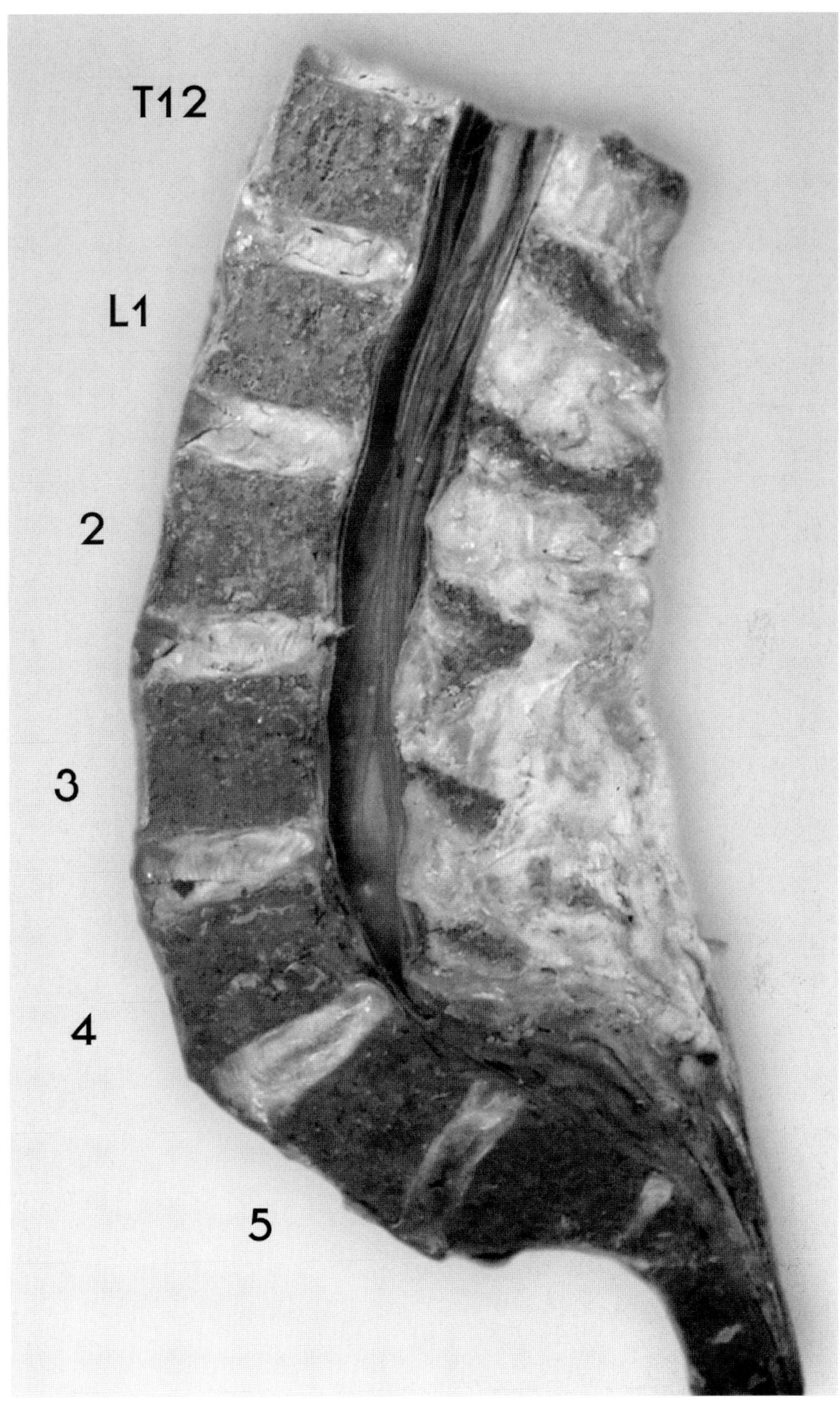

brown degeneration. L3 is antro to L4 with anterior brown degeneration and tearing. L4 is slightly antro to L3 with brown degeneration, tearing. L5 is slightly retro to L4 with brown degeneration, tearing, and wedging. The sacrum is retro to L5 with significant tearing, cavitation, and some loss of disc height.
Note the absence of even moderate A to P subluxations in the lumbar spine.

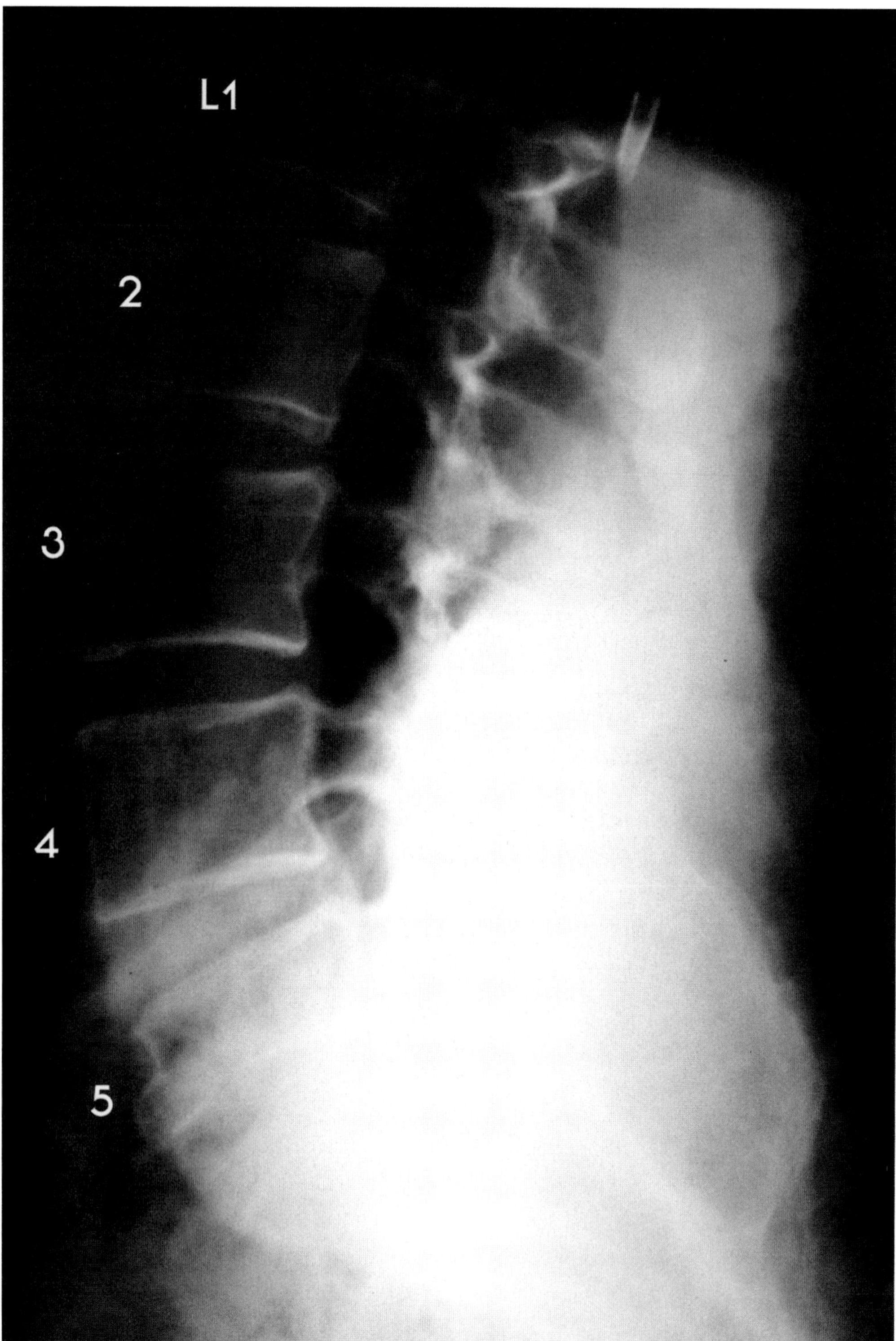

Plates 5-3 A & B

LUMBAR SPINE - L5 has a compression fracture with sclerosis and healthy discs.
This specimen has suffered a trauma with a resulting compression fracture of the L5
vertebral body. This fracture repaired and the L4-5 and L5-S1 discs have taken the loss of
volume for the L5 vertebral body. L1-4 look nearly aligned with slight anterior disc brown

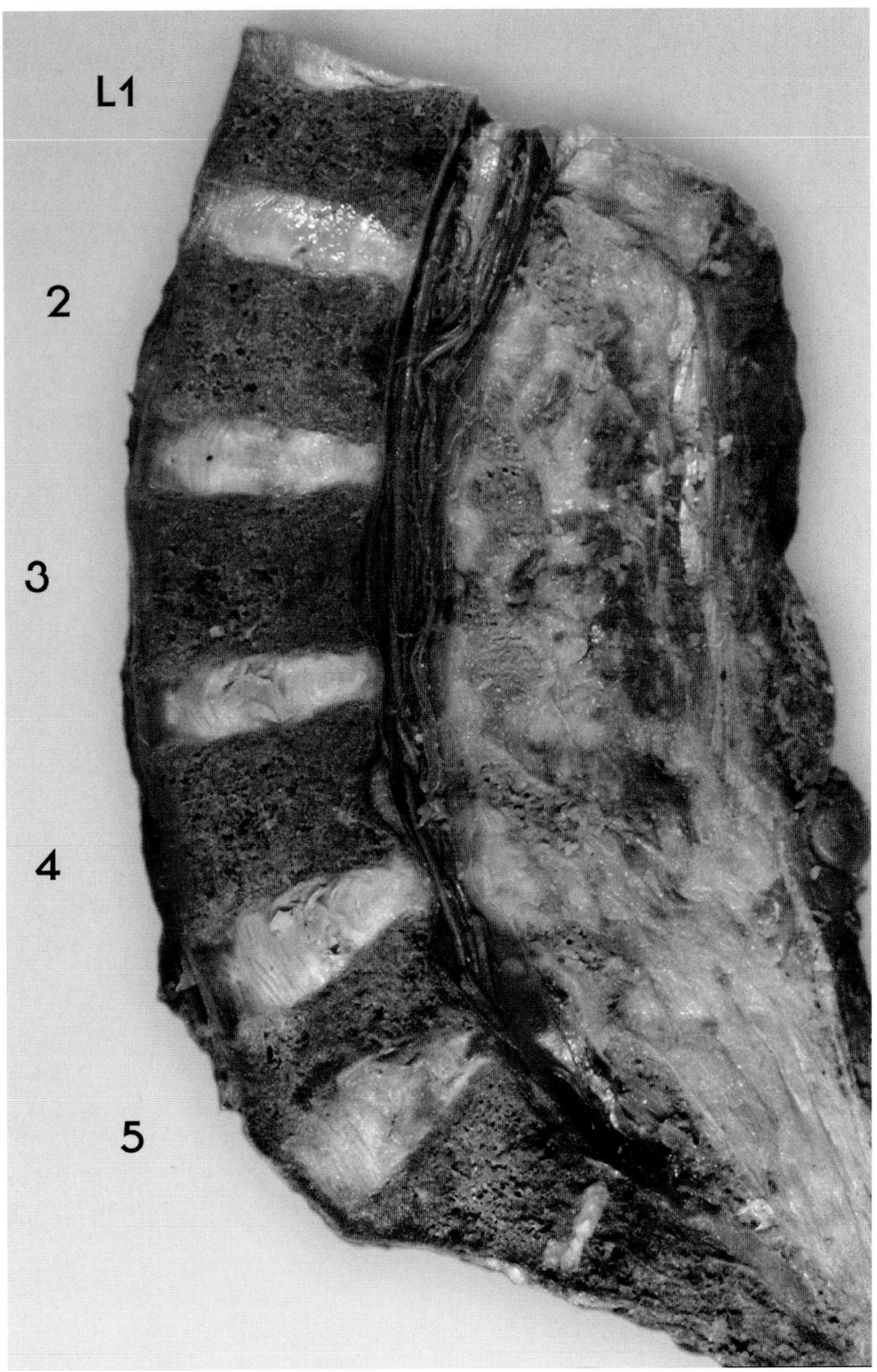

degeneration; L4-5 and L5-S1 have wedging accompanying compression fracture of L5.
There is a slight, but complete retro of L5 with a L4-5 posterior disc bulge.
This specimen has only minor signs of degeneration because the curve is maintained.
This is another example of the vertebral body absorbing the shock.

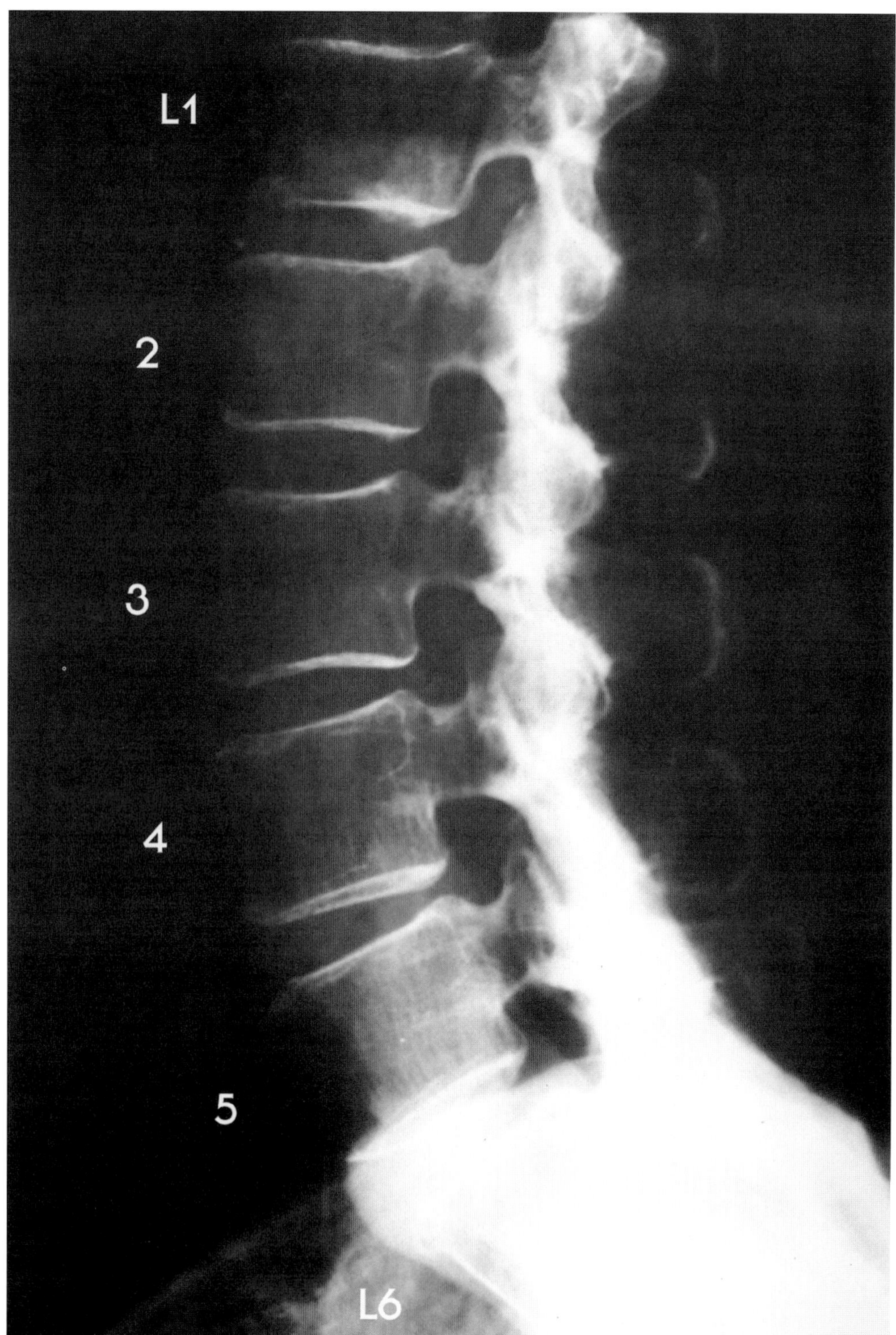

Plates 5-4 A & B
LUMBAR SPINE - Variations in the "normal" lumbar curve
This specimen has a lordotic curve with six lumbar vertebrae with disc degeneration that
corresponds to the degree of subluxation. L1 is slightly retro to L2 with slight disc bulging.

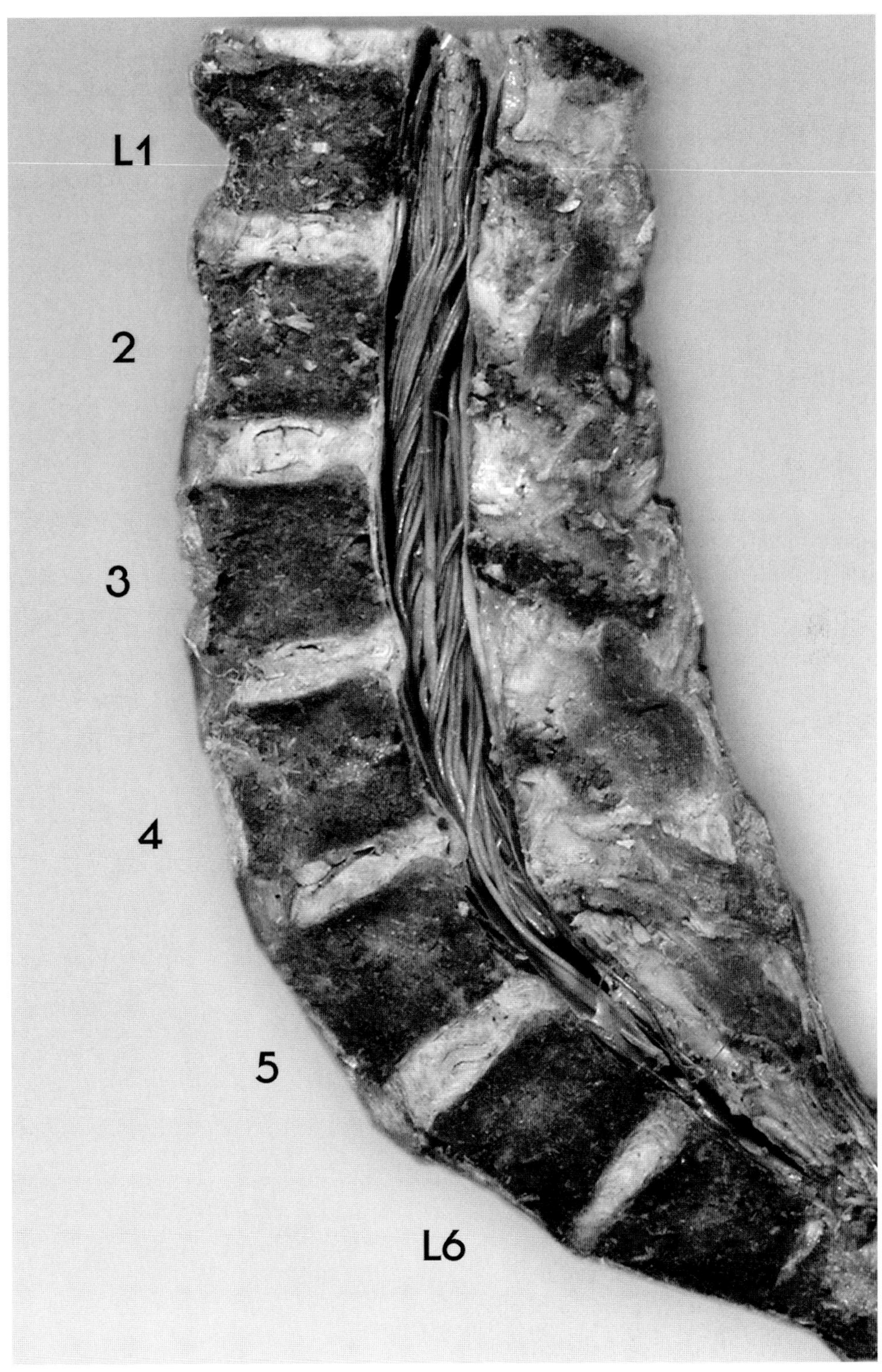

L2 is retro to L3 with slight disc tearing. L3 is retro to L4 with slight tearing and bulging. L4 is retro to L5 with disc tearing, wedging, and bulging. L5 is slightly antro to L6 with moderate wedging and slight tearing. L6-S1 look aligned.

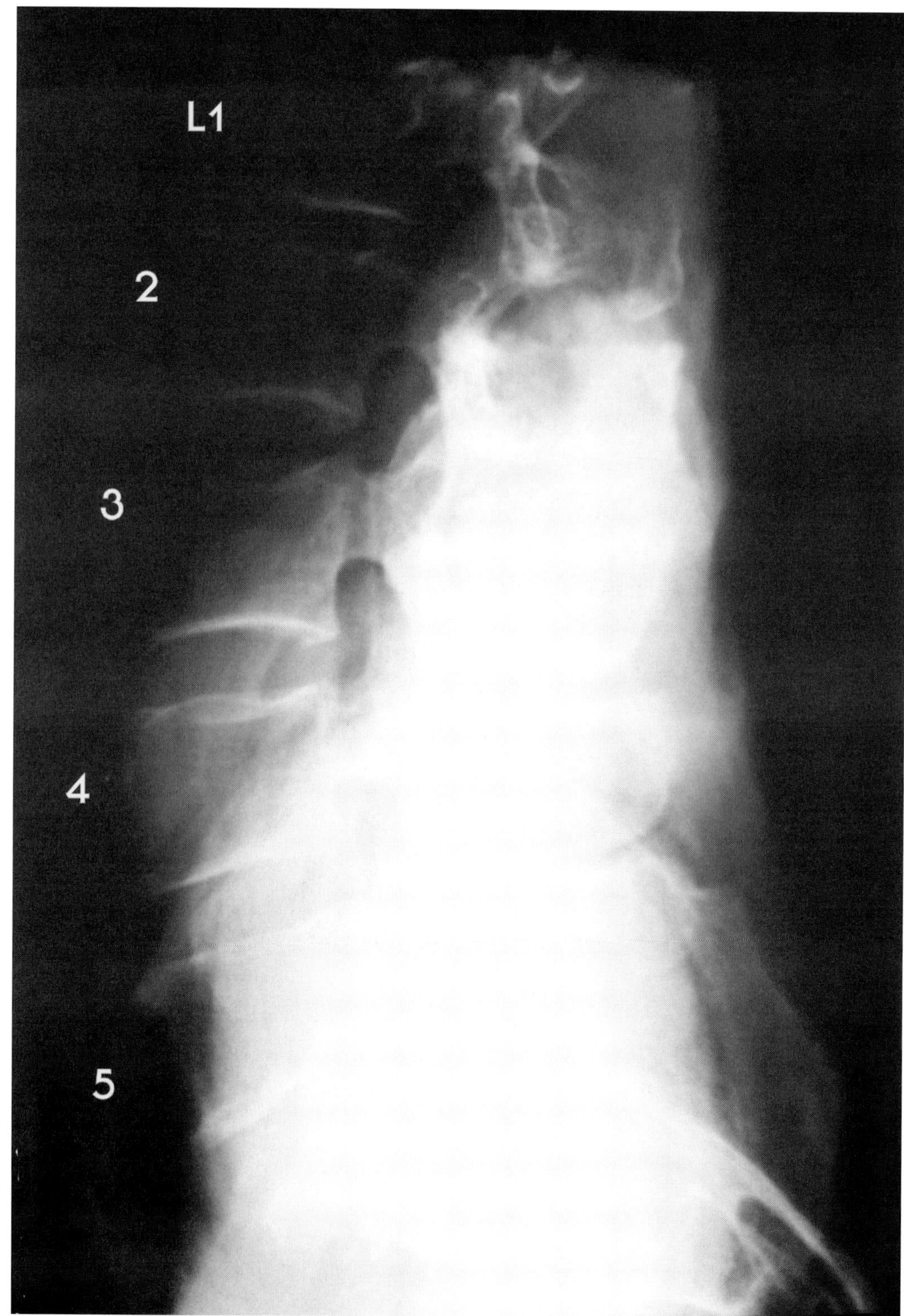

Plates 5-5 A & B

LUMBAR SPINE - A near normal lordotic curve with L5-sacral wedging
This person had a near normal alignment with the sacrum angled or subluxated posteriorly. The contracture of the thoracolumbar fascia can make permanent this "sacral apex posterior" subluxation. L1 is retro to L2 with disc tearing, and anterior and posterior bulging; L2-3 are aligned with slight wedging; L3-4 is normal; the L4-5 alignment is near normal, while the

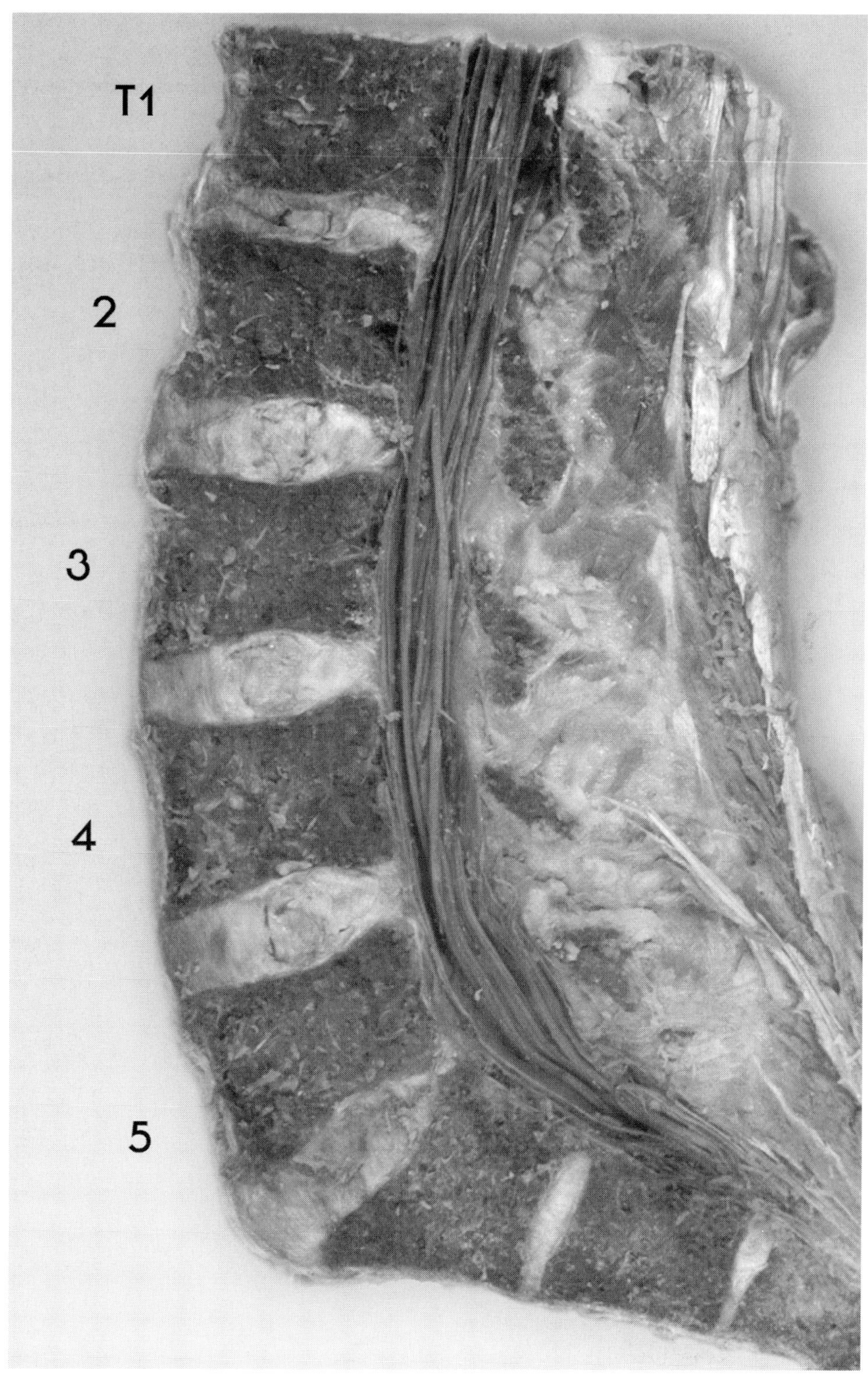

sacrum is only slightly retro to L5 with significant posterior disc height loss,anterior and posterior bulging, and tearing. Lack of A to P subluxation results in less DJD (degenerative joint disease).

Note: The sacral discs show that sacral motion was persistent. This lumbar spine is a good example of DJD associated with subluxation and normal discs associated with alignment and a normal curve.

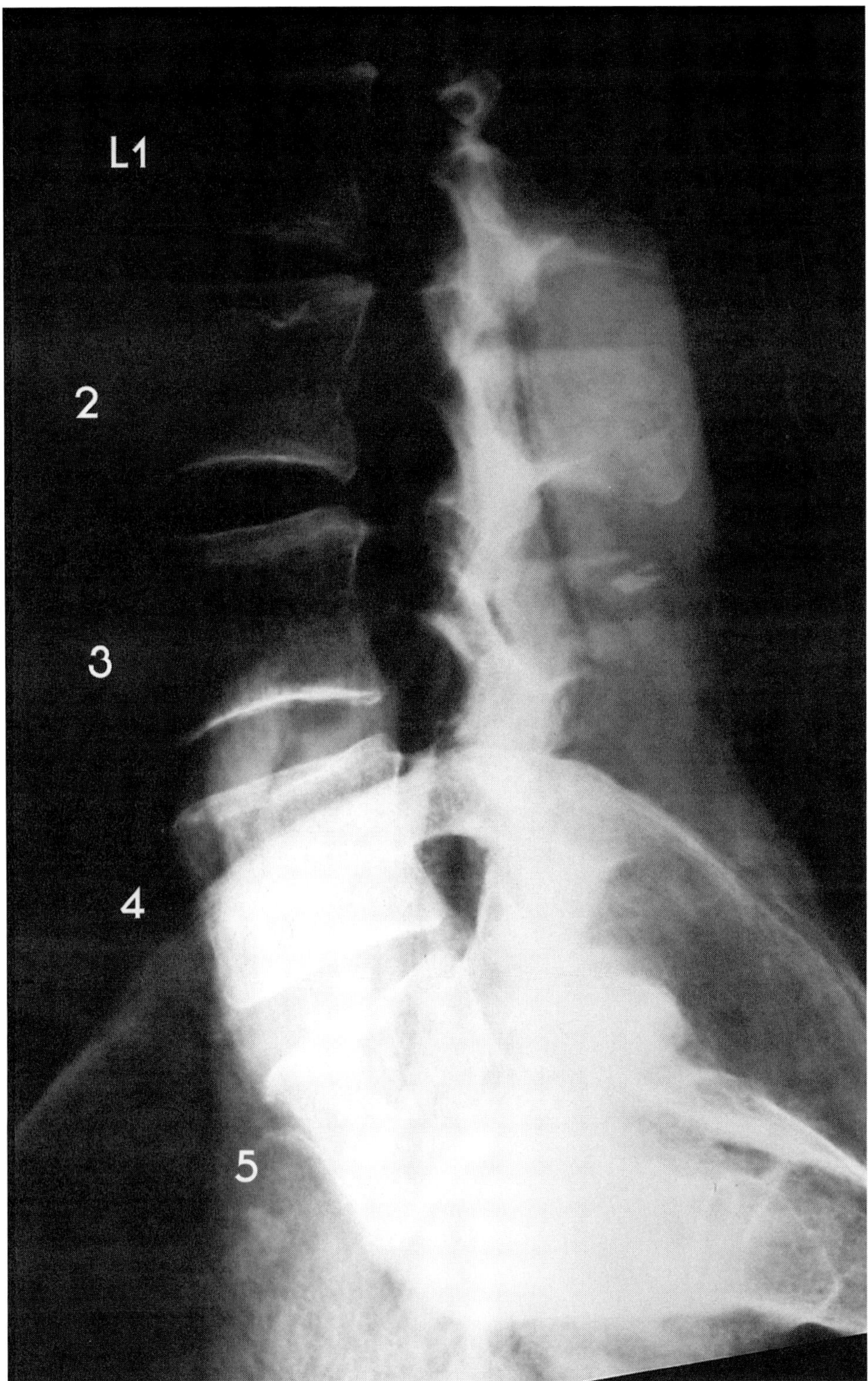

Plates 5-6 A & B

LUMBAR SPINE - This shows variations in a"normal" lumbar curve
L1-2 look aligned but the endplates appear damaged and repaired with a Schmoral's node of the superior L2 endplate, with some disc tearing. L3 is aligned with L2 but has endplate damage with repair to both.

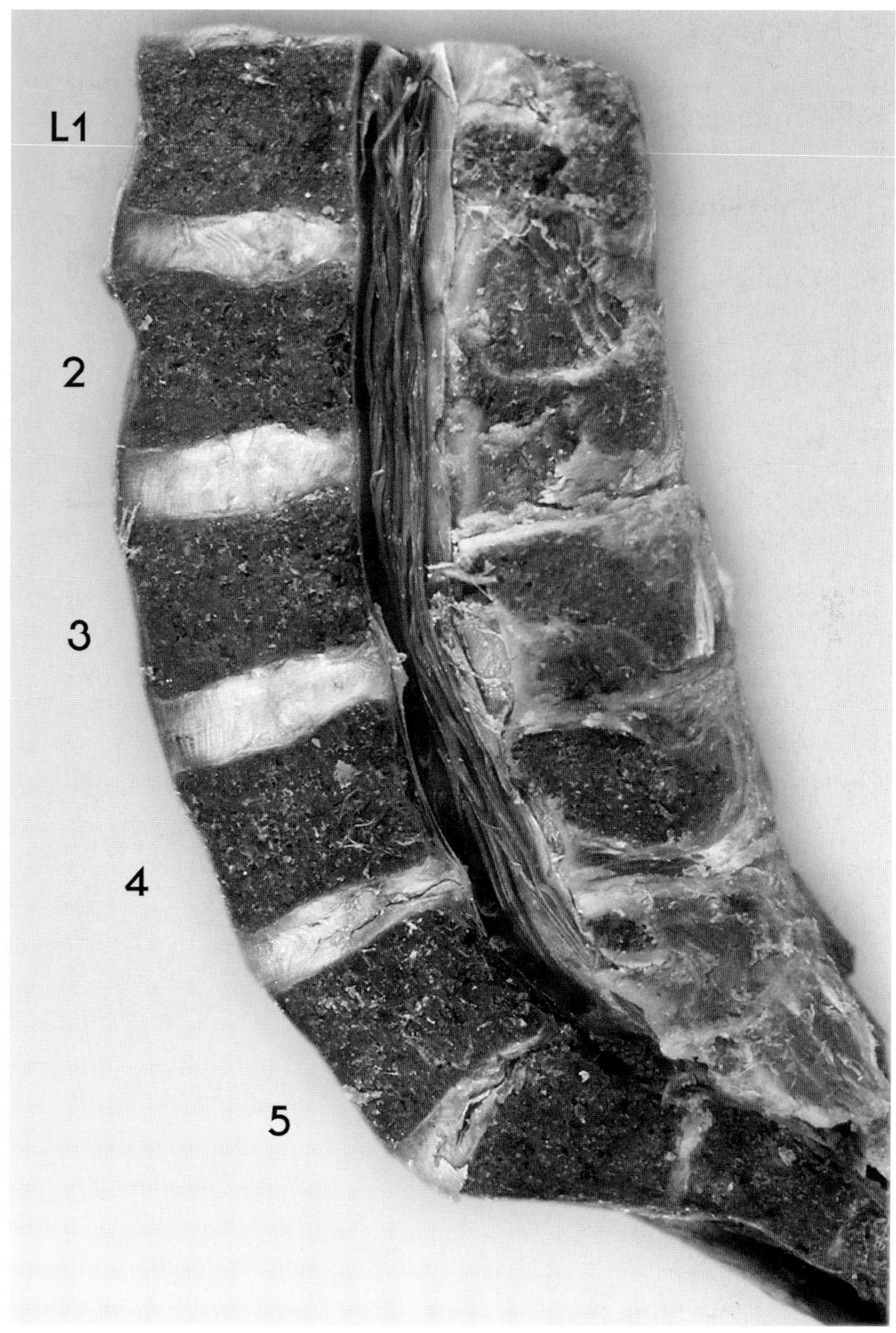

NOTE: The nucleus has expanded into the body of both L2 and L3 with near normal disc. L4 looks aligned with L3 with some endplate damage, repair, posterior disc bulging, and slight tearing. L5 is antro to L4 with disc tearing, posterior bulging, and loss of disc height. The sacrum is antro to L5 with significant disc tearing, wedging, and loss of disc height.

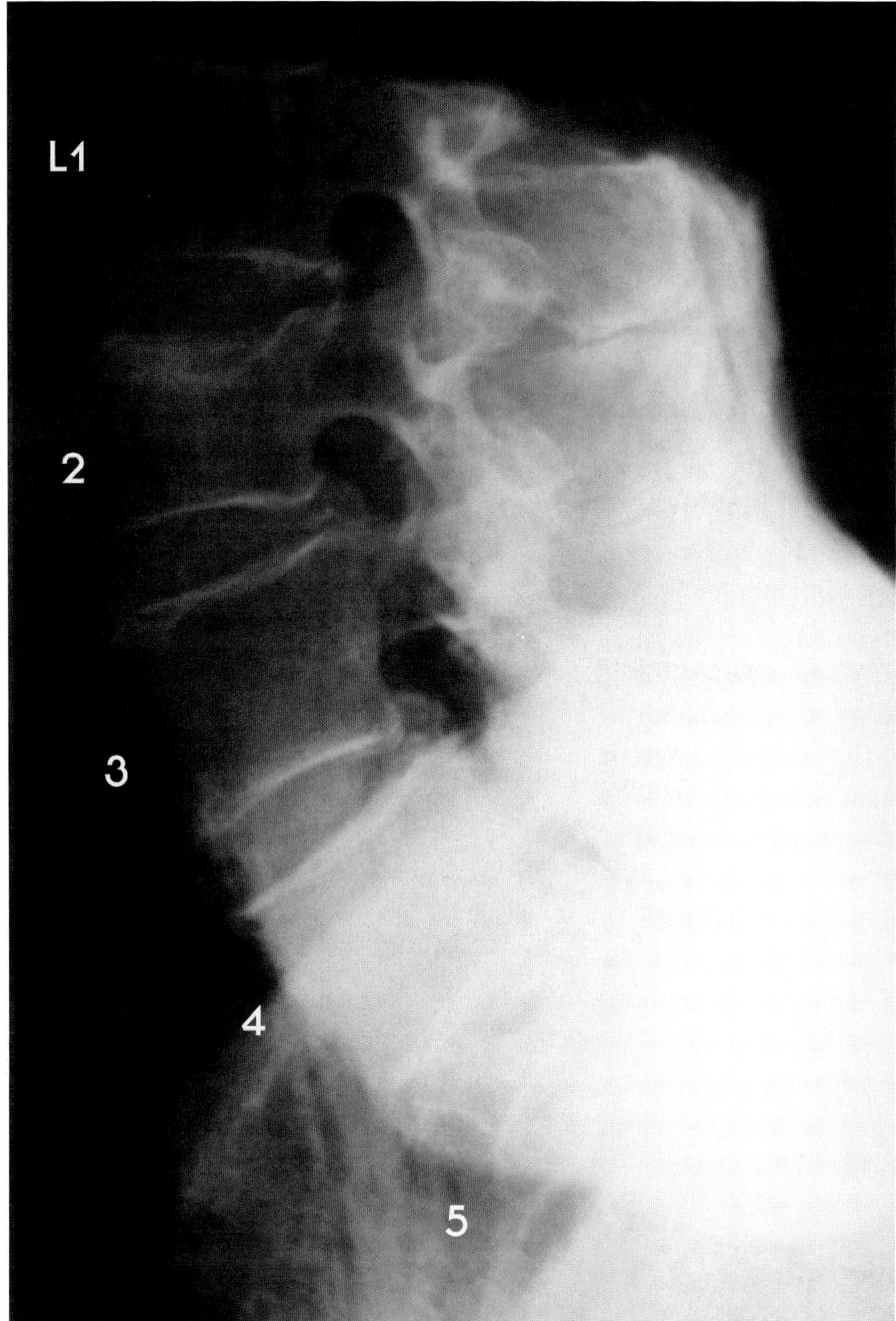

Plates 5-7 A & B

LUMBAR SPINE - This specimen has subluxated segments with the curve maintained
This shows there are signs of trauma with repair in the vertebral bodies. There is minor to moderate A to P subluxations but the normal lordotic curve is present. L1-2 look aligned with compression fracture of L2. There is disc wedging and expansion of nucleus pulposus into vertebral body of L2. L3 is retro to L2 with disc tearing, wedging, and slight posterior bulging.

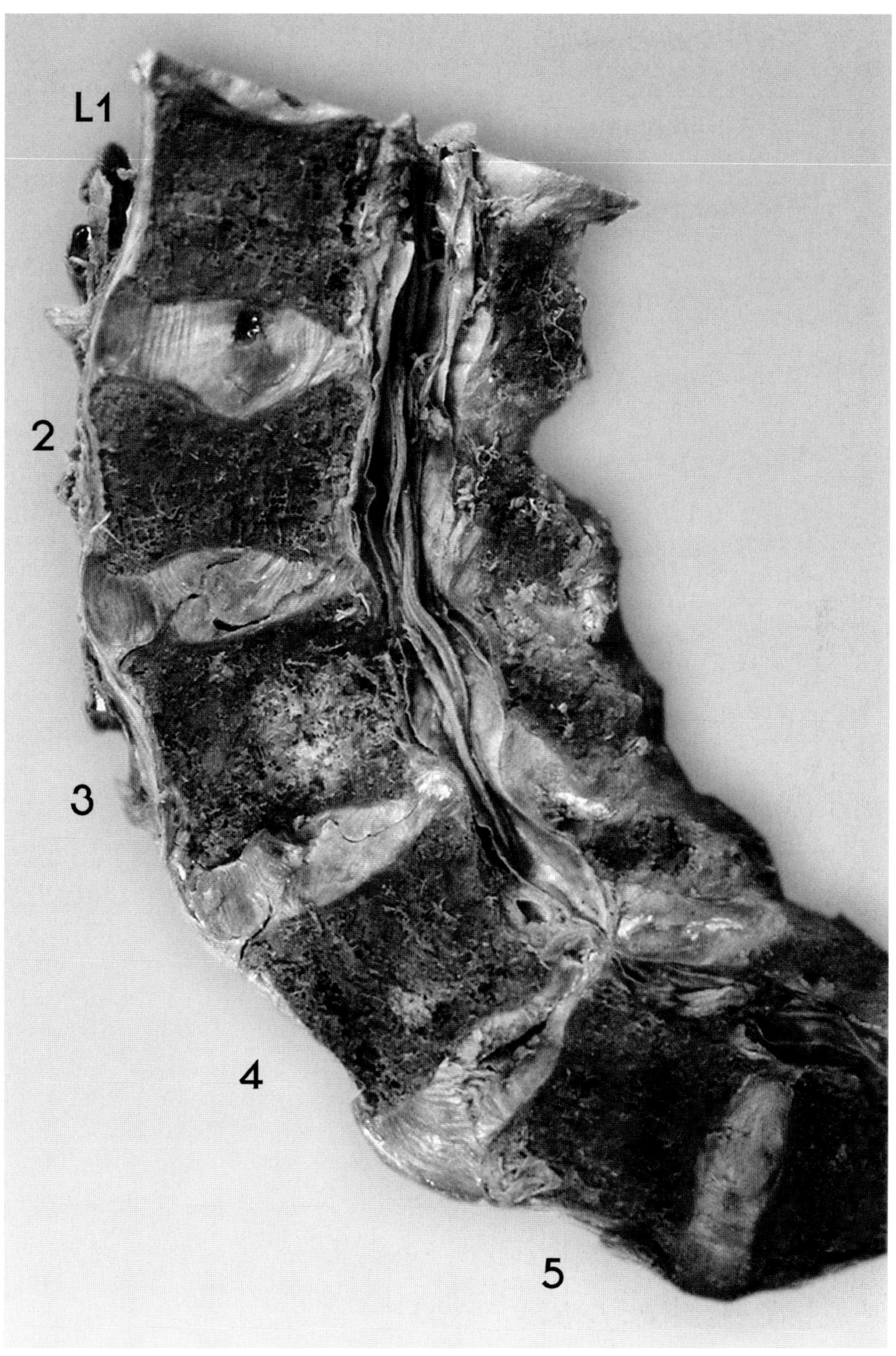

L4 is retro to L3 with disc tearing, wedging, and posterior bulging. L5 is retro to L4 with disc tearing, slight cavitation, wedging, and bulging. The L5-sacrum alignment looks normal. Note: The L2 vertebral body deformation with compressive force indicates it took the absorption of the shock, not the disc.

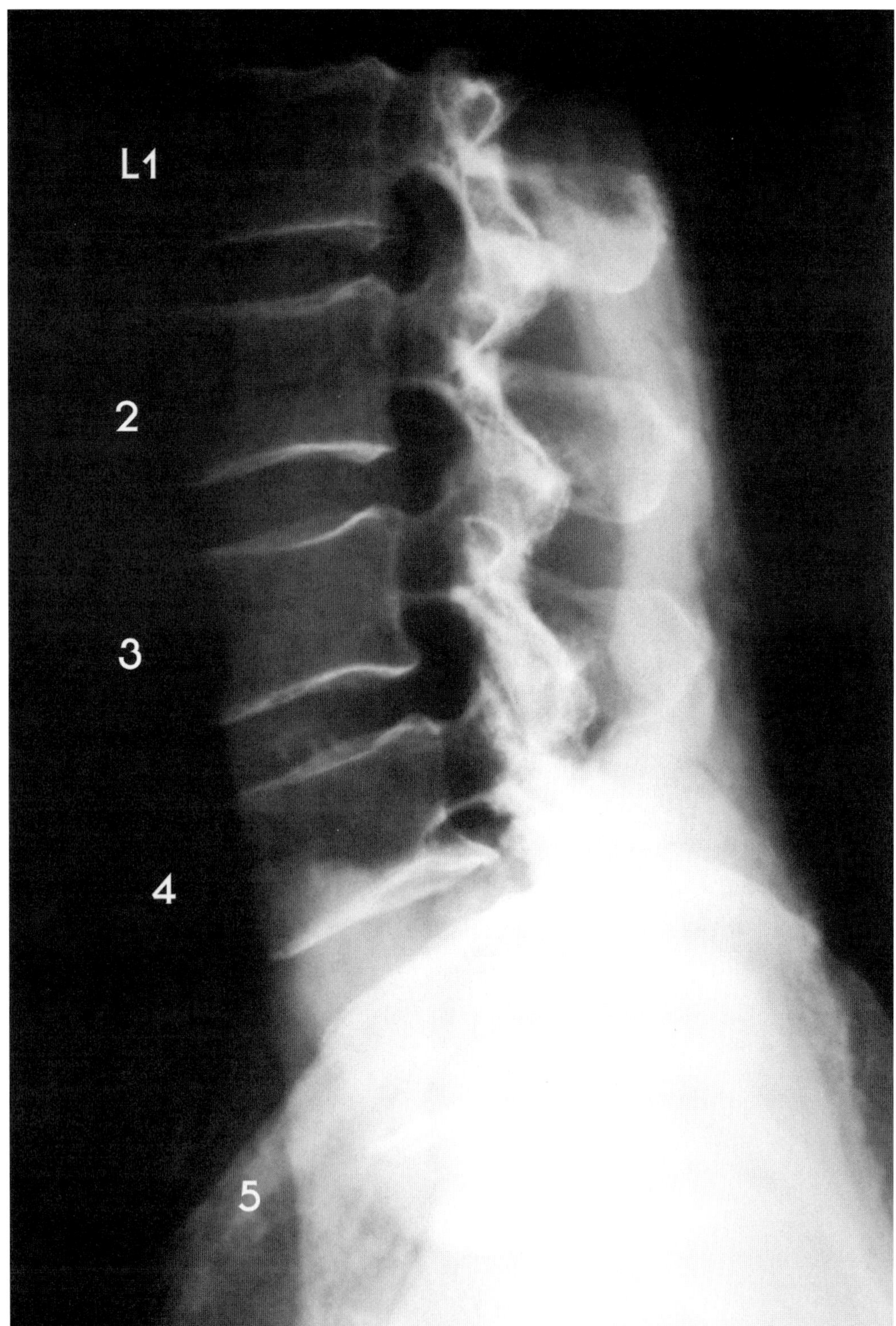

Plates 5-8 A & B
LUMBAR SPINE - variations in "normal" lumbar curve -I
In this specimen L1-L4 has good alignment with slight anterior brown degeneration. L5 is slightly retro to L4 and the sacrum, making L5 a complete retrolisthesis.

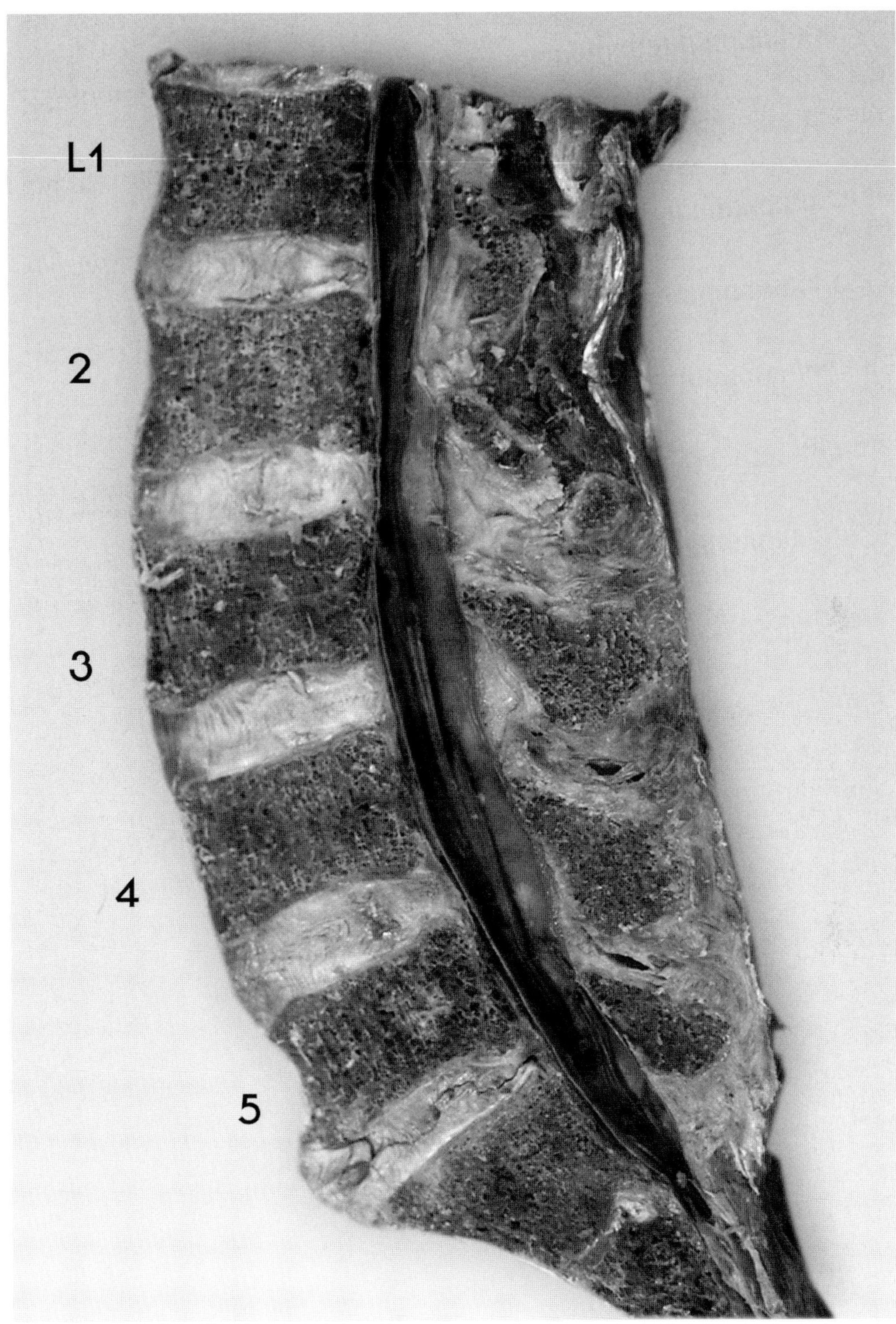

The L5-S1 disc is wedged, bulging anteriorly, and with disc tearing.
Note the presence of a lordotic curve.

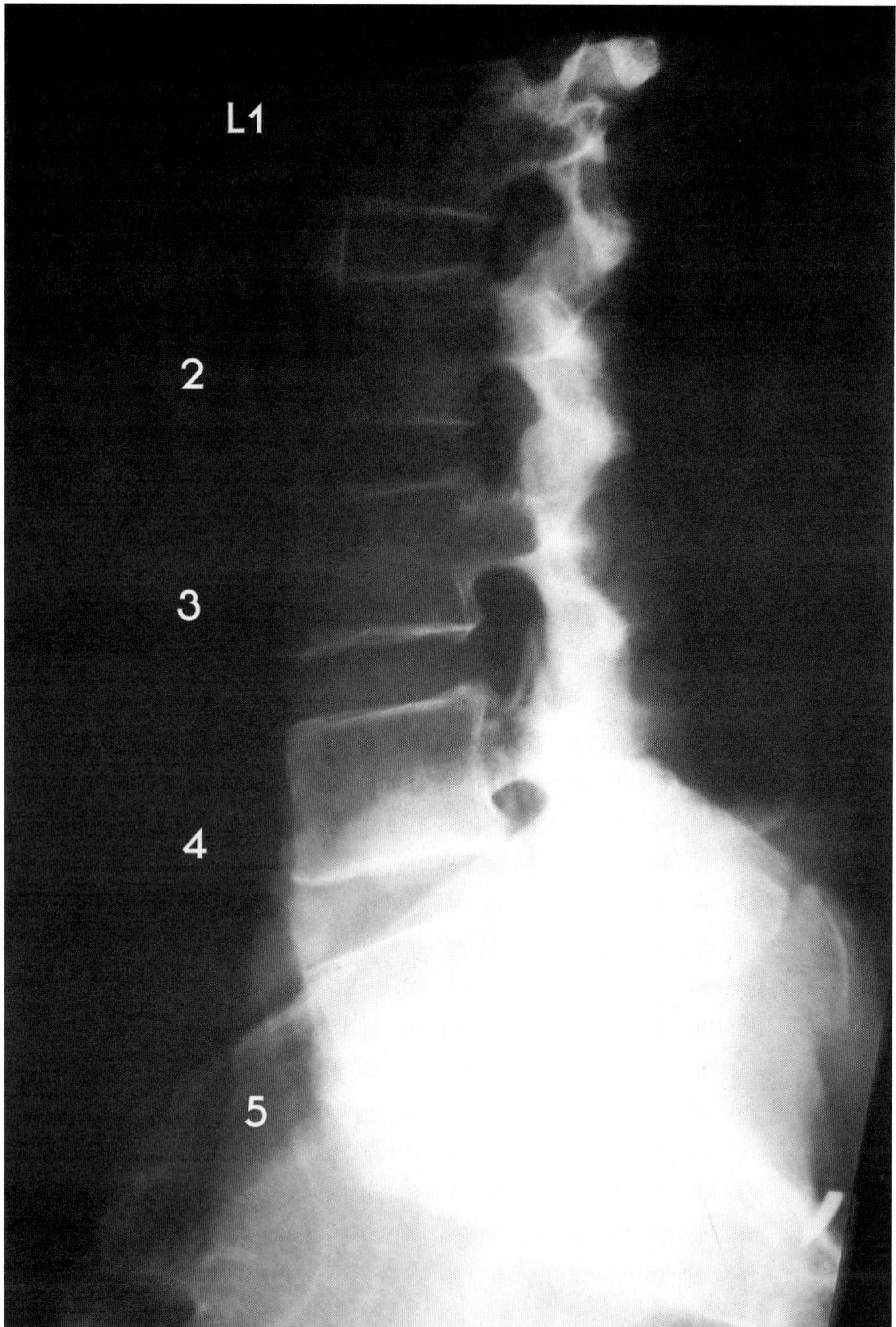

Plates 5-9 A & B

LUMBAR SPINE - Normal discs above a major subluxation with damaged discs

This specimen has maintained a moderate lordotic curve and the subluxations of L5 and the sacrum did not generate major osteophytic changes. L1 through L4 have normal alignment. L5 is slightly antro to L4 with nucleus desiccation, tearing and cavitation.

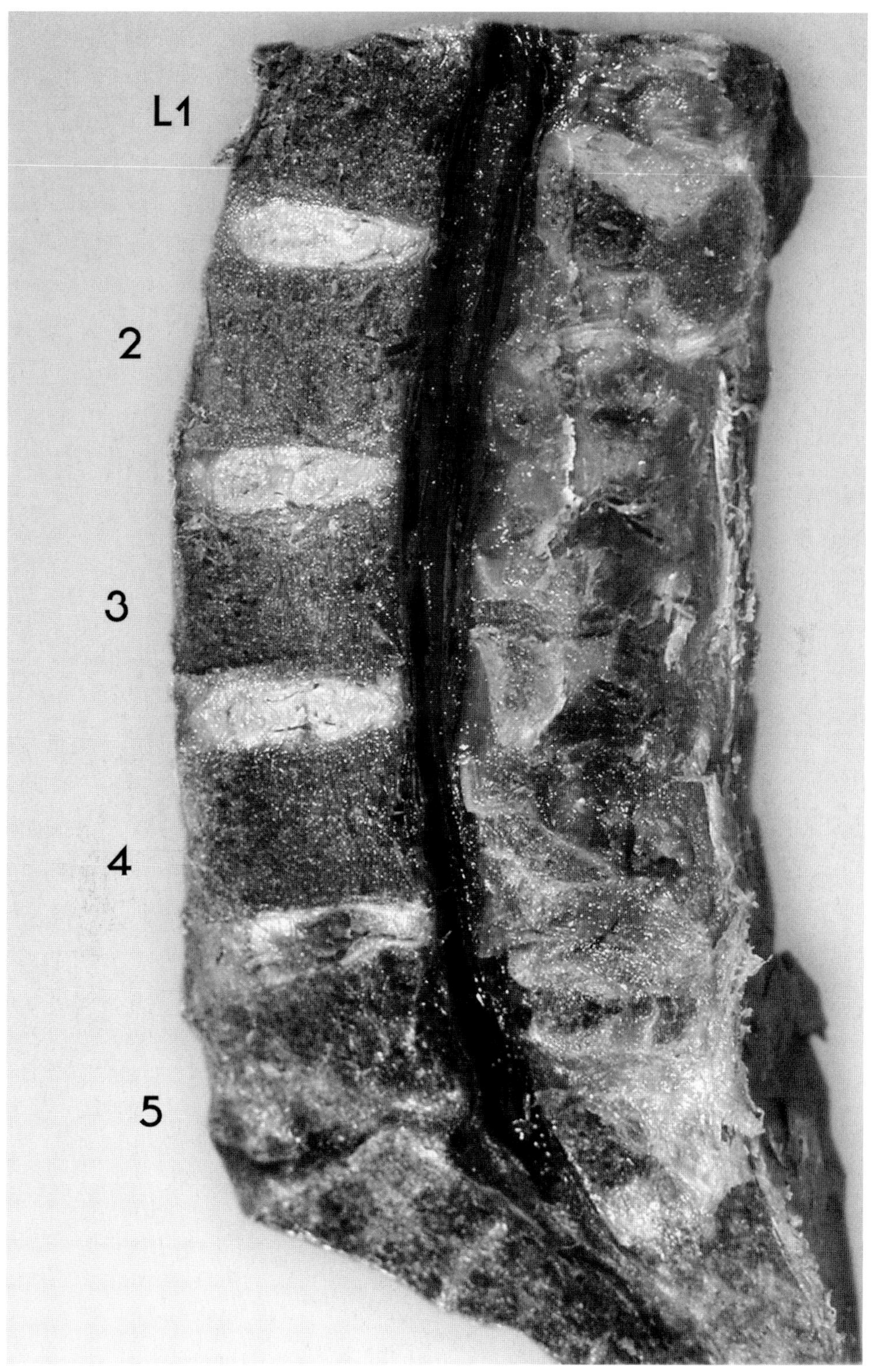

The sacrum is significantly antro to L5 with major degenerative changes, desiccation of the disc, and near fusion.

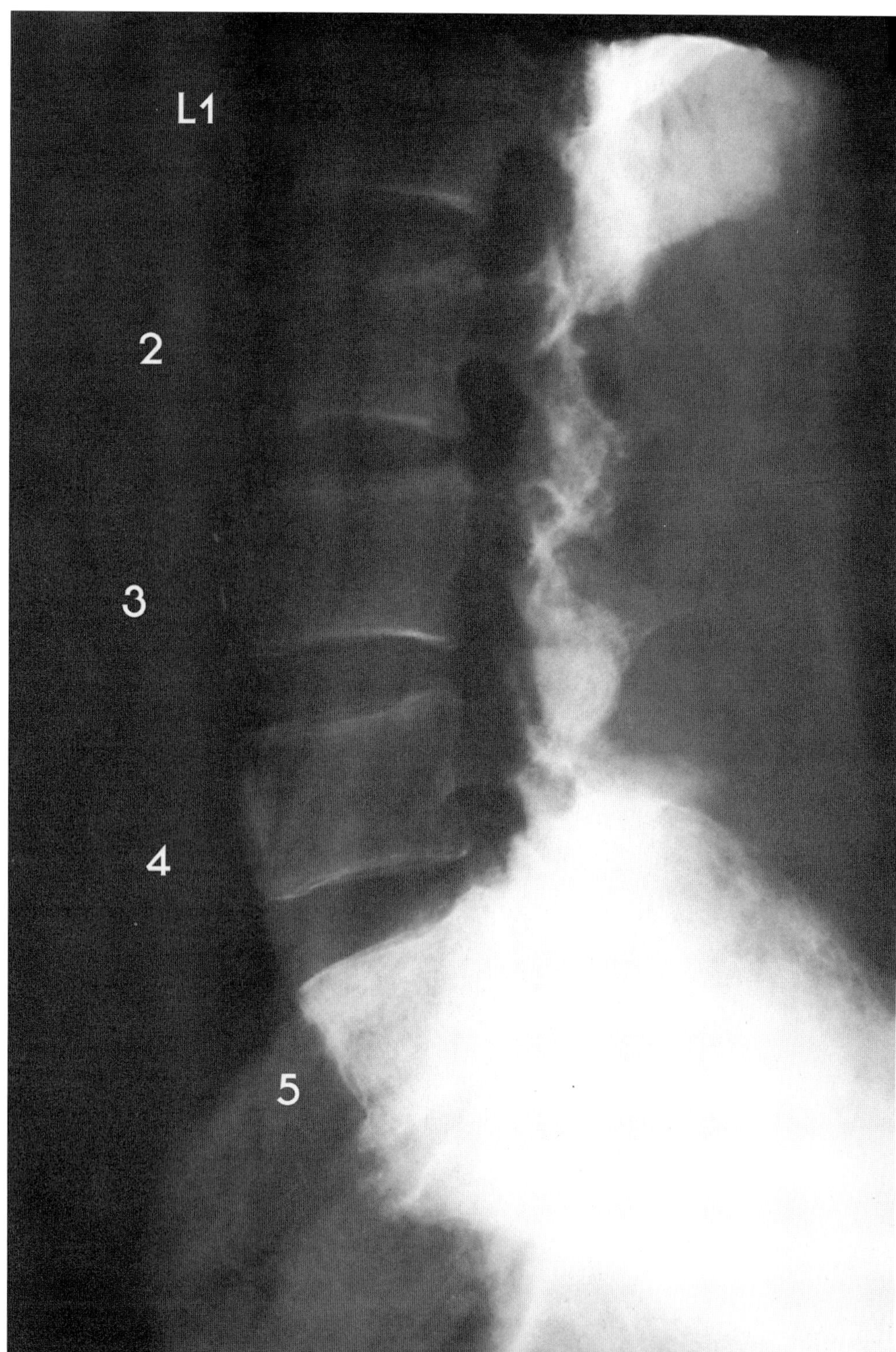

Plates 5-10 A & B
LUMBAR SPINE - This demonstrates L5-sacrum wedging
with anterior displacement of the sacrum

This specimen has significant disc degeneration in the presence of normal and near normal discs. L1-2 are near normal with the beginnings of brown degeneration. L3 is retro to L2 and

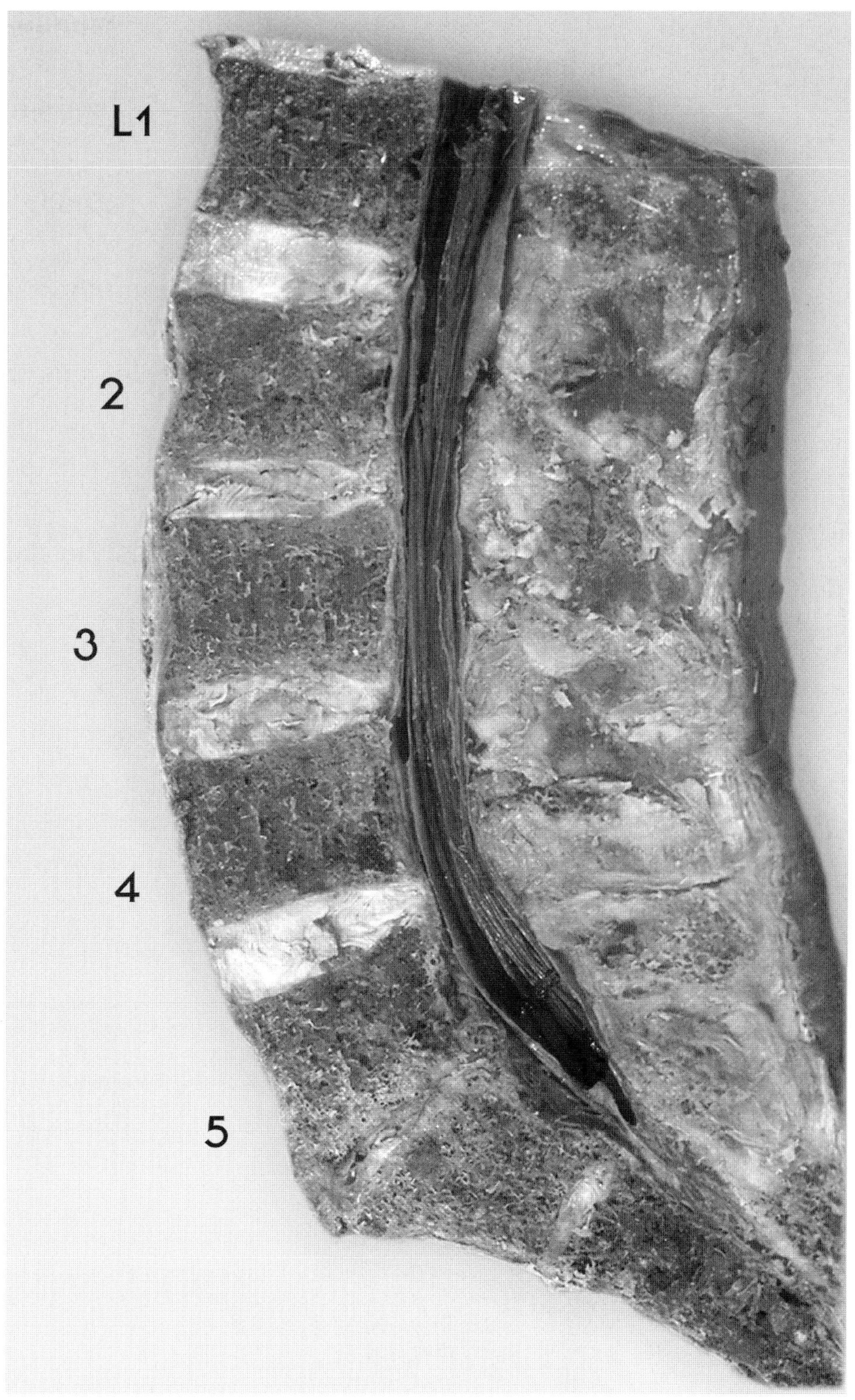

L4 with L2-3 disc tearing and loss of height. L4-5 looks good with slight wedging and tearing, the sacrum is antro to L5 with fusion of posterior aspect of both segments. The disc has anterior bulging, tearing, and cavitation. The A to P subluxation of the sacrum stopped normal motion and doomed the disc. Contracture of the thoracolumbar fascia fixes the subluxation.

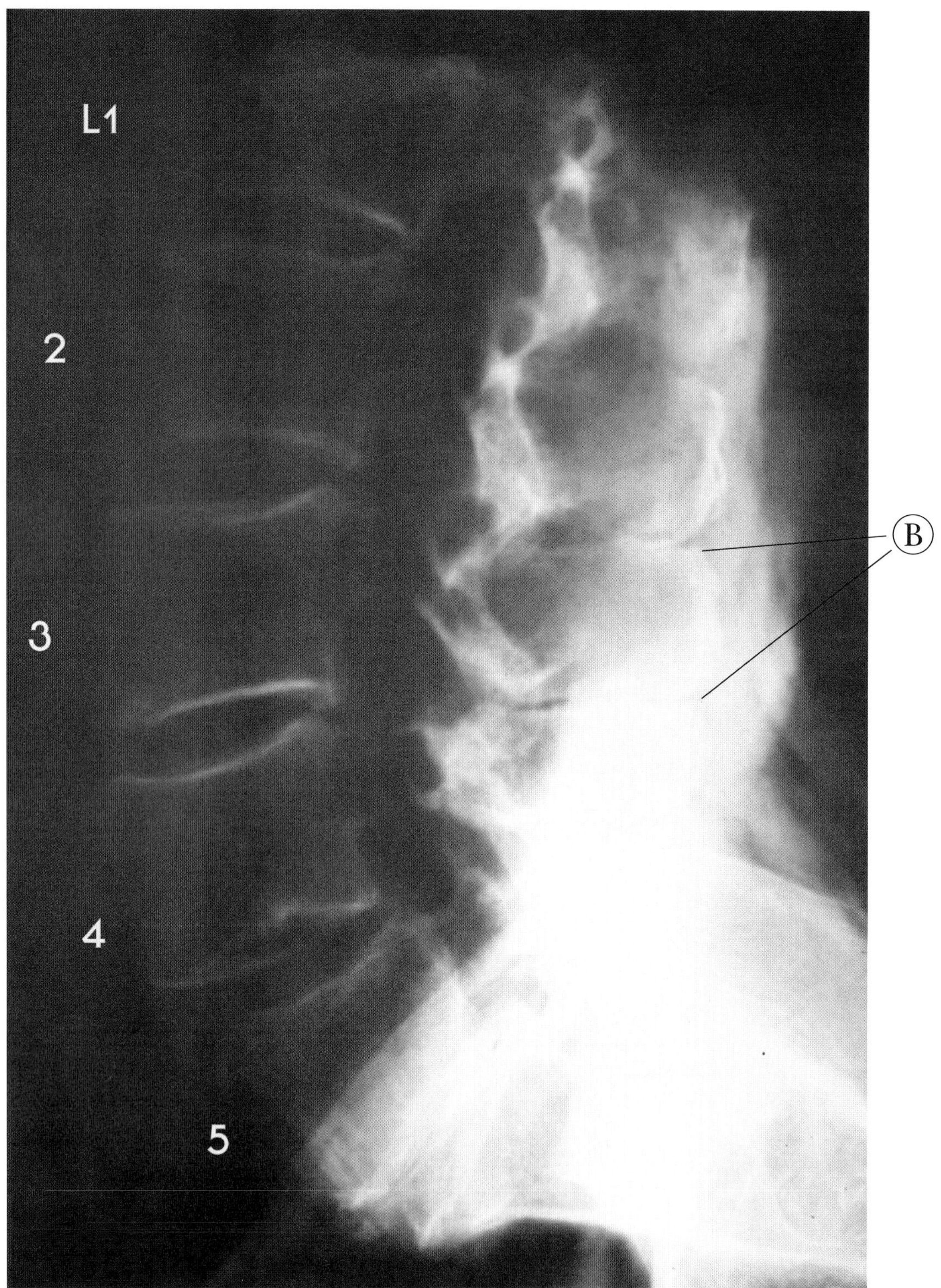

Plates 5-11 A & B
LUMBAR SPINE - This shows complete anterolisthesis of L4 and
partially of L5 and S1 with end stage fusion

This is a specimen that has every segment subluxated with the lordotic curve maintained.
An L1 compression fracture with repair has occurred. L2 is antro to L1 with disc wedging,
tearing, and posterior bulging; L3 is antro to L2 with slight wedging, tearing, and bulging. L4 is

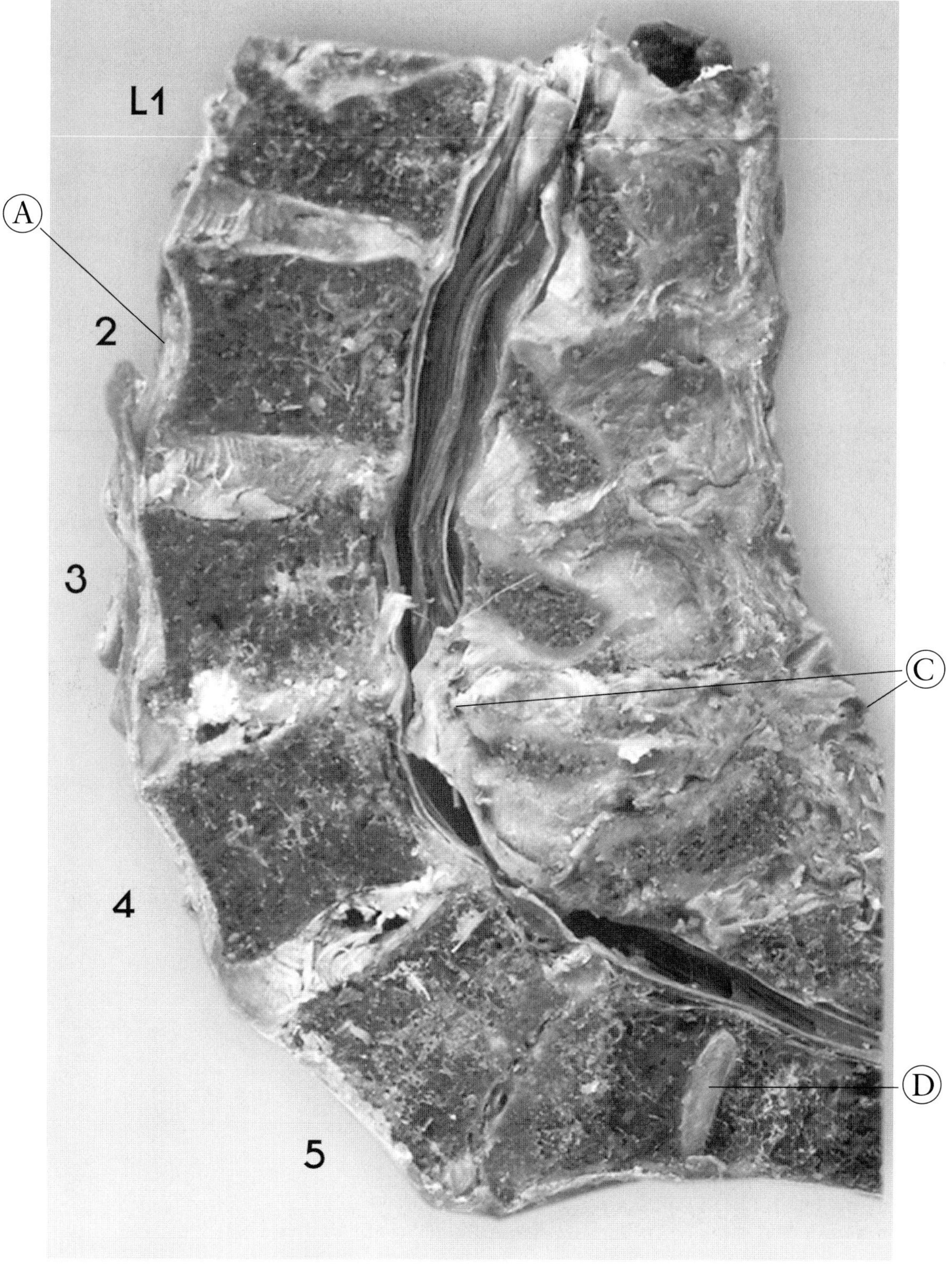

antro to L3 with disc tearing, cavitation, slight bulging, and significant posterior disc height loss. L5 is retro to L4 with disc tearing, cavitation, anterior and posterior bulging. The sacrum is significantly retro to L5 with fusion.

  (A) A.L.L. hypertrophy
  (B) L1-5 spinous process proximity
  (C) Loss of midsagittal plane at L3
  (D) Sacral disc

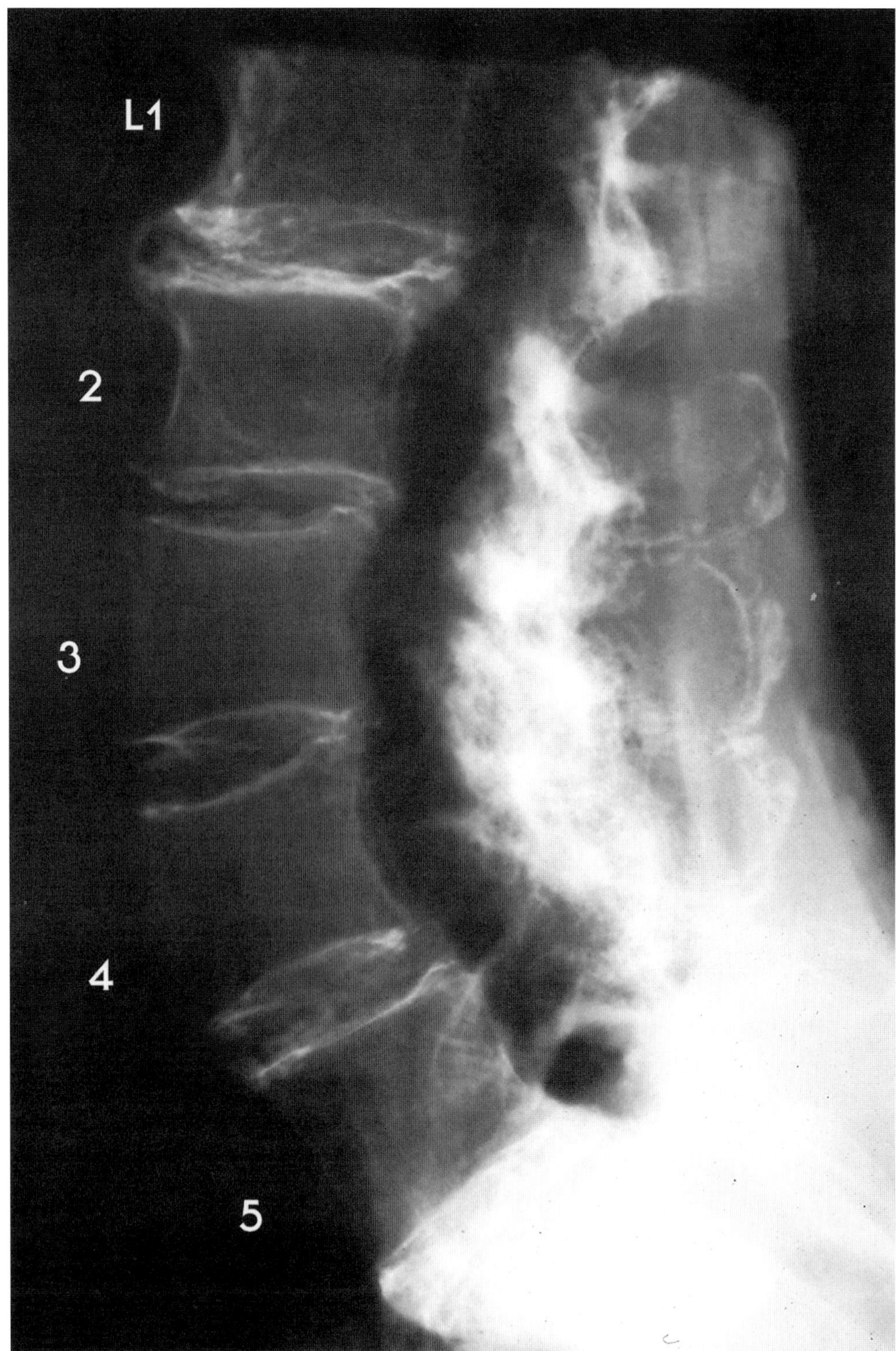

Plates 5-12 A & B
LUMBAR SPINE - This illustrates normal discs below damaged discs
with lordosis maintained
In this specimen there are degrees of subluxation with corresponding degenerative changes.
L1 is retro to L2 with significant endplate disturbance, loss of height, and anterior and

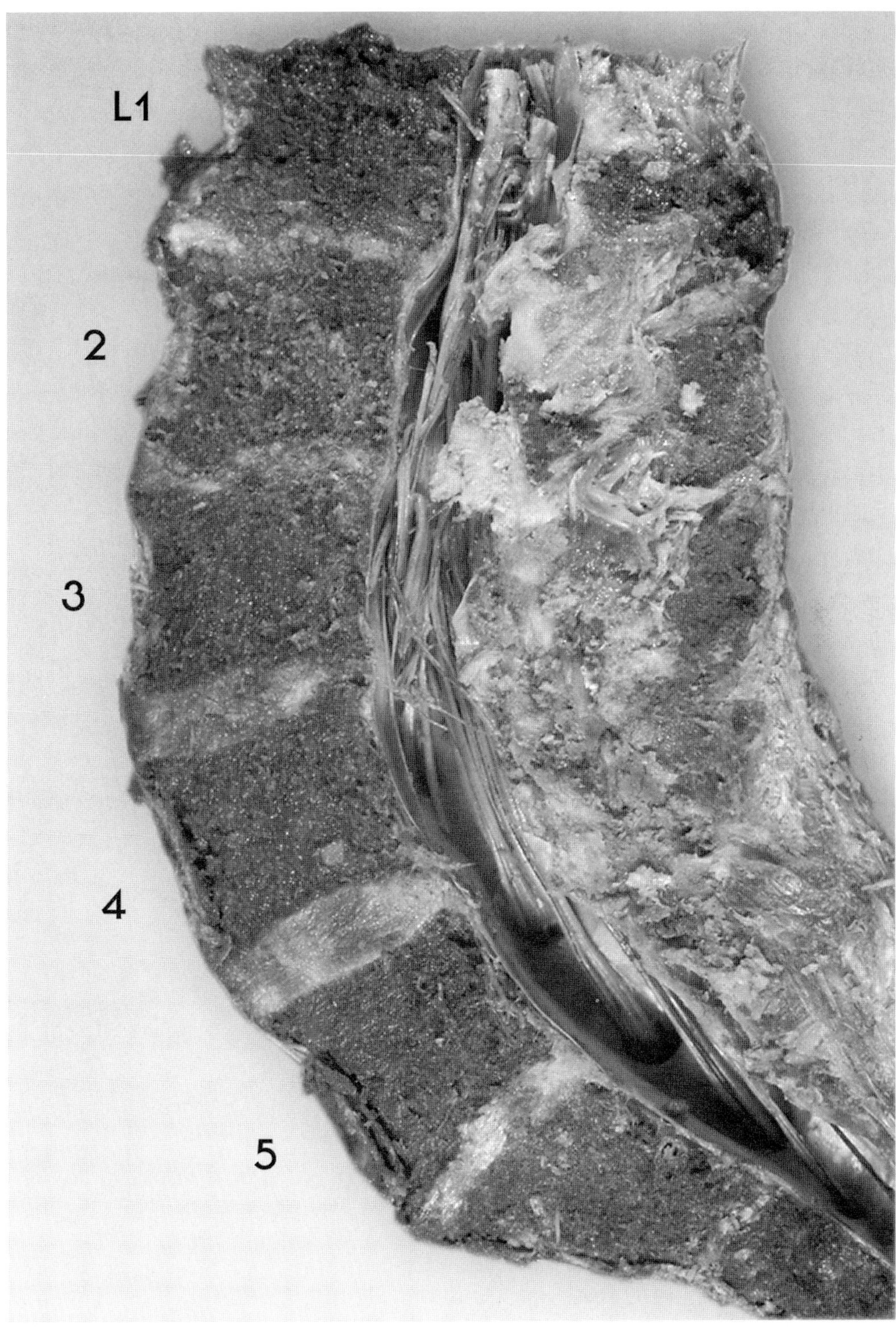

posterior disc bulging. L2 is retro to L3 with spurring and loss of disc height. L4 is anterior to L3 and L5 with disc wedging, bulging, and brown degeneration. The sacrum is slightly retro to L5 with loss of the disc height and calcification.
Note the lordotic curve is maintained and there is significant sclerosis of the facets and some of the spinous processes.

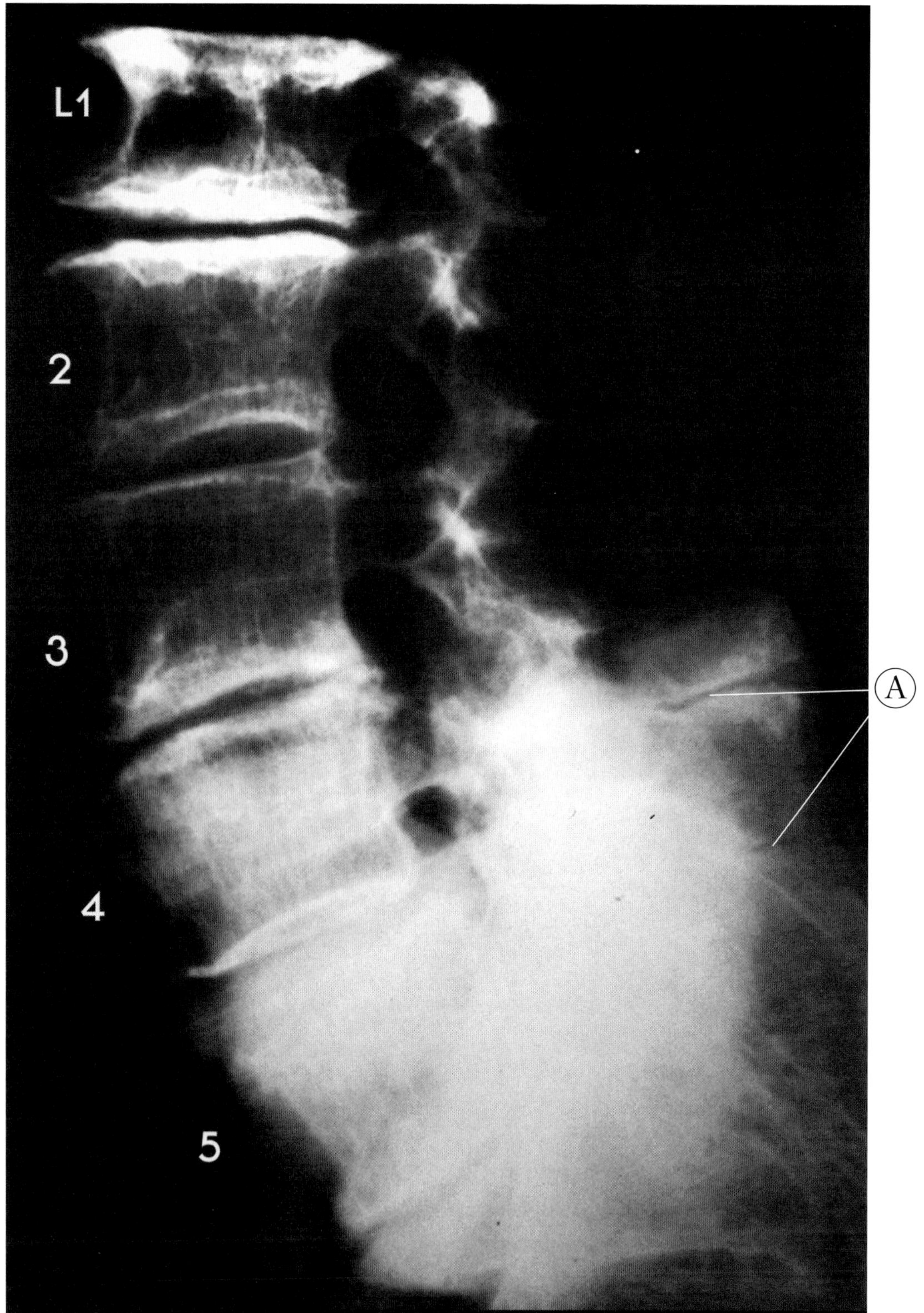

Plates 5-13 A & B
LUMBAR SPINE - The end-stages of degeneration, post trauma
L1 has significant endplate repairs with anterior and posterior spurring. L2 is antro to L1 with
significant loss of disc height, bulging anterior and posterior, tearing, and endplate repairs.
L3 antro to L2 with disc tearing, bulging, loss of height, and impression into the inferior
endplate of L2. L4 is antro to L3 and L5 with endplate repairs, anterior and posterior

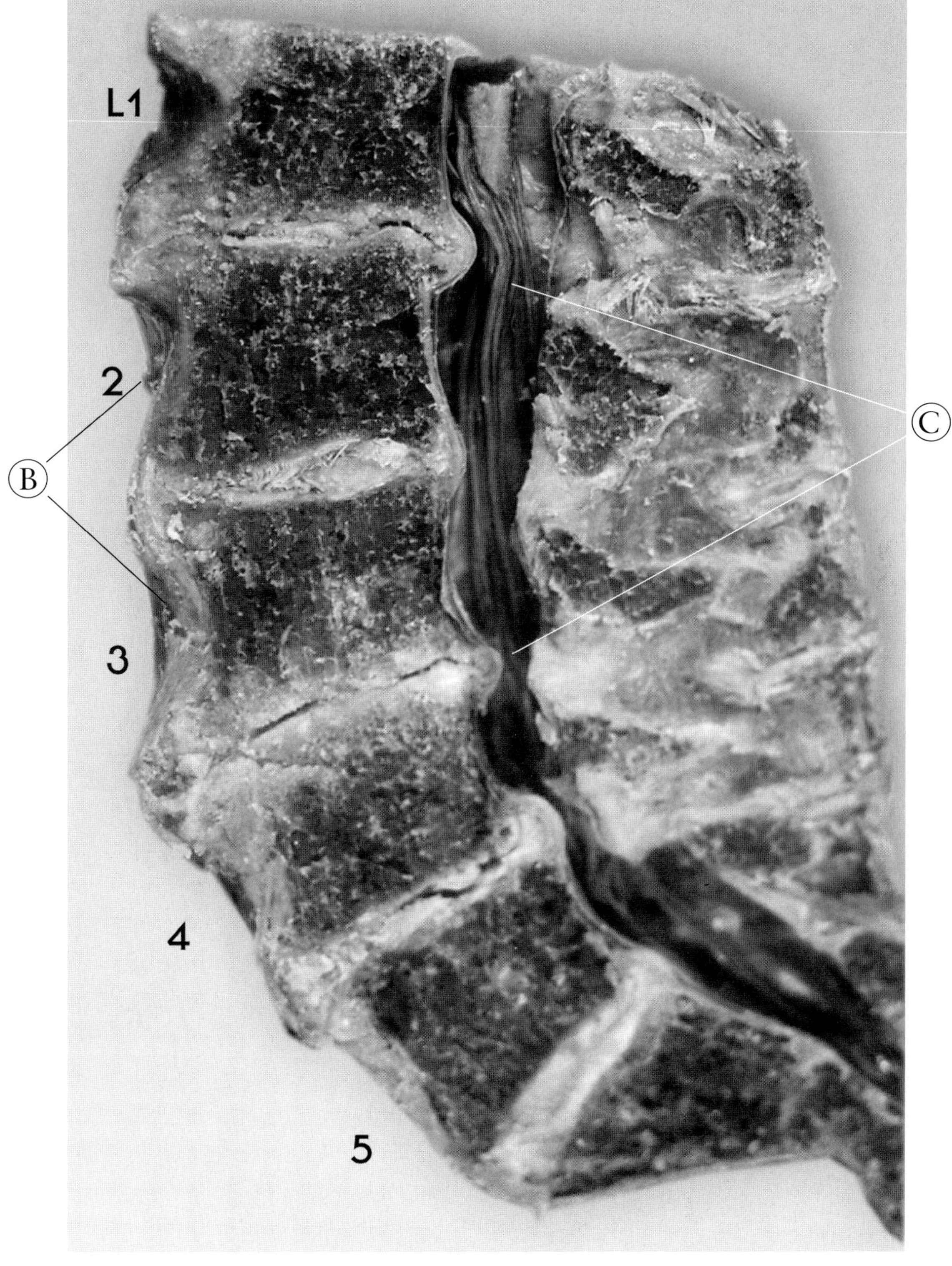

spurring, disc tearing, and anterior and posterior bulging. L4-5 has slight anterior and posterior spurring, disc tearing, anterior and posterior bulging, and loss of disc height. The sacrum is slightly antro to L5 with disc tearing, anterior and posterior bulging, loss of height, and anterior spurring.

  (A) Spinous process contact forming pseudo-joints
  (B) Hypertrophy of anterior longitudinal ligament
  (C) Narrowing of spinal canal due to spurring and disc bulging

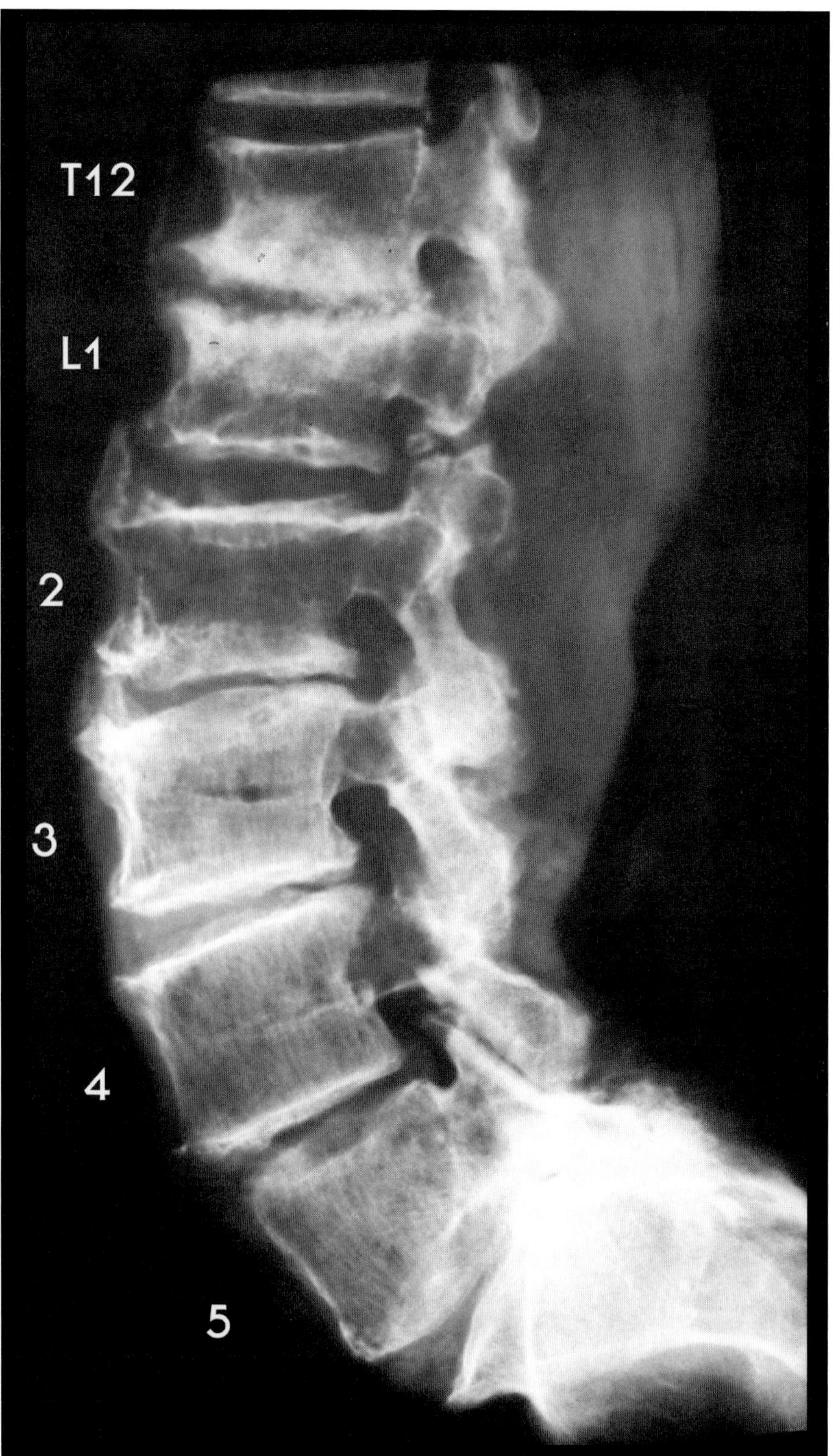

Plates 5-14 A & B

LUMBAR SPINE - This has subluxated segments with the curve maintained, sequential retrolisthesis to the segment below, or stairstepping This specimen has a subluxation at every level. The degenerative changes are limited because the lordotic curve is maintained. L1 is antro to T12 with spurring anterior and posterior, disc bulging, and loss of height. L2 is antro to L1 with disc tearing, calcification of disc, and the anterior longitudinal ligament.

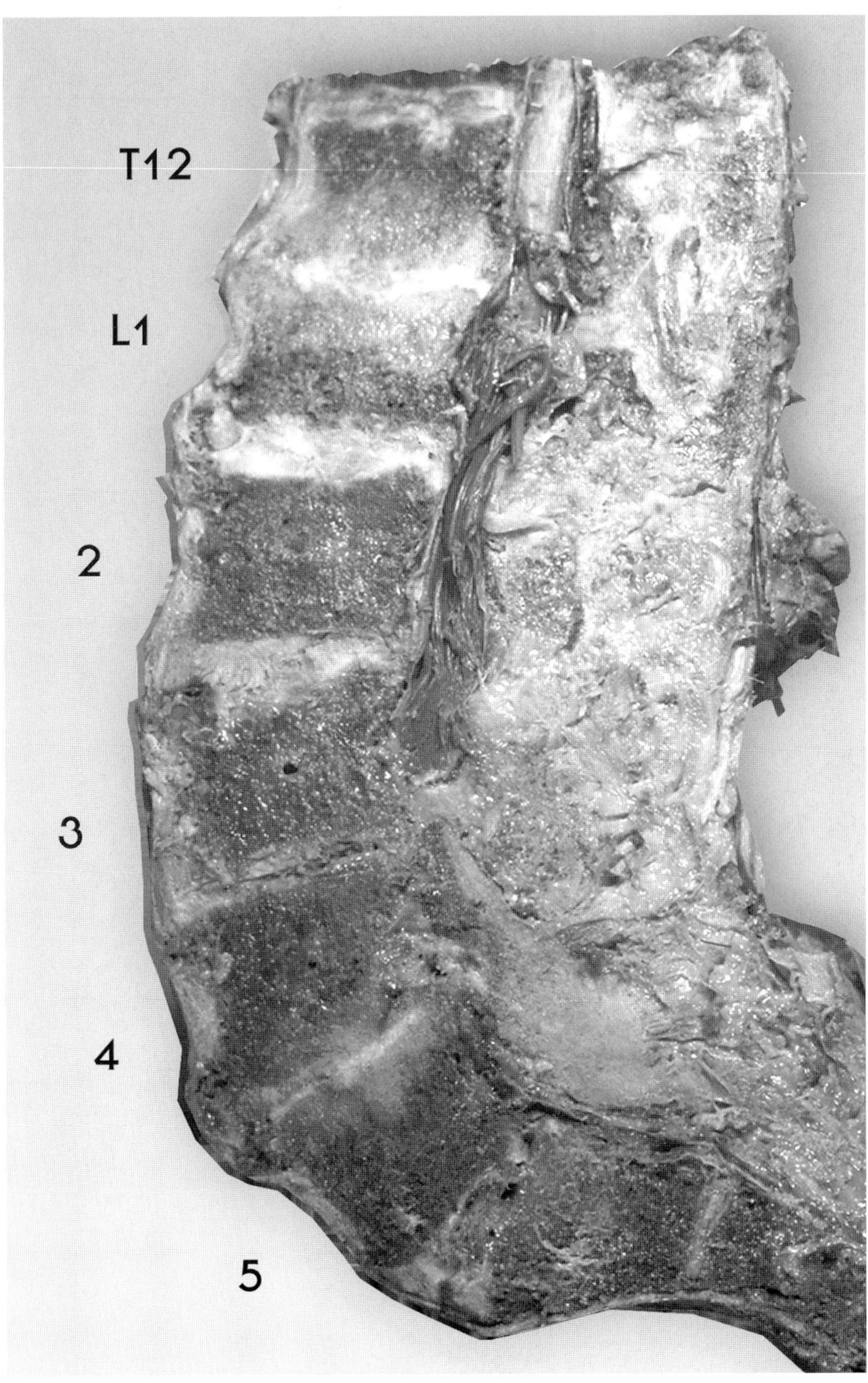

Note fracture of L1 inferior facet. L3 is antro to L2 with disc tearing, loss of height, calcification of anterior disc, and anterior and posterior spurring; L4 is antro to L3 with disc tearing, cavitation, and anterior and posterior spurring; L5 is retro to L4 with anterior and posterior disc bulging and loss of disc height. The sacrum is retro to L5 with disc tearing, cavitation, wedging, and near fusion of the posterior aspect of L5 and S1. Note lack of spinous processes on X-ray due to perisagittal plane of the specimen.

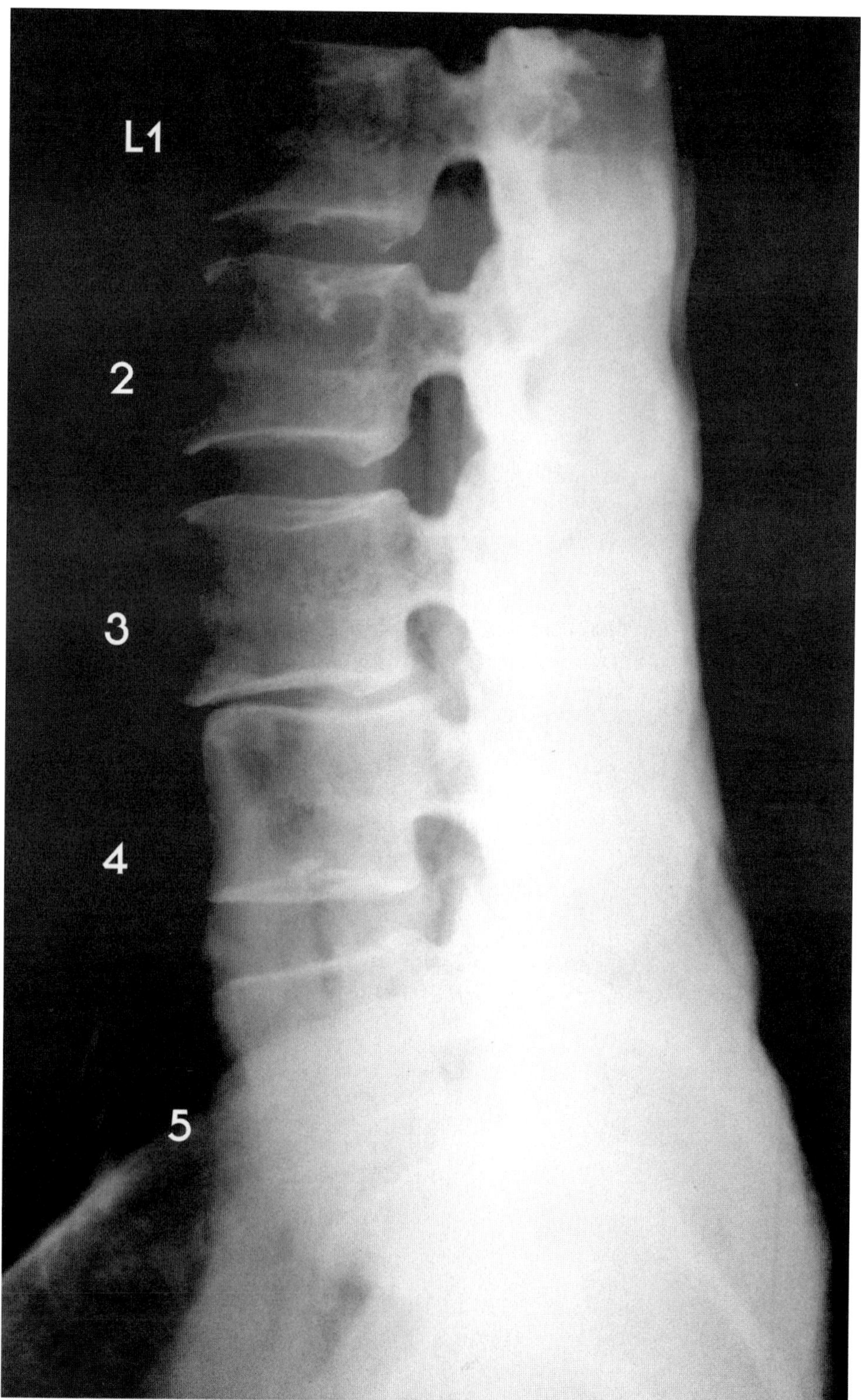

Plates 5-15 A & B
LUMBAR SPINE - This shows hypolordosis with one significant subluxation
This specimen has near normal alignment and joints with the presence of one significant subluxation. L2 is slightly anterior to L1 with slight disc tearing, anterior and posterior bulging, and endplate damage. L3-2 has good alignment with a normal disc. L4 is significantly retro to L3 with anterior disc bulge, loss of disc height, and near fusion.

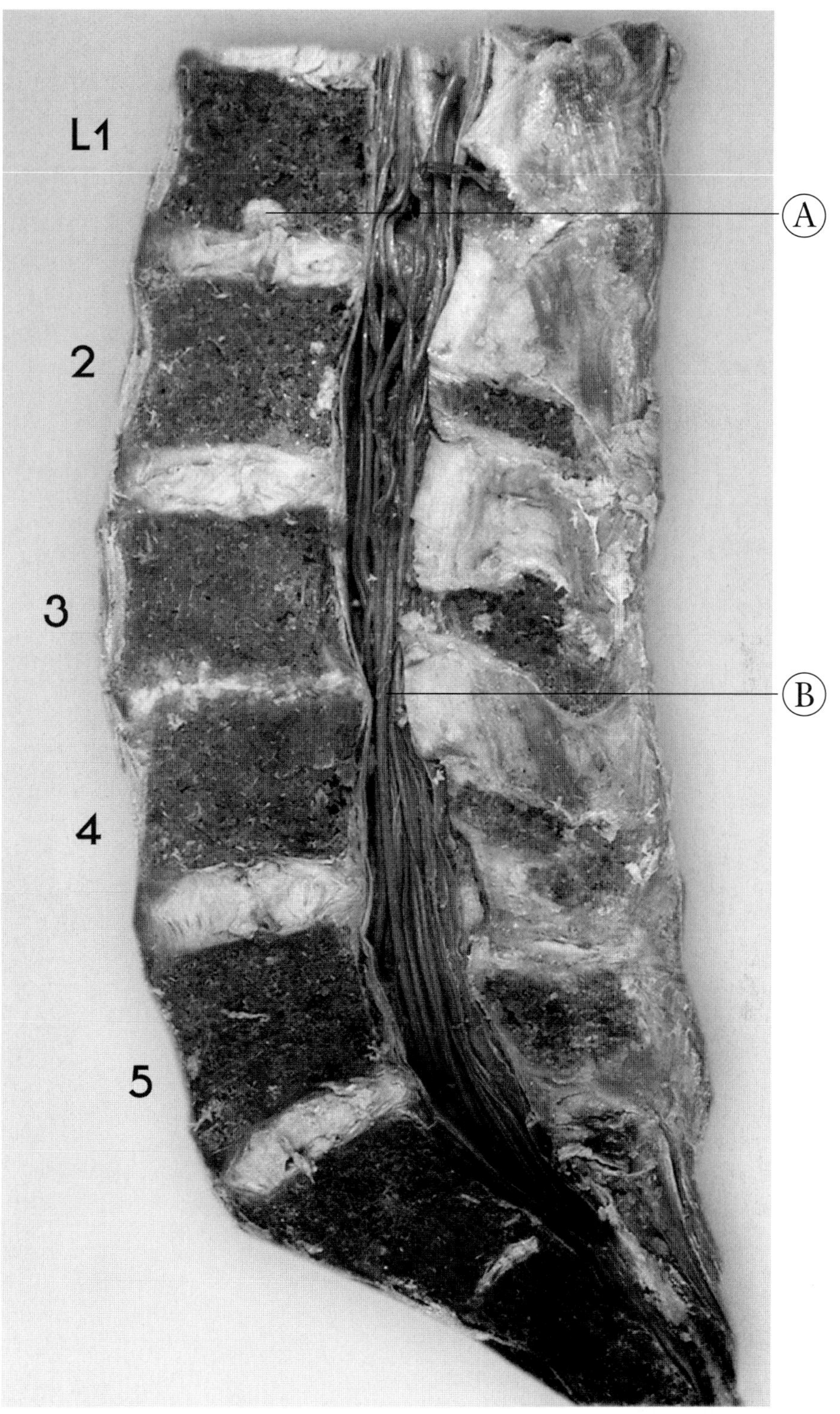

L5 is antro to L4 with a slight posterior disc bulge. L5 and sacrum
alignment is near normal with slight anterior and posterior disc bulging.
(A) Schmoral's Node (invagination of nucleus pulposus into vertebral
       body) of inferior L1 endplate
(B) Canal stenosis at L3-4

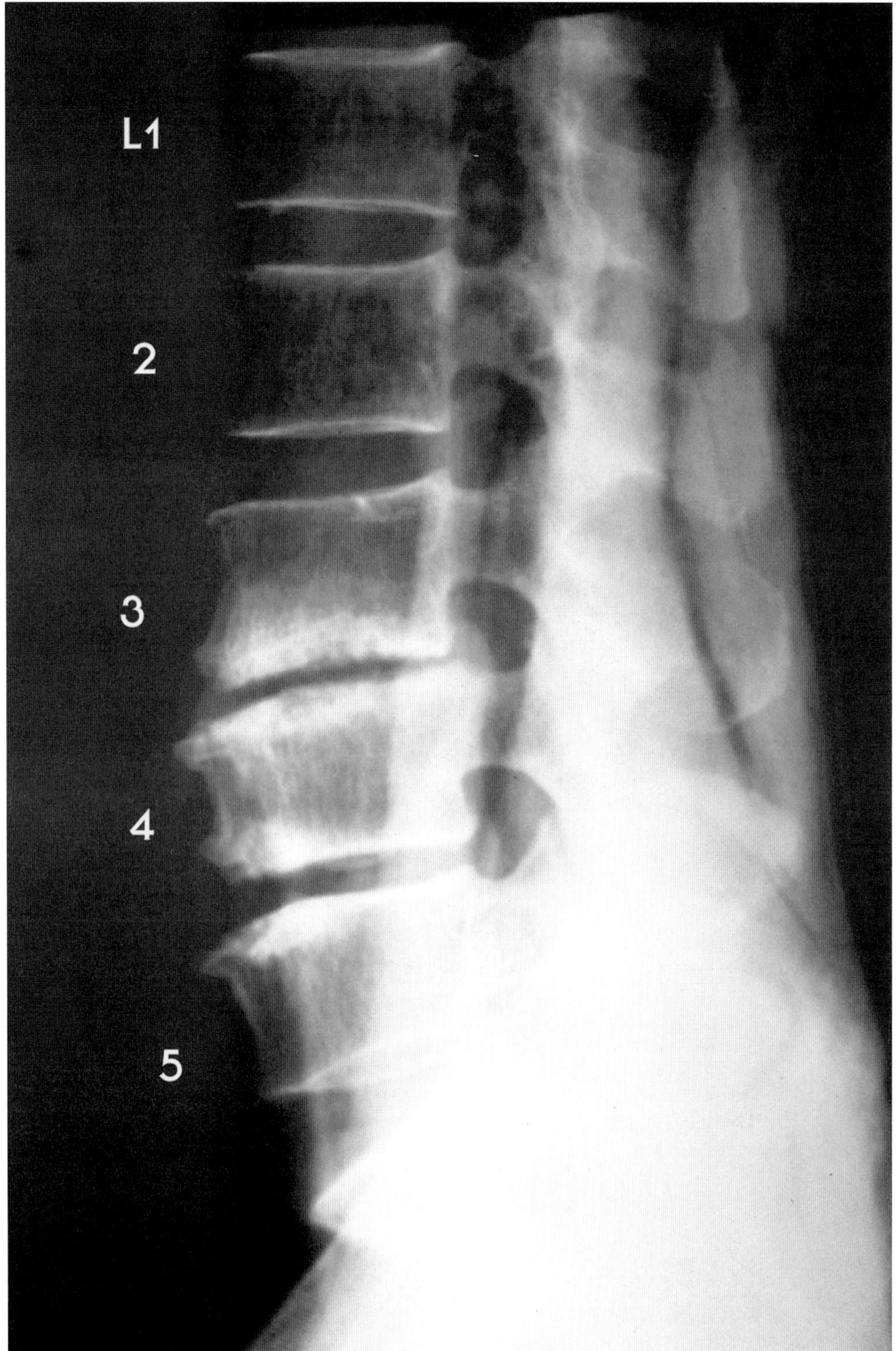

Plates 5-16 A & B
**LUMBAR SPINE - This illustrates subluxations with a loss of lordotic curve
and various stages of disc degeneration**
Subluxation results in degeneration. The loss of lordotic curve has resulted in the increase
in the vertebral body width in these subluxated segments. L1-2 and L2-3 look nearly normal
with the beginning of brown degeneration. L4 is retro to L3 with signs of a compression
fracture, anterior and posterior spurring, disc tearing, and anterior and posterior bulging.

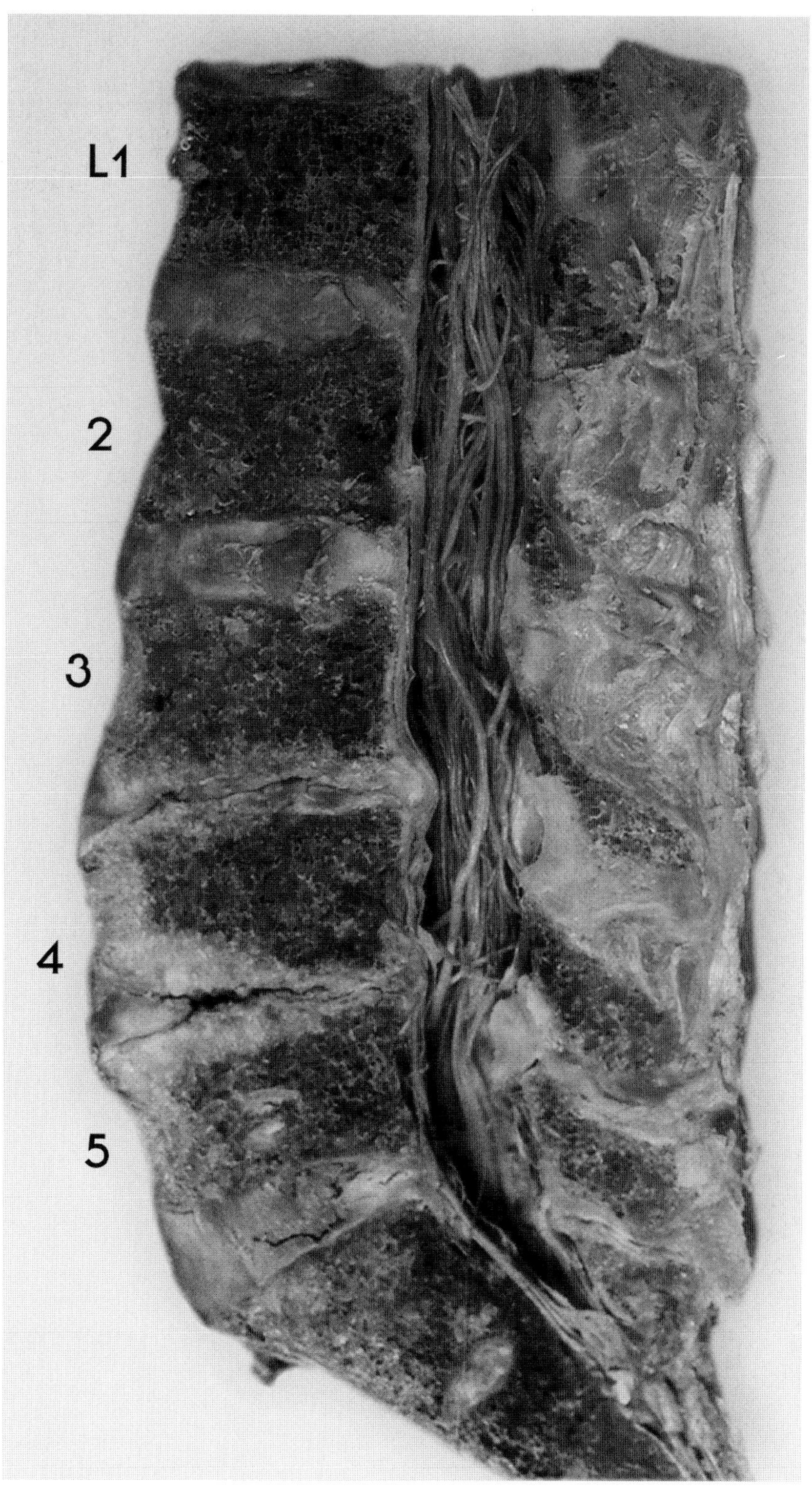

L4 is a complete retrolisthesis; L5 is antro to L4 but posterior to the sacrum, with anterior spurs. The L4-5 disc has tearing, cavitation, and separation of the posterior longitudinal ligament from L5 because of the posterior disc migration. The L5-S1 disc has wedging, tearing, and posterior bulging over the back of the sacral base. The endplates of L3, 4, and 5 indicate trauma with repair and L4 has loss of anterior body height.

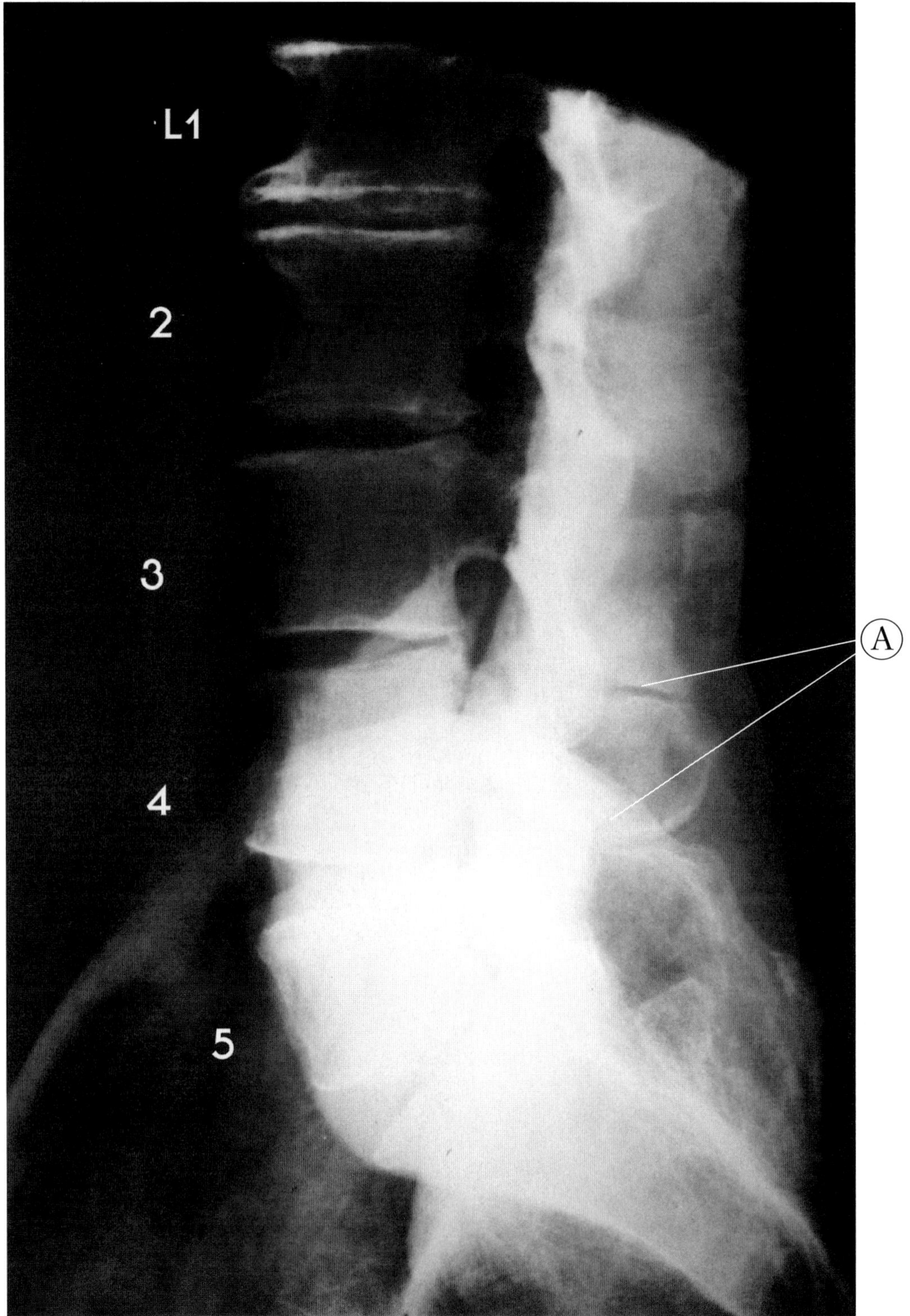

Plates 5-17 A & B
LUMBAR SPINE - The subluxation complex of this specimen
involves the entire lumbar spine

There is stairstepping of each segment posteriorly to the one below, eliminating the lordotic curve. This a common feature of the standing posture with the pelvis being translated anteriorly to the thorax. L1 is retro to L2 and has major endplate spurring and repair processes indicating a chronic long-term condition. L2 is retro to L3 with significant spurring, tearing, loss of height, and endplate changes. L3 is retro to L4 with disc tearing,

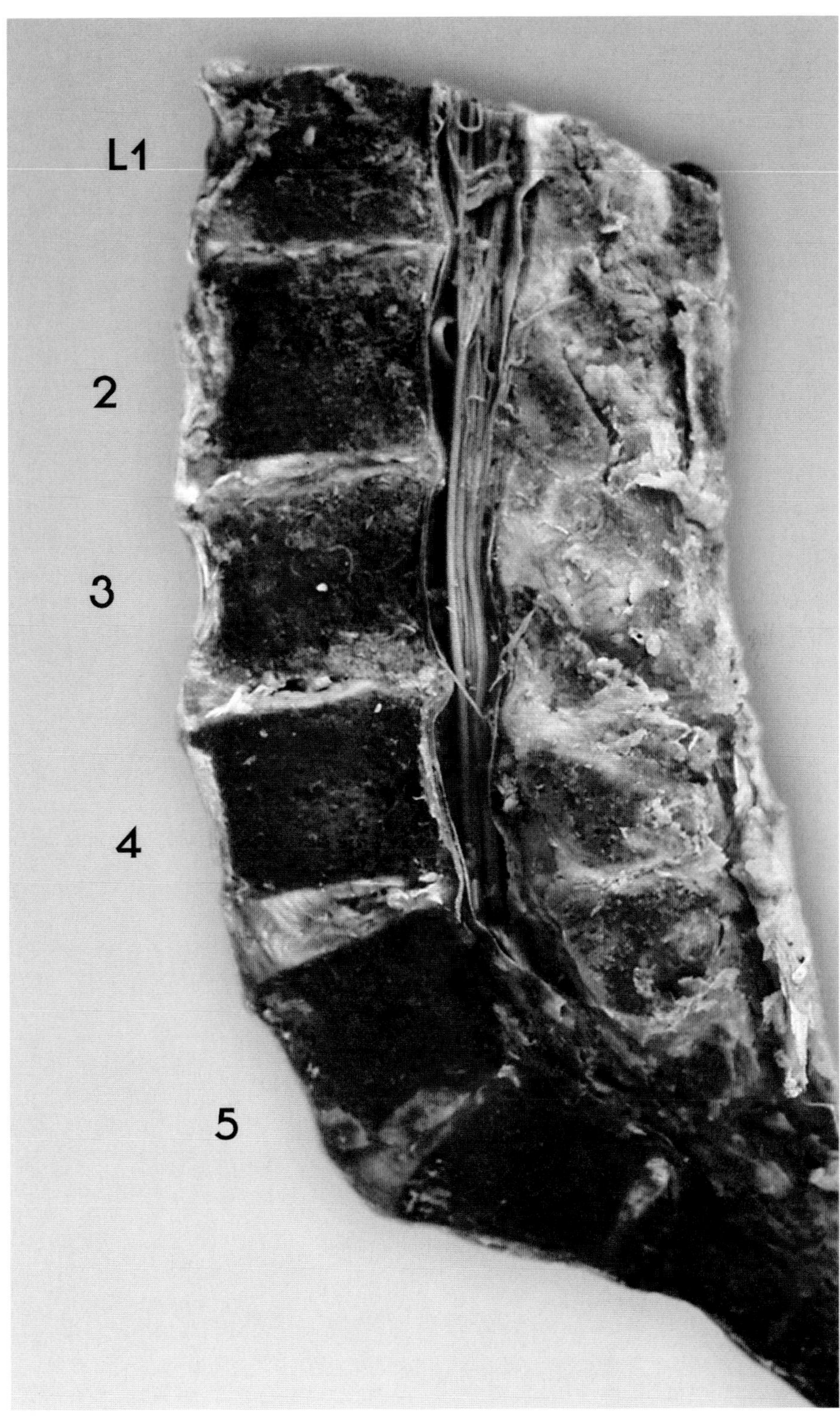

minor anterior bulging, and loss of height. There is anterior longitudinal ligament hypertrophy. L4 is retro to L5 or L5 is antro to L4 and the sacrum with disc tearing, wedging, slight cavitation, and bulging. L5-S1 has disc wedging, loss of disc height, and near fusion. The sacral disc S1-2 has wedging, slight posterior bulging, and angulation of S1-2 segments.

Note that every joint is subluxated in this example.

(A) Spinous process pseudo-joint formation due to loss of disc height

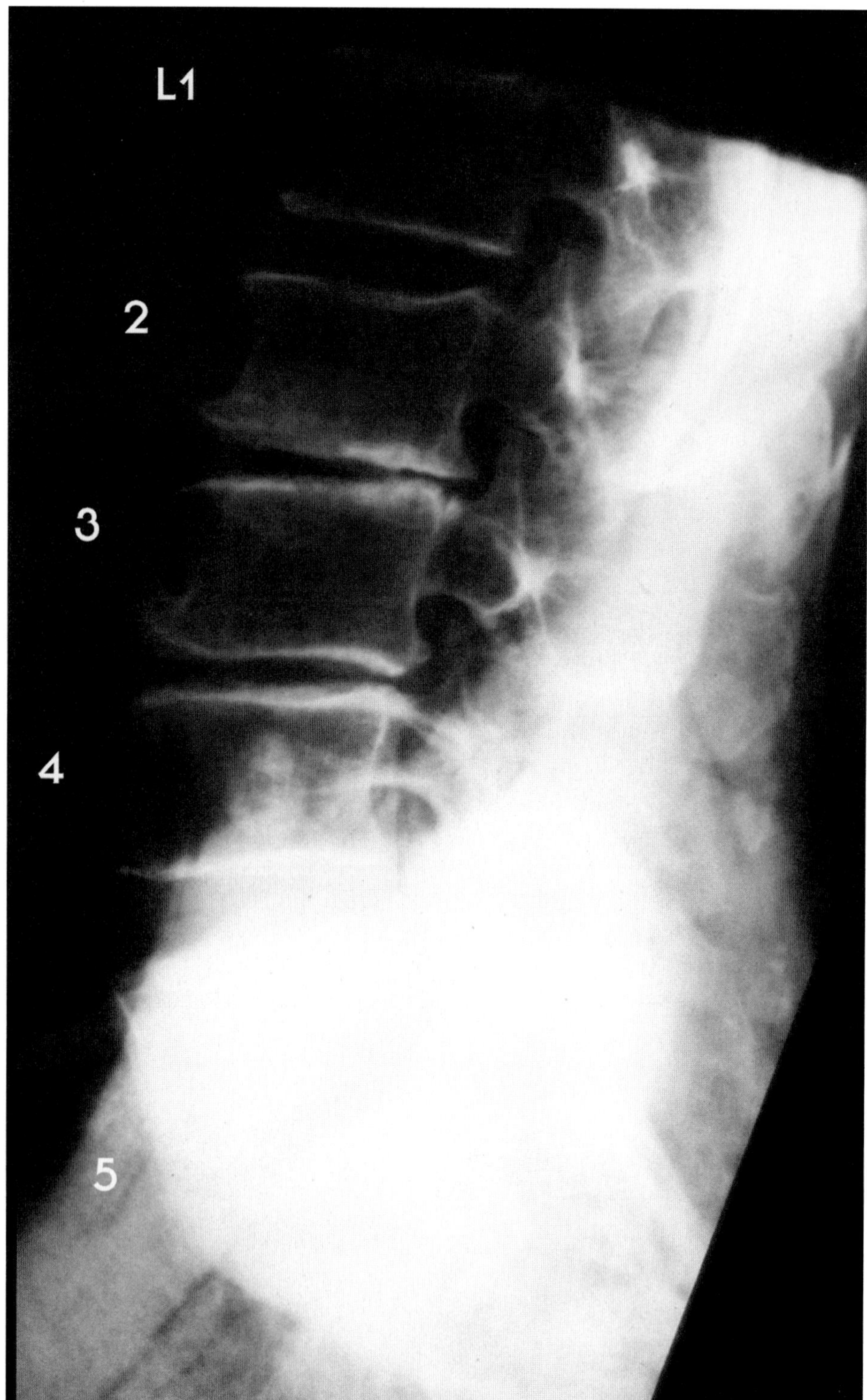

Plates 5-18 A & B
LUMBAR SPINE - This shows multiple subluxations with loss of curve
This specimen has chronic posterior stairstepping of vertebrae L2-4 to the segment above. L1 is retro to L2 with disc tearing, cavitation, and endplate repair, and has a slight compression fracture. L2 is retro to L3 with posterior spurring, end plate repair, disc wedging, tearing, anterior and posterior bulging, and loss of disc height. L3 is

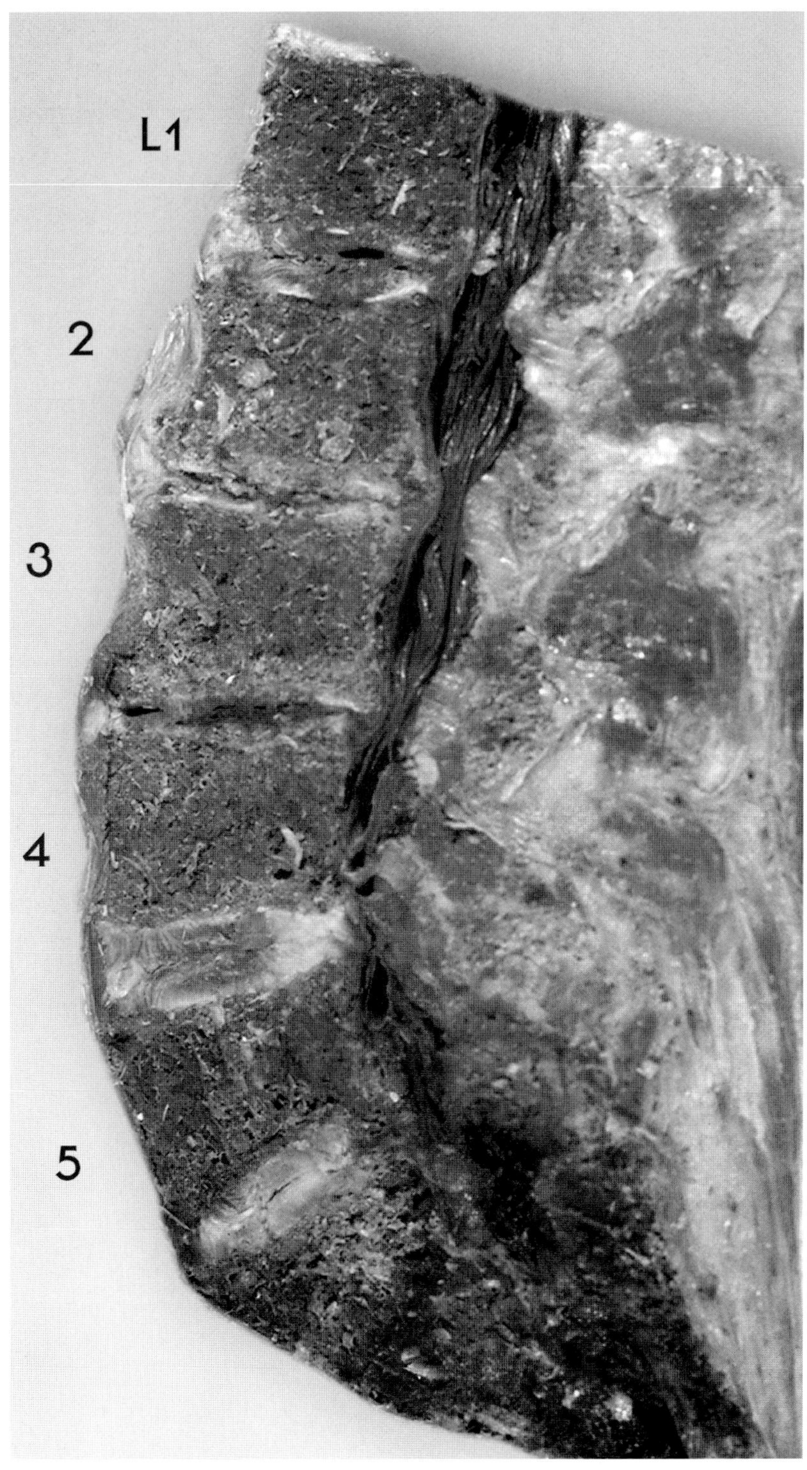

retro to L4 with disc tearing, cavitation, loss of disc height, slight wedging, and spurring. L4-5 are aligned with slight tearing, wedging, and inferior endplate repair, with the L5 compression fracture indicating trauma to these joints. The sacrum appears slightly antro to L5 with disc expansion into the L5 vertebral body, disc wedging, loss of disc height, and near fusion of L5-S1. This pattern of a subluxation complex is found in individuals with an anterior pelvis posture.

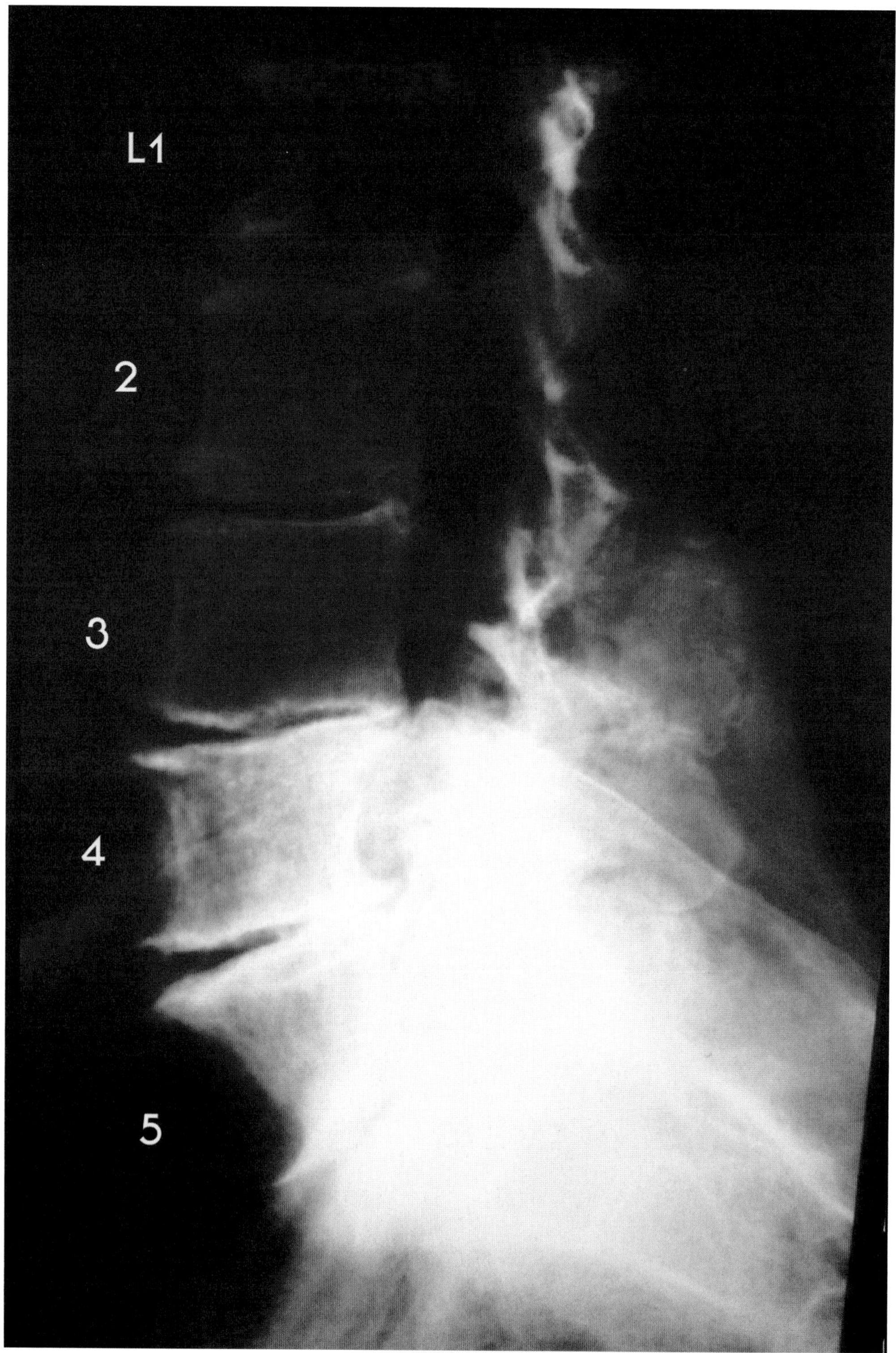

Plates 5-19 A & B
LUMBAR SPINE - This illustrates subluxations in end-stages
of degeneration with a loss of lordotic curve

L1 is retro to L2 and has inferior endplate anteriorly and repairs with anterior spurring, disc tearing, and anterior and posterior bulging. L2 is retro to L3 with anterior and posterior spurring, near fusion with anterior and posterior disc bulging, and loss of height.

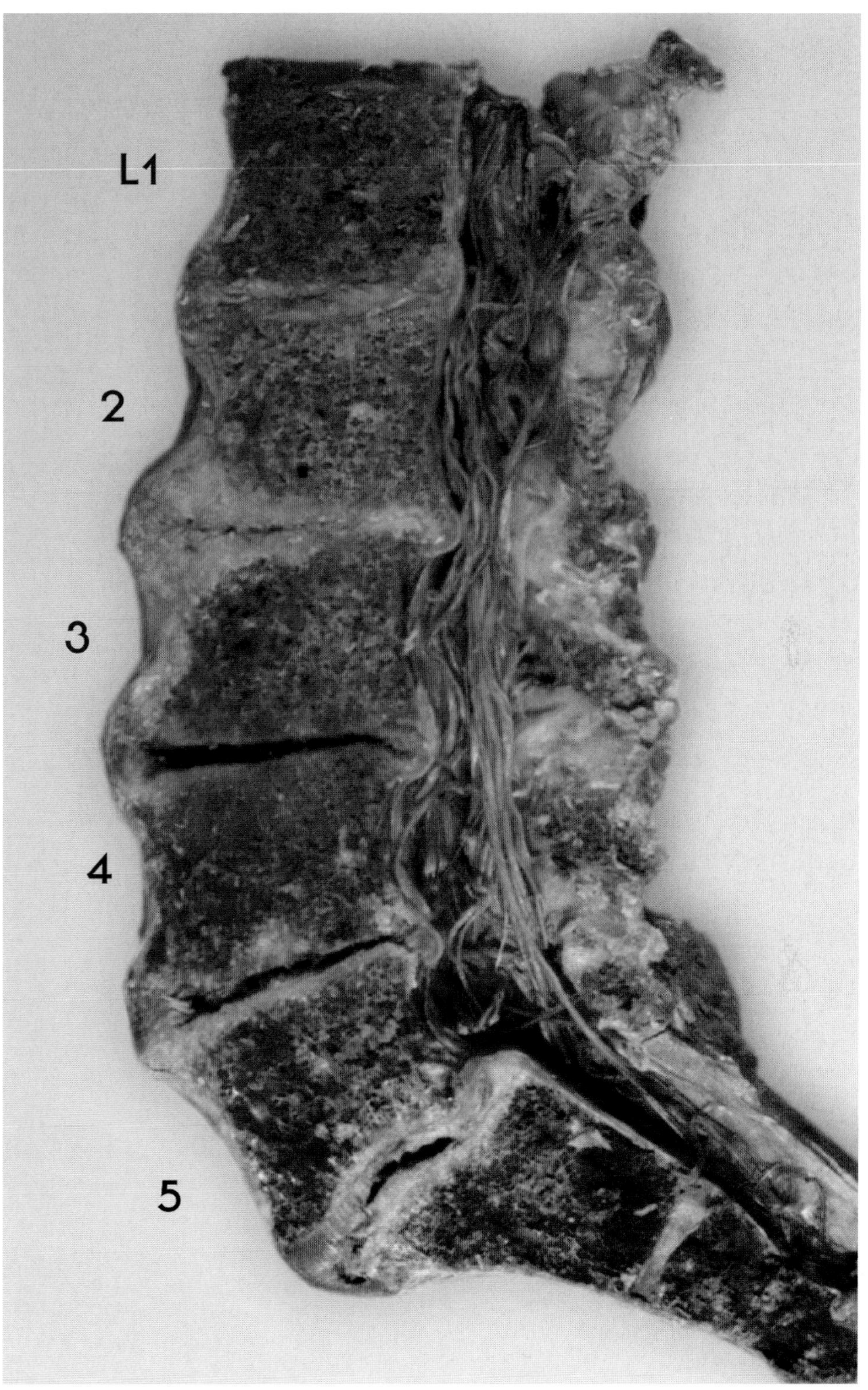

L3 is retro to L4 with anterior and posterior spurring, significant cavitation, total loss of disc matrix, and wedging of the space; L4 is retro to L5 with some anterior disc annulus remaining with cavitation, anterior and posterior spurring, loss disc height and matrix. L5 is antro to L4 and to the sacrum with disc tearing, cavitation, anterior and posterior bulging, and loss of height. This subluxation pattern of L5 and the sacrum can be described as a "sacral base posterior."

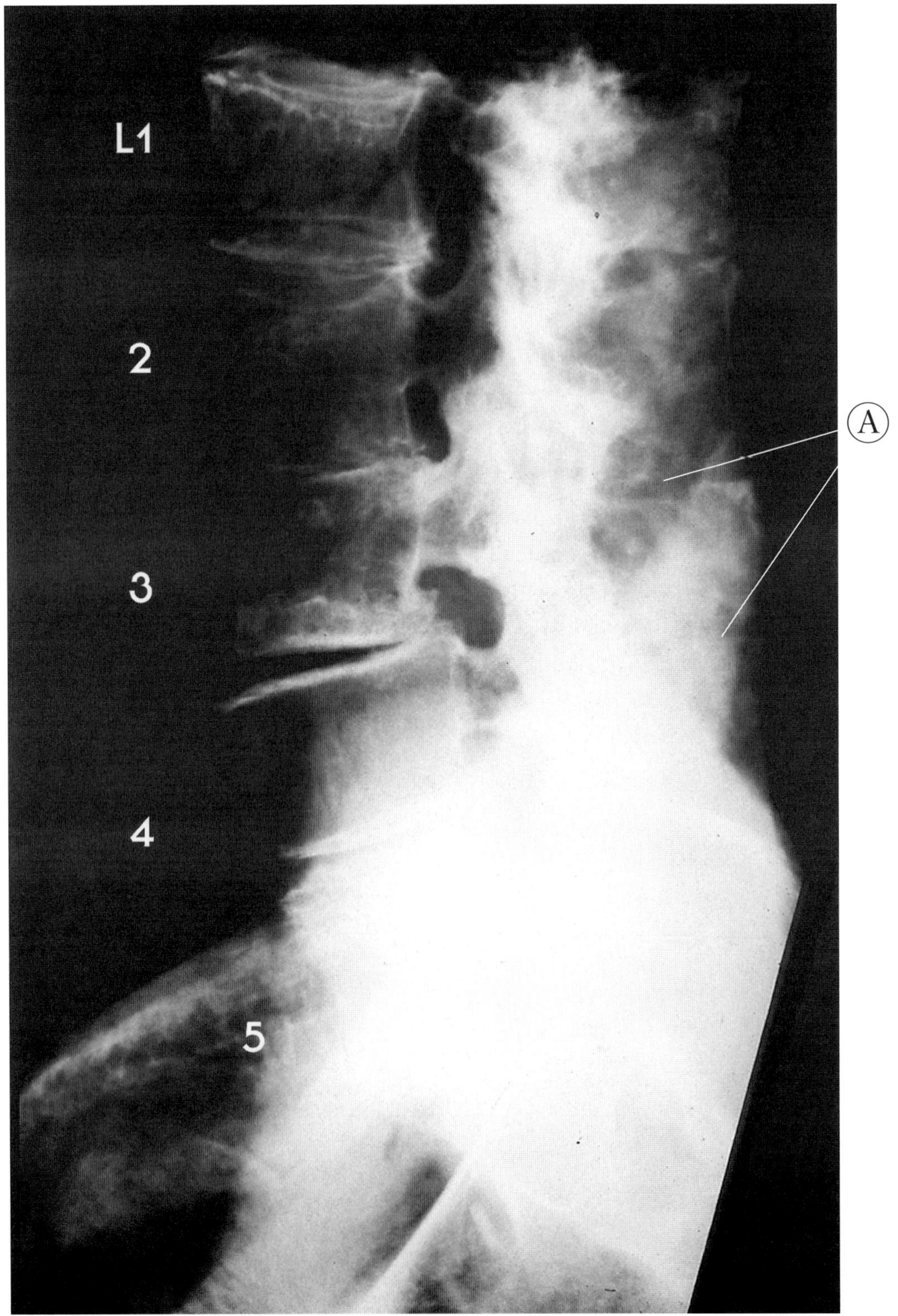

Plates 5-20 A & B
**LUMBAR SPINE - This specimen has multiple subluxations
and the end-stages of degeneration**

It has a reduced lordosis with chronic loss of joint integrity from L1 to L4. Note the increased vertebral body width due to the altered weight bearing produced by the subluxations. L1 is retro to L2 and has inferior and superior endplate damage, and spurring with disc tearing, anterior and posterior bulging, and loss of disc height.

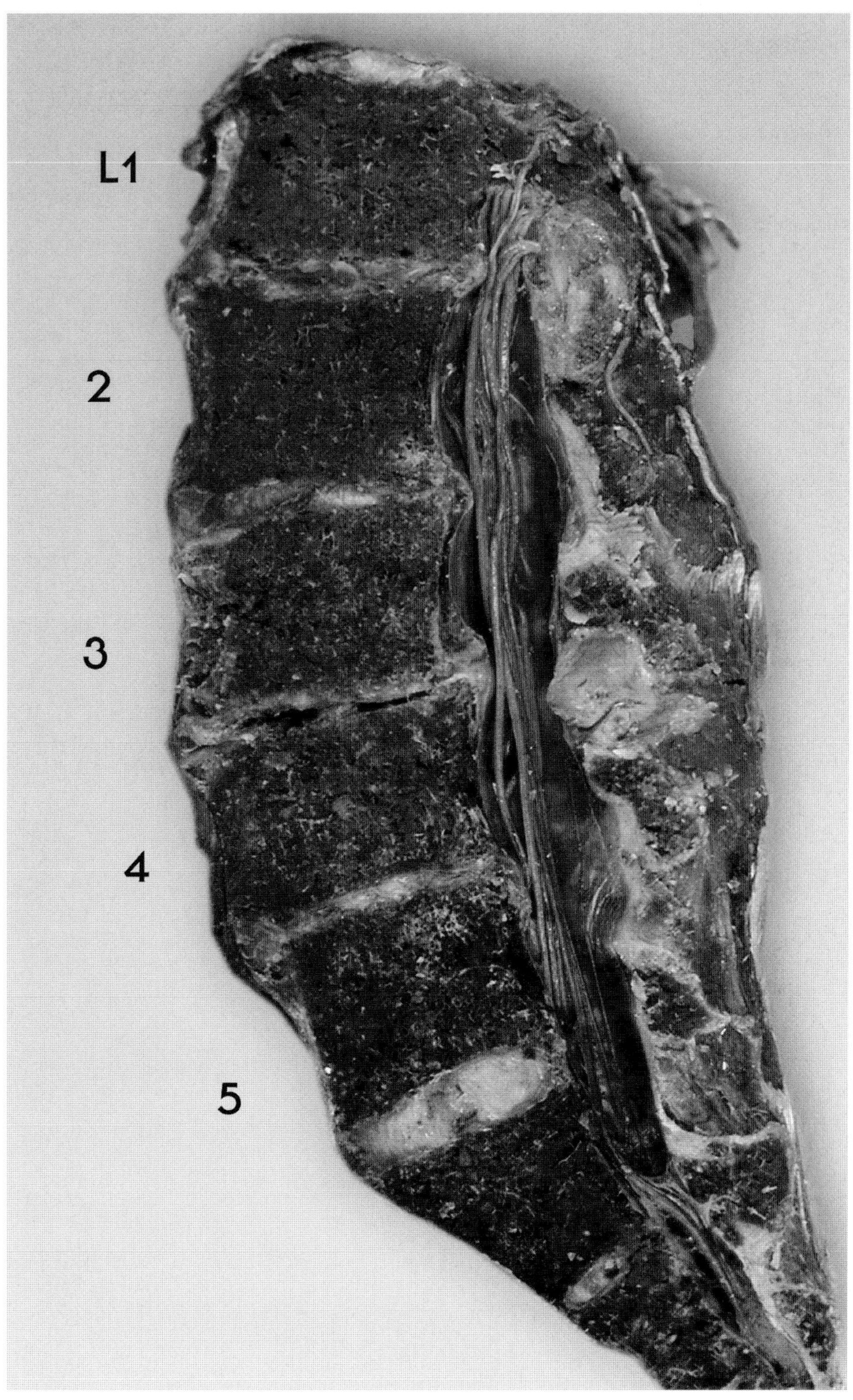

L3 is retro to L2 with posterior spurring, disc tearing, bulging, wedging, and loss of disc height. L4 is retro to L3 with disc cavitation, anterior and posterior bulging, near fusion, and anterior and posterior spurring. L5 is retro to L4 with disc tearing, loss of height, and anterior bulging. The sacrum-L5 segments are aligned with a near normal disc. This illustrates how subluxation results in chronic degenerative changes of the involved vertebrae.

(A)   Spinous process contact from loss of disc height

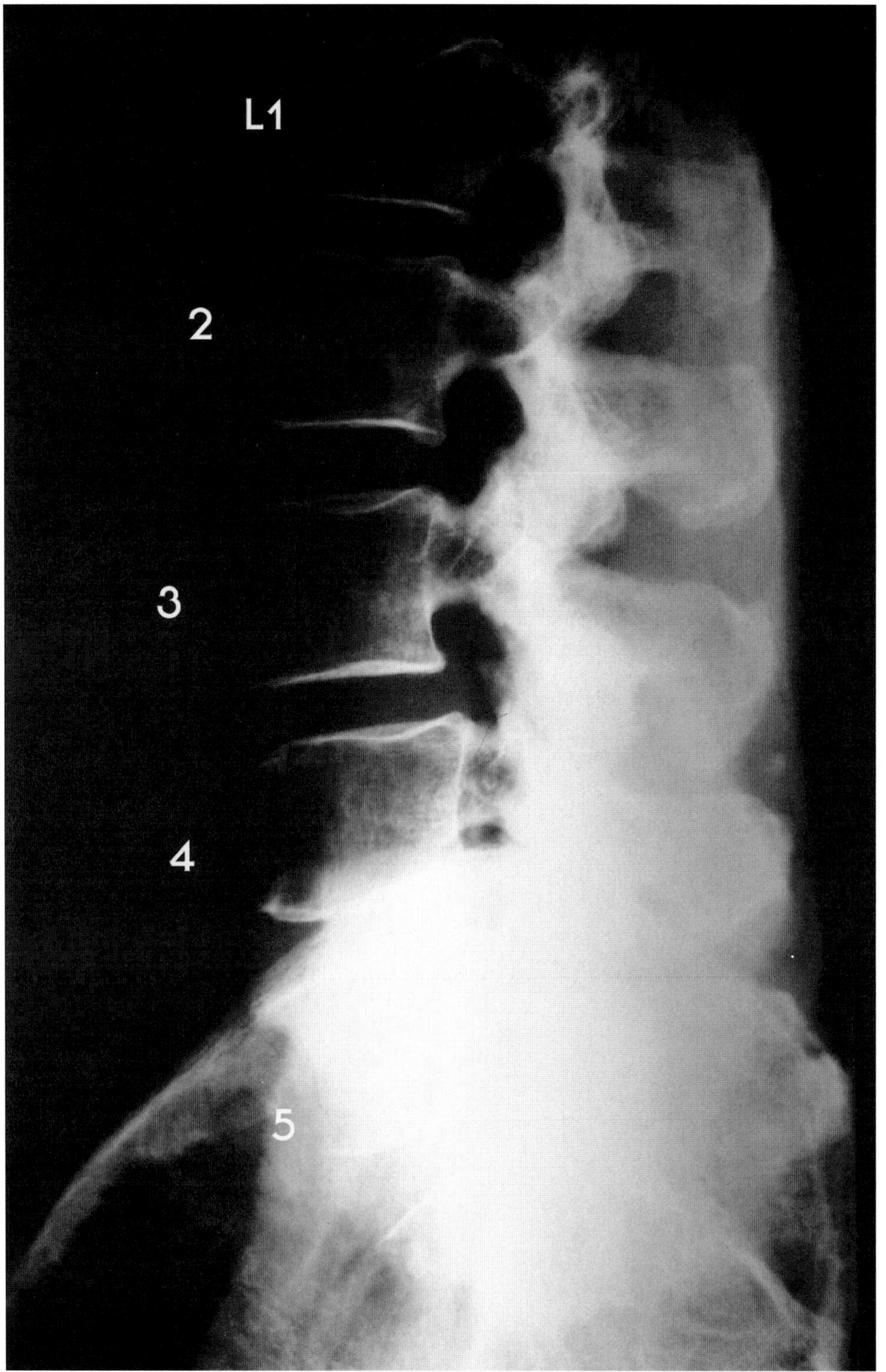

Plates 5-21 A & B
LUMBAR SPINE - This individual has a reversal of
lumbar lordotic curve with complete retrolisthesis of L4

This specimen has significant posterior displacement of L4 which causes loss of curvature. L1 and L2 have near normal alignment. L4 is retro to L3 and L5 (complete retrolisthesis) with tearing and loss of normal disc height.

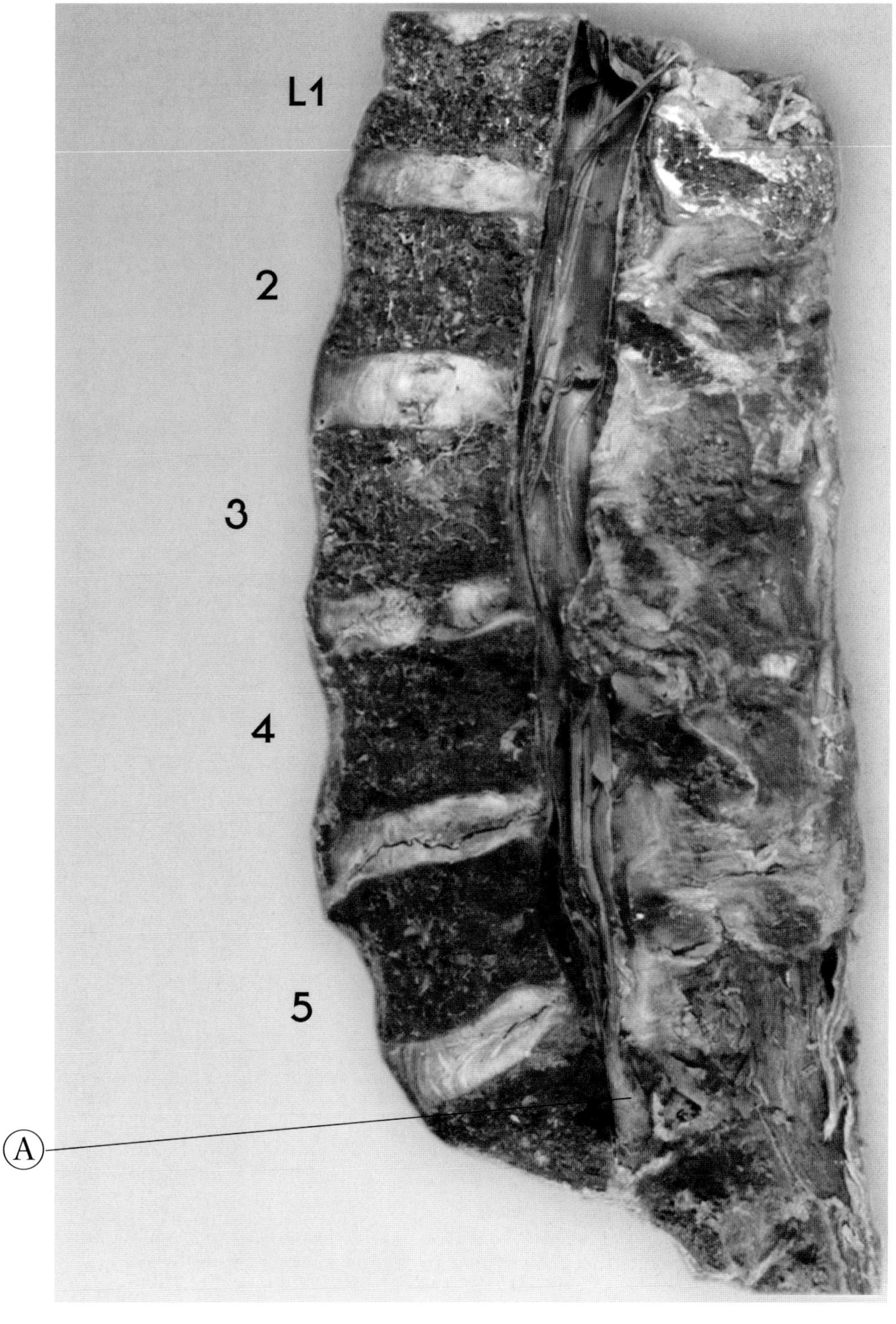

L5 is antro to L4 with tearing of the disc and a slight disc bulge posteriorly, loss of disc height and anterior and posterior spurring of the L5 superior end plate. The sacrum is slightly retro to L5 with slight wedging and tearing.

(A) The sacrum view is perisagittal with the first sacral nerve descending from the caudae equinae

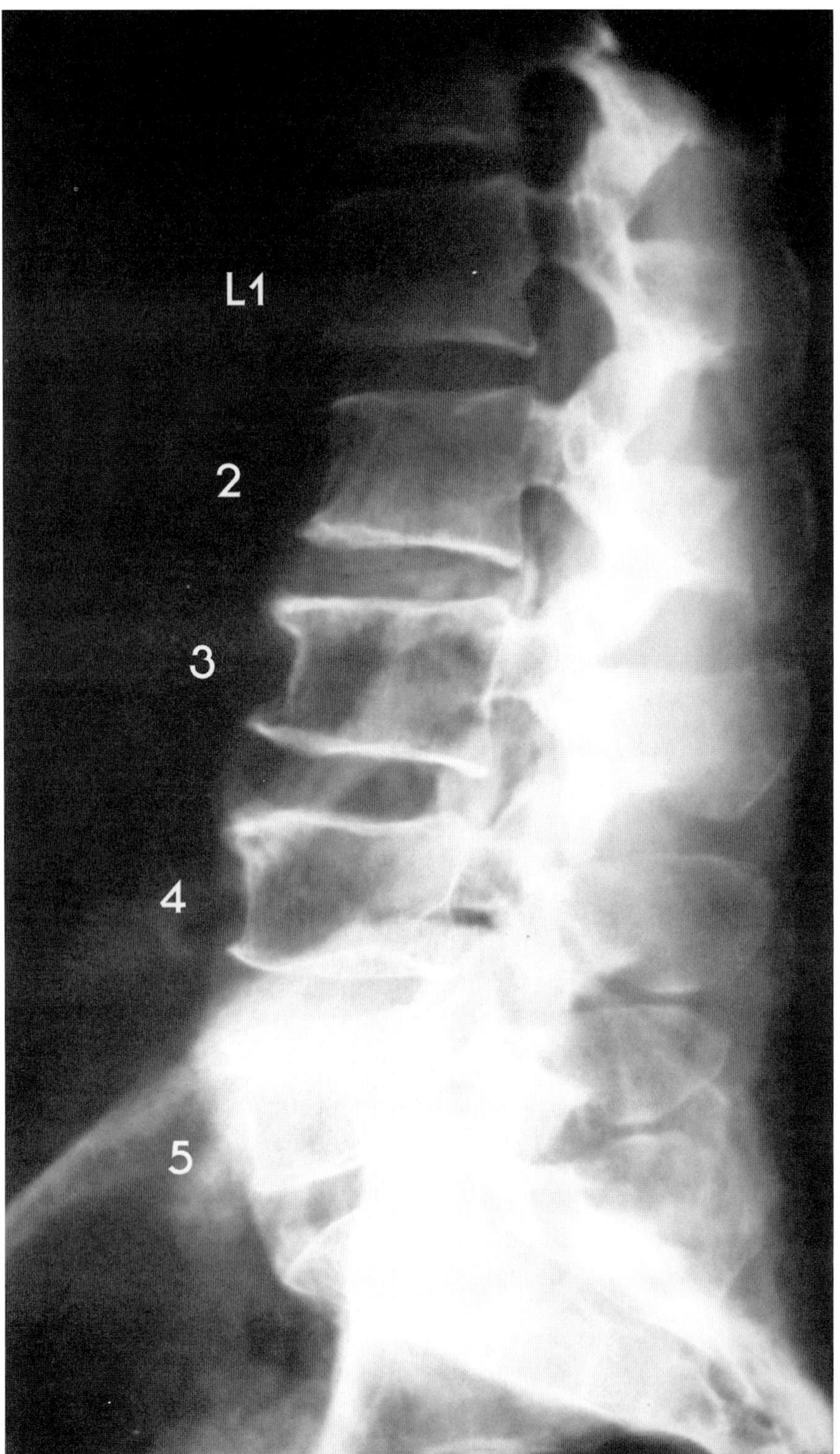

Plates 5-22 A & B
LUMBAR SPINE - Sequential retrolisthesis forming a "stairstepping"
of L1-L5 into a reversal of the lordotic curve

This specimen's lumbar spine is a subluxation complex. L1 is retro to T12 with slight DJD. L1 is slightly retro to L2 with anterior L1 spurring, disc tearing, and anterior and posterior disc bulging. L2 is retro to L3 with anterior spurring,

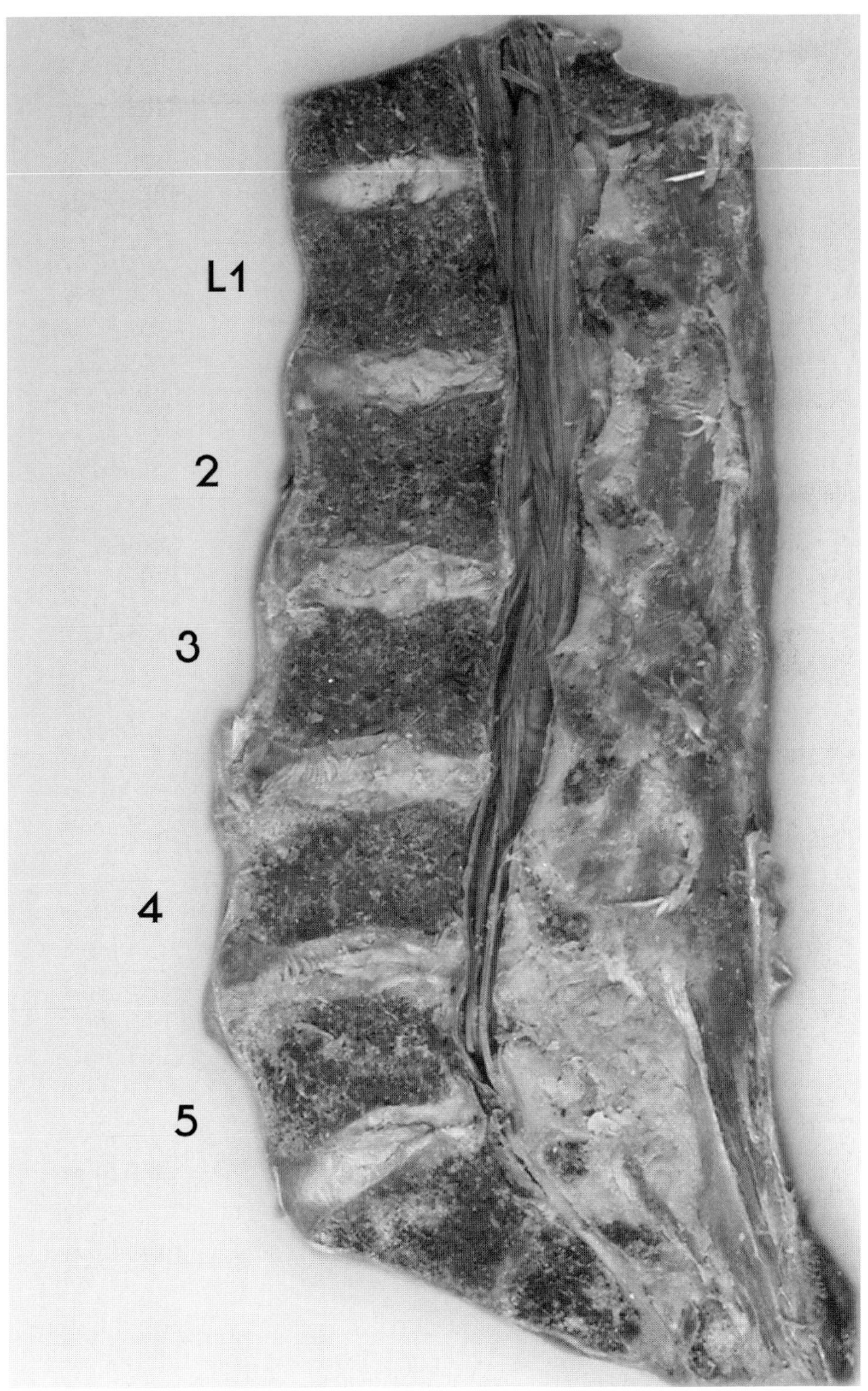

thickening of the anterior longitudinal ligament and wedging of the vertebral body of L3 with signs of end plate repair, and anterior and posterior disc bulging. L3 is retro to L4 with anterior spurring and wedging of disc, tearing, anterior and slight posterior bulging. L4 is retro to L5 with disc tearing and slight posterior bulging, anterior spurring, loss of disc height, and spinous process approximation. The sacrum and L5 are misaligned (sacrum anterior) with minor disc tearing and slight bulging and wedging.
Note the increase in the length of the spinal canal.

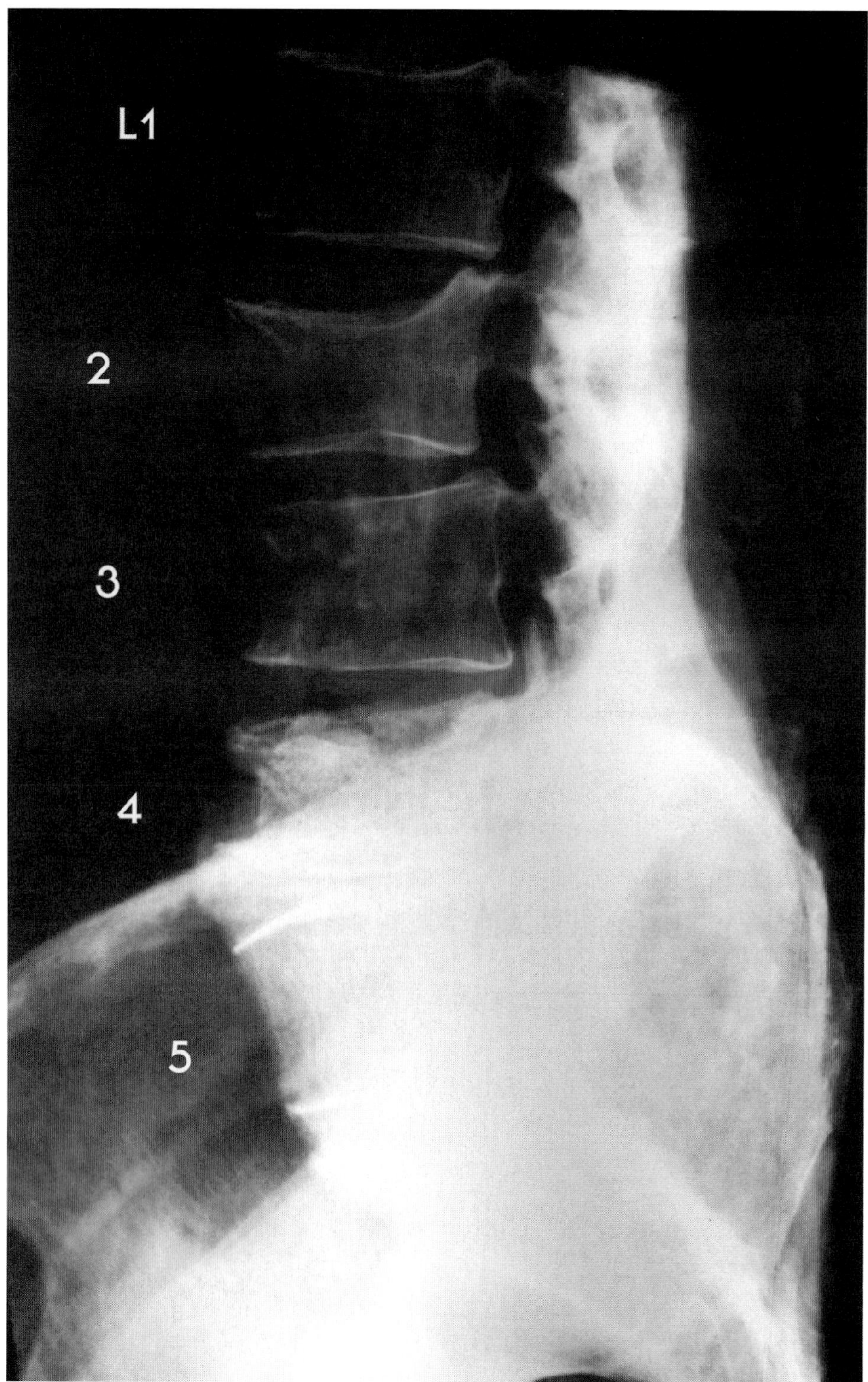

Plates 5-23 A & B
LUMBAR SPINE - L3 is a complete retrolisthesis creating
a reversal of the lordotic curve

This specimen has suffered an injury that subluxated and damaged L2 through L4. Notice the altered length and width of the spinal canal. L2 is slightly retro to L1 with significant end plate destruction indicating a compression fracture of L2 with anterior and posterior disc bulging, tearing, wedging, and anterior and posterior spurring.

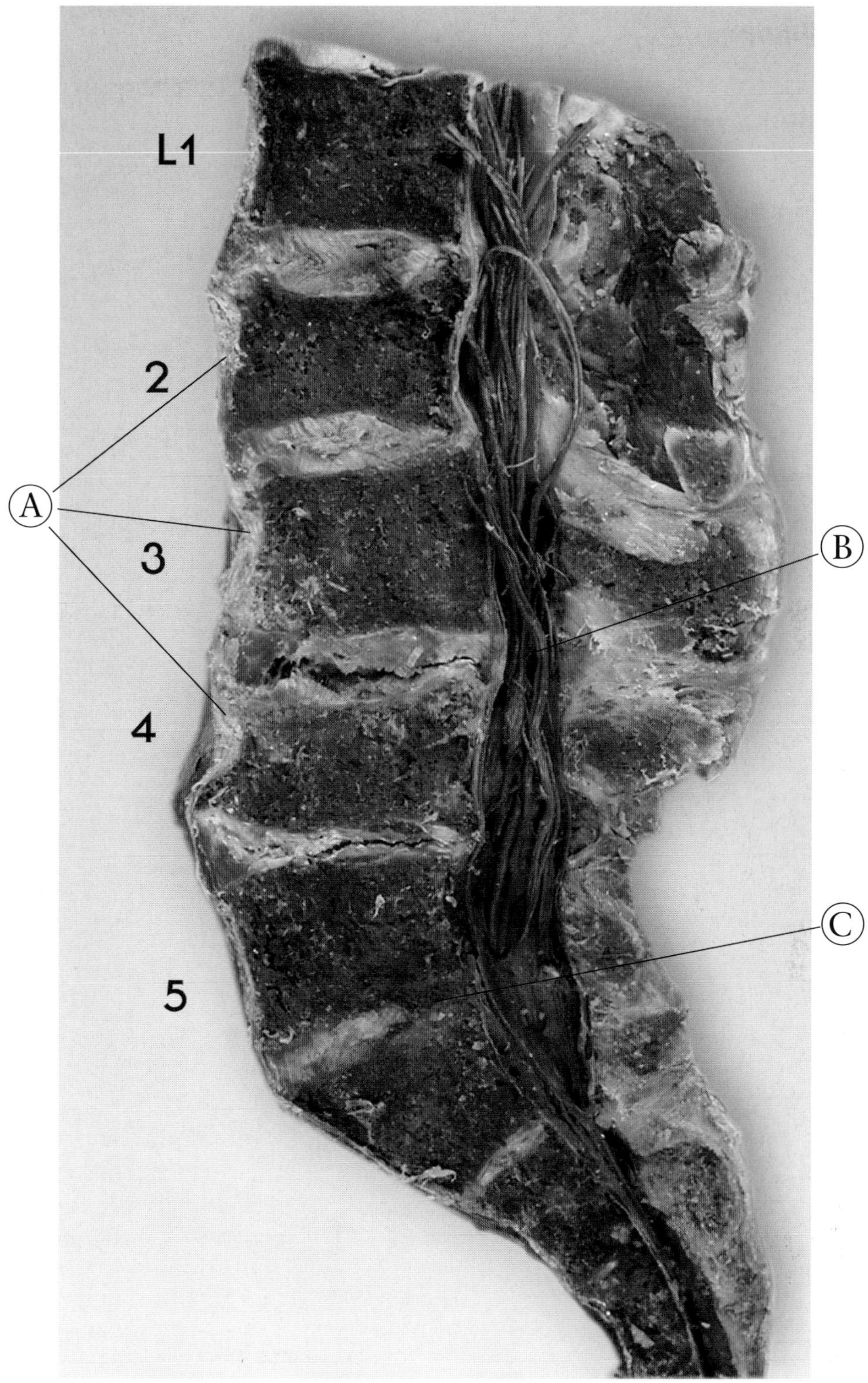

L3 is retro to L2 with disc tearing and wedging. L3 is a complete retro. L3 is retro to L4 with disc tearing, cavitation, wedging, bulging with compression fracture of L4, and anterior spurring. L4 is retro to L5 with disc tearing and significant loss of height. The sacrum is slightly antro to L5 with near fusion of segments.

(A) Thickening of A.L.L. over L2-4
(B) Spinal canal narrowing
(C) End-stage wedging of L5-S1

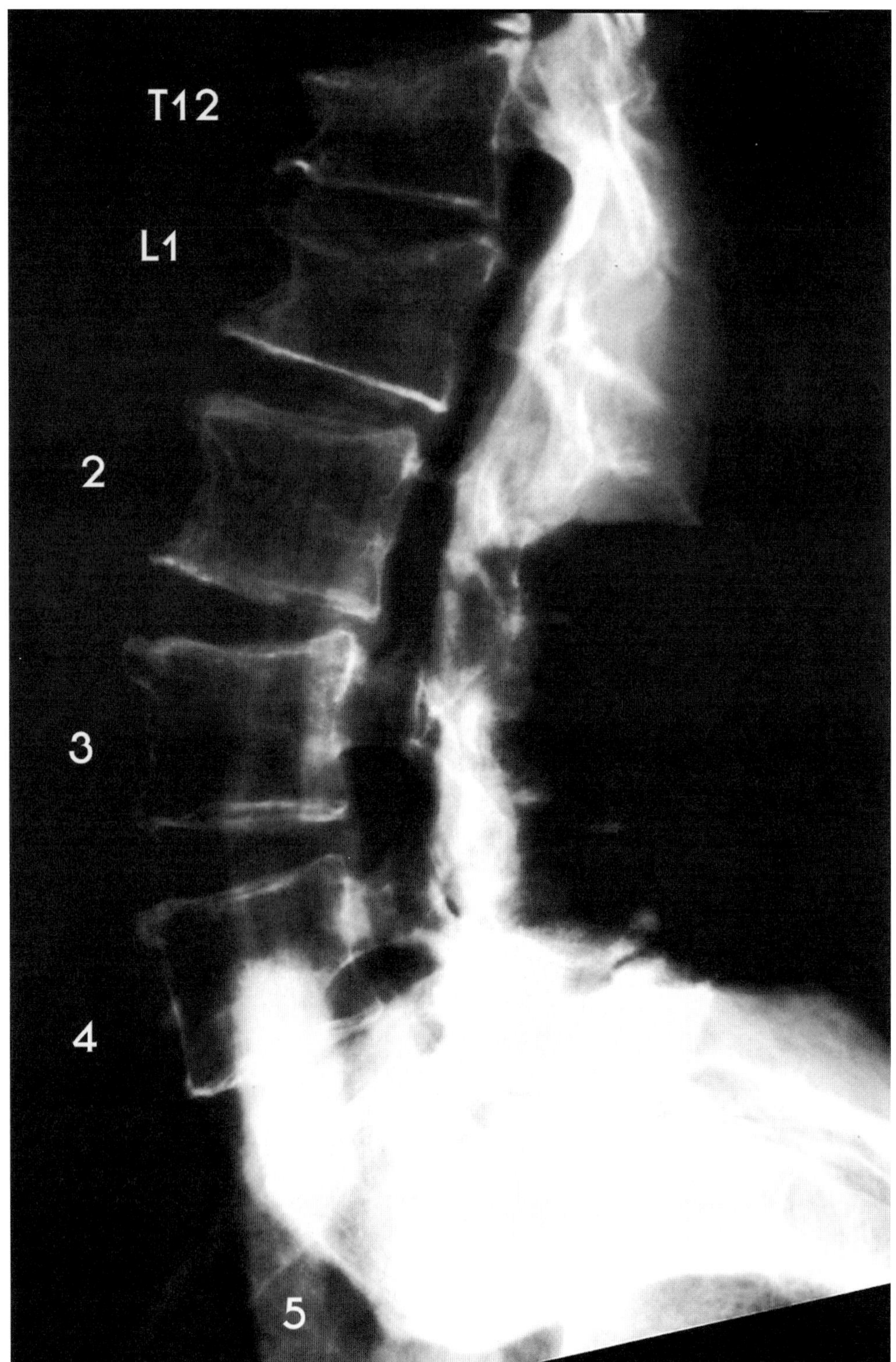

Plates 5-24 A & B
LUMBAR SPINE - This shows a reversal of the
lordotic curve in the upper lumbar spine
This specimen has suffered compressive force causing anterior vertebral damage of T12 and L1. L1 is a complete retrolisthesis. T12 has an anterior compression fracture with loss of the anterior vertebral body height. L1 is retro to T12 with disc wedging, tearing, anterior and posterior bulging, and an anterior compression fracture with loss of vertebral body height. L1 is retro to L2 with disc tearing, bulging, and anterior spurring. L2 is retro to L3 with disc

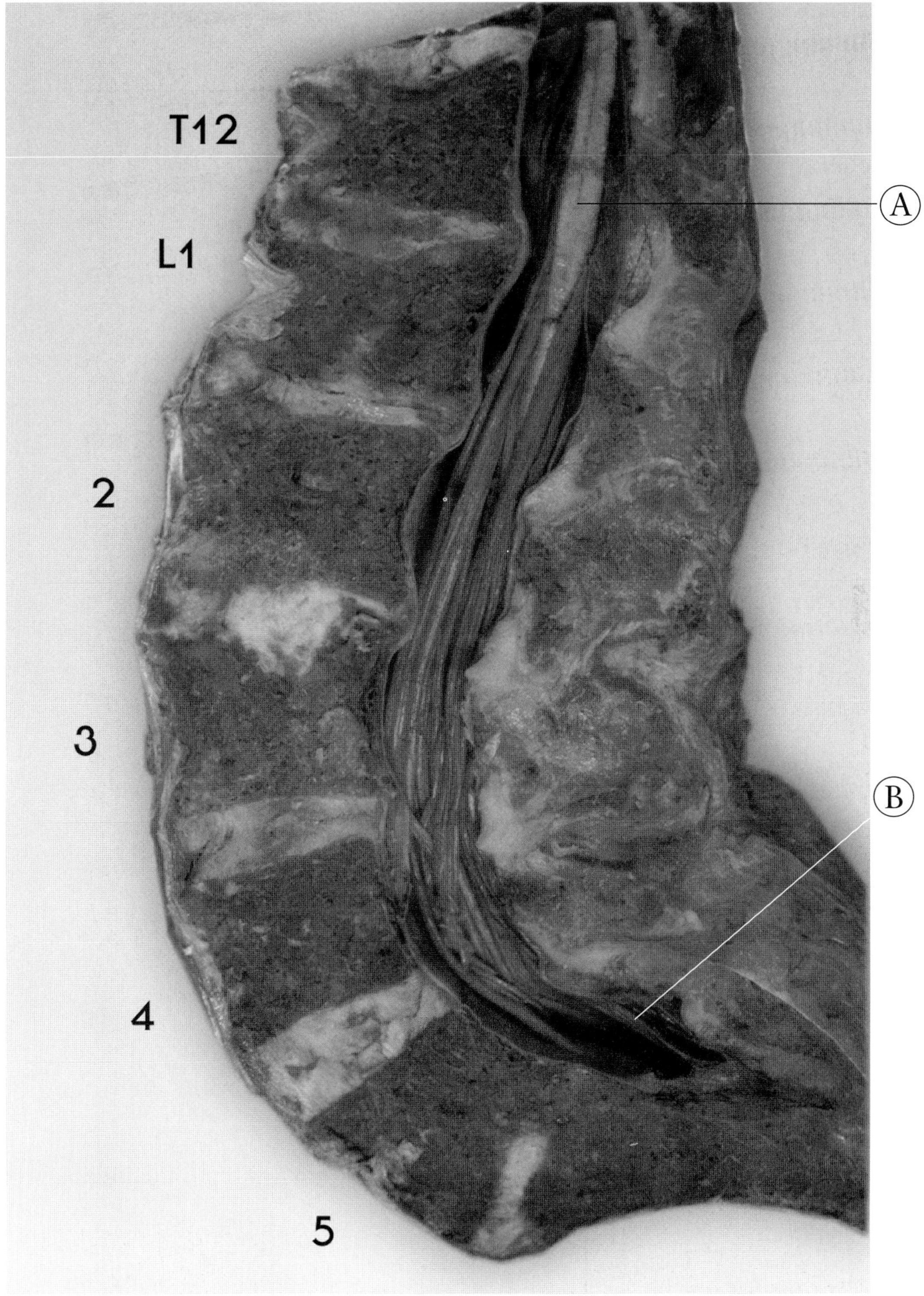

wedging and anterior spurring and bulging posteriorly (with some kind of change in the L2-3 disc that is not radiographic). L3 is retro to L4 with tearing of the disc and posterior bulging and some end plate damage. L4-5 look aligned with slight tearing and wedging. The sacrum is retro to L5 with near fusion.

(A) Sagittal section of conus medularis and caudae equinae
(B) Note how caudae equinae components are pulled around posterior canal to the sacrum
    Cervical flexion can make this worse.

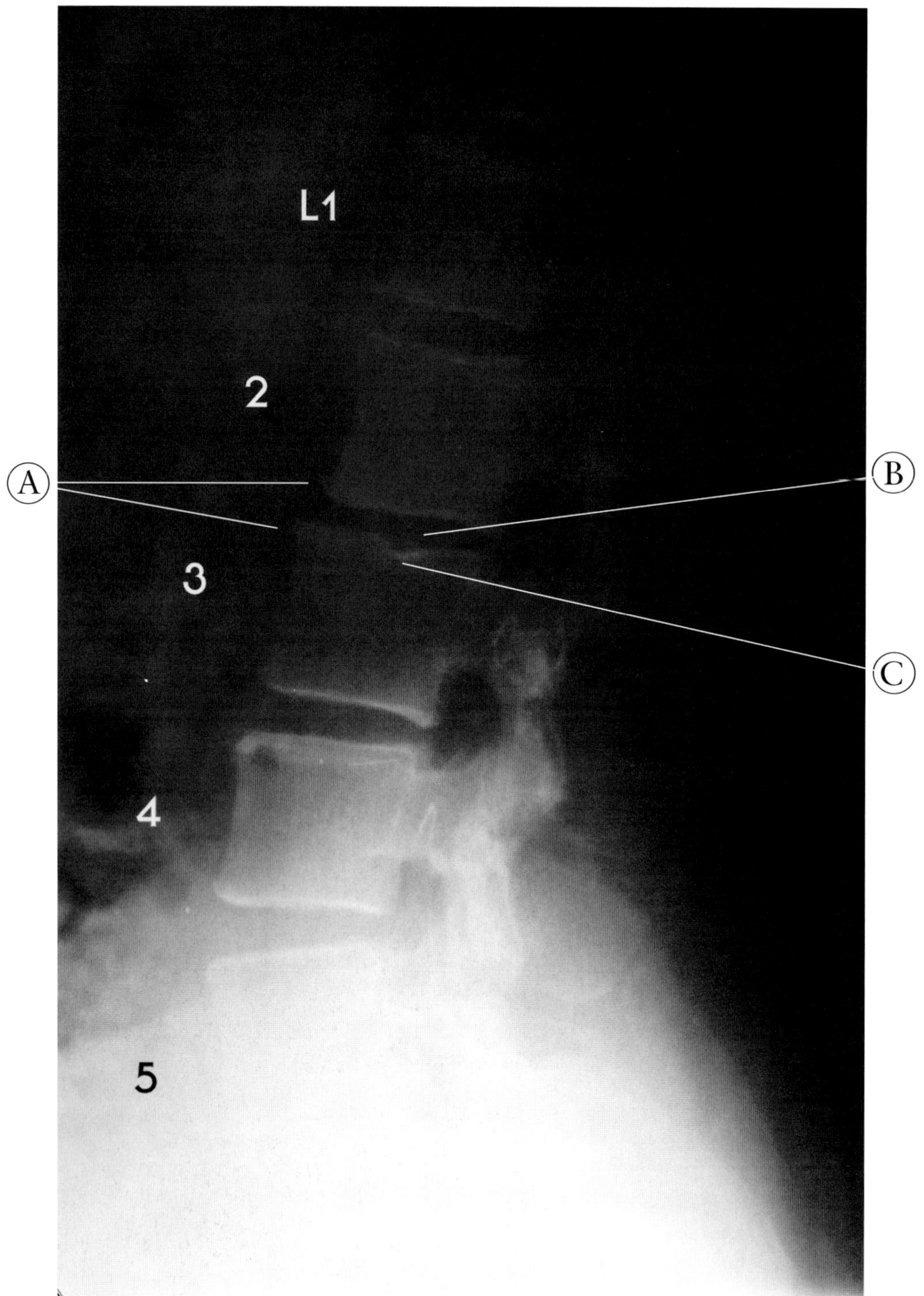

Plates 5-25 A & B
SUBLUXATIONS WITH A LOSS OF LORDOSIS
An X-ray and MRI comparison

This individual has suffered a subluxation of L2: a complete retrolisthesis to L1 and L3. L3, L4, and L5 are all posterior to the segment below. This loss of lordotic curve has a significantly damaged disc at its apex. The vertebrae with the most A to P displacement have degenerative changes. Note the osteophyte formation at

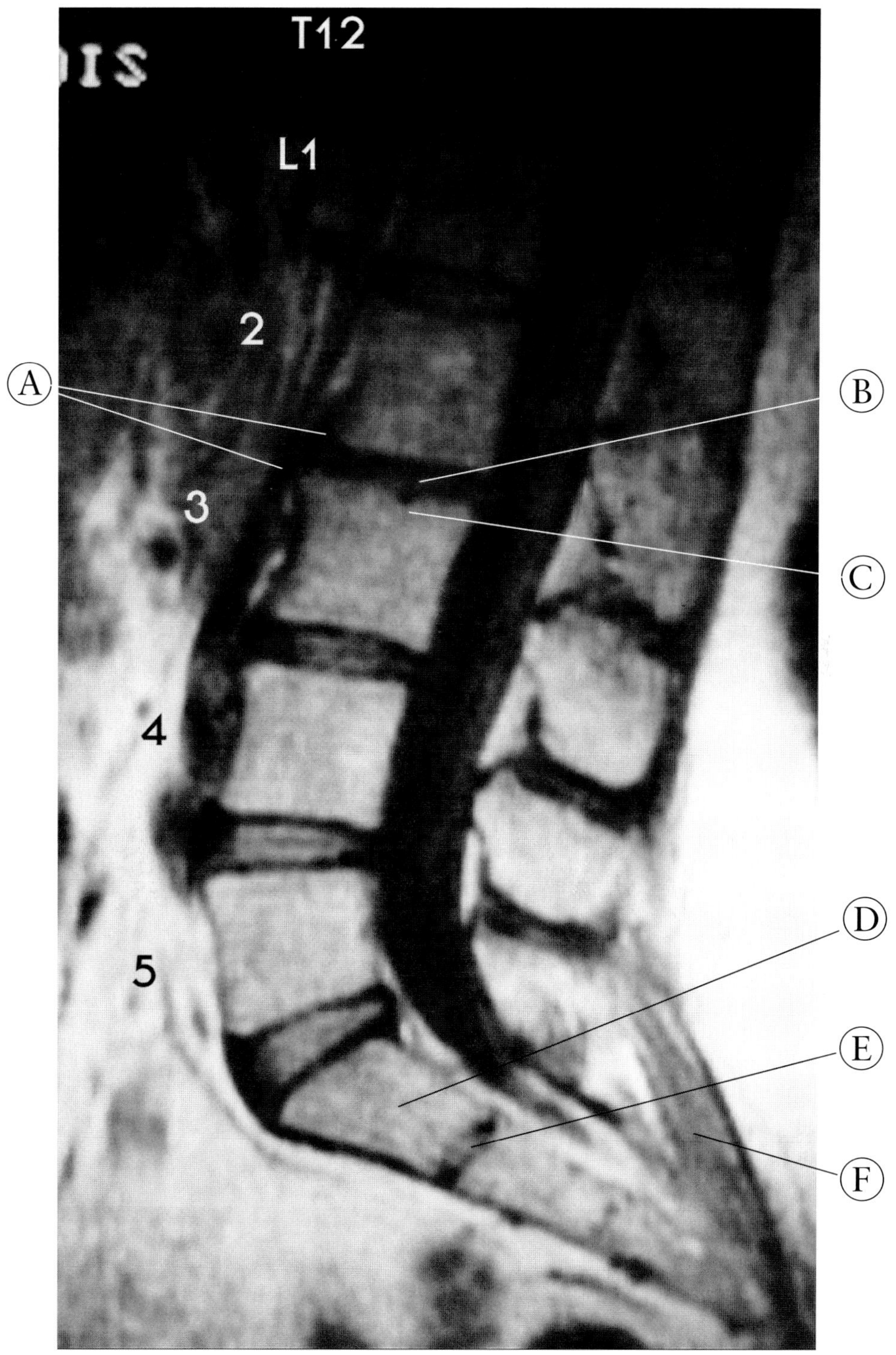

only L2 and L3. The end plate damage indicates old trauma. The sacrum is anterior to L5 and there is a sacral disc at the S1-2 level. The sacrum has lost its kyphotic shape and the lower sacral discs are gone. The sacral origins of the erector spinae are taut in the supine position, indicating their relaxed state has more superior sacral apex translation.

(A) Osteophytes	(D) Sacrum
(B) Degenerating disc	(E) S1-2 disc
(C) Endplate	(F) Erector spinae

CHAPTER SIX
Subluxations Of The Pelvic Girdle

Discussion

In the adult, the pelvic girdle is a three-bone complex including the sacrum and the right and left innominates. ("Innominate"is a Latin word meaning "no-name," referring to its embryonic origin as three separate bones: the ilium, ischium, and pubis.) Three joints unite the bones of the pelvic girdle; the two sacro-iliac joints and the pubis symphysis. The sacrum is the base of the spine and the pelvic girdle, as a whole, is the anchor for quite a substantial part of the muscular system of the spine, legs, thorax, and abdomen. All of the abdominal, hip, and thigh muscles originate from the pelvic girdle, as do the two large back muscles, the erector spinae, and the latissimus dorsi (**See Figure 6-1**). So it is not difficult to see how subluxations of the pelvic girdle can affect any or all of these muscle groups, causing them to contract, become hypertonic, or go into spasm. The key to understanding the etiology of much "low back pain" is the integrity and function of the three pelvic joints.

In **Figure 6-1** some of the muscles directly involved with sacroiliac joint and pubic symphysis motion and integrity are illustrated. The abdominal wall musculature has its inferior attachment from the pubic symphysis, medially, to the posterior aspect of the iliac crest. Innominate subluxation involving the SI joint and pubic symphysis will adversely affect the rectus and transverse abdominus, and internal and external abdominal oblique muscles. The

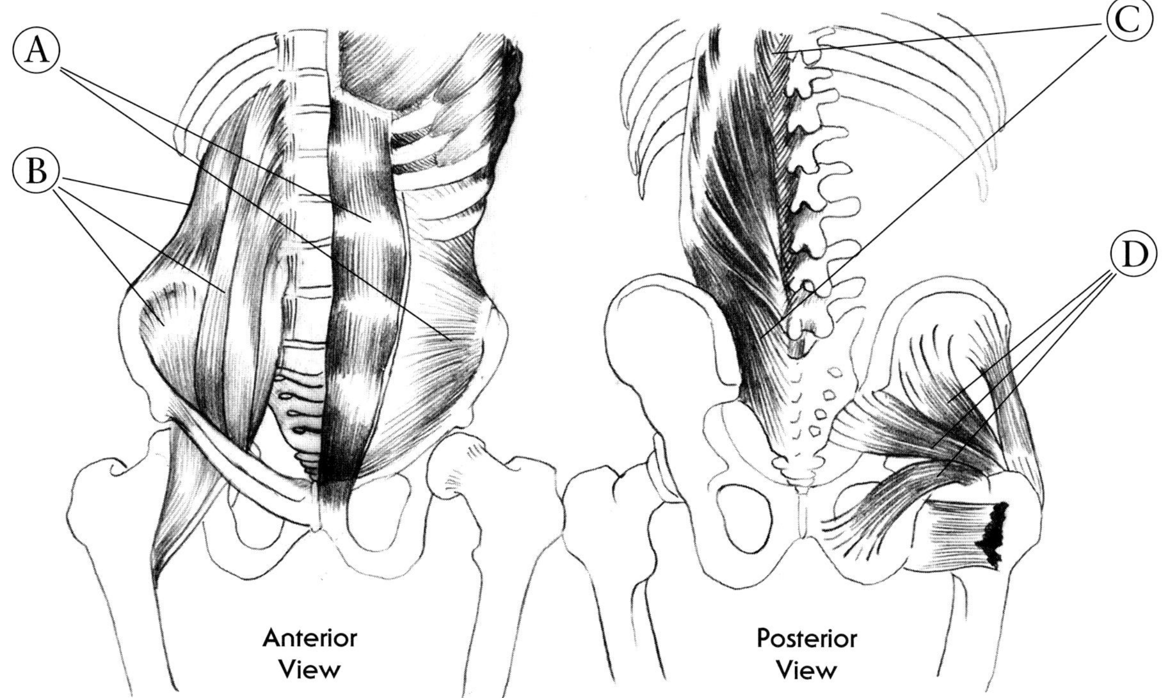

Figure 6-1

These illustrations are anterior and posterior views of the pelvis and the major muscle groups of the back, hip, and abdomen. All the muscles depicted have proprioceptive links to the sacroiliac joints and pubic symphysis. The figure on the left is the anterior view and the right is the posterior view of the pelvis.
  (A) The abdominal wall which include rectus and transverse abdominus, internal and external oblique muscles
  (B) The major hip flexors psoas and iliacus and quadratus lumborum
  (C) The erector spinae muscles
  (D) The deep hip muscles include gluteus minimus and medius, piriformis, gemellus inferior and superior, obturator internus, and quadratus femoris

psoas and iliacus muscles will be recruited neurologically to guard and protect the injured joint by limiting their range of motion. The posterior muscles will be in the same altered state. These muscles are the erector spinae, latissimus dorsi, and the deep hip muscles. The deep hip muscles, as well as others, experience distress when pelvic subluxation causes the acetabulum to shift relative to the femoral head, trochanter, and shaft. As the hip joint alters these relationships, the bottom of the foot must still contact the ground. Analysis of these problems is complicated by the variety of pelvic tilts encountered (**See Figure 6-15**). Muscular distress, pain, and limited range of motion will be only some of the clinical symptoms. The loss of motion, normal joint space, and fluid exchange initiates degenerative processes.

The neurology involved is very complex and will be discussed only in general terms. All the tissues are embedded with neurological sensors of various types. However, it is extremely important to understand that the guarding (spasmed) muscles around the symphysis pubis can, like any other muscles, be relieved only by correcting the subluxation and removing the noxious proprioceptive input into the central nervous system. The nervous system may never adapt to neurological input from noxious proprioceptive stimuli arising from joint distress (subluxation). This neurological phenomenon is present in all the studied mammalian neuromusculoskeletal systems. The sacrum gives rise to the sacral nerves and the internal iliac arteries contribute the arteries to the pelvic organs. They are retroperitoneal and are adhesed to the back or dorsal surface of the abdominal lining. Mechanical distress can displace abdominal tissues away from the origins of their nerves and arteries.

Visceral Implications of Pelvic Subluxations.

A variety of complaints can result from subluxations of the pelvic joints, including urogenital and intestinal problems. In a normal female pelvis, the broad ligament stretches between the two ilia, suspending the ovaries and the uterus. (**See Figure 6-2**). When the pelvic girdle subluxates, the broad ligament skews as the ilia displace with respect to one another. This changes the position of the ovaries and the uterus in the abdominal cavity, and can exacerbate any problem that might exist. The pelvic examination can reveal tight and tender musculature on one side and the uterus tractioned to one side. I think that a large percentage of gynecological pathology may be the result of unresolved pelvic trauma. Correction of the subluxation complexes of the pelvic girdle has been shown clinically to relieve or reverse these conditions.

I have also encountered instances of testicular pain, ensuing from subluxation of the pubic symphysis. This can be explained anatomically by the fact that the testicular nerve, artery, and vein traverse the top of the pubic rami before they descend into the testicles, creating a neurovascular bundle that can become entrapped in some individuals.

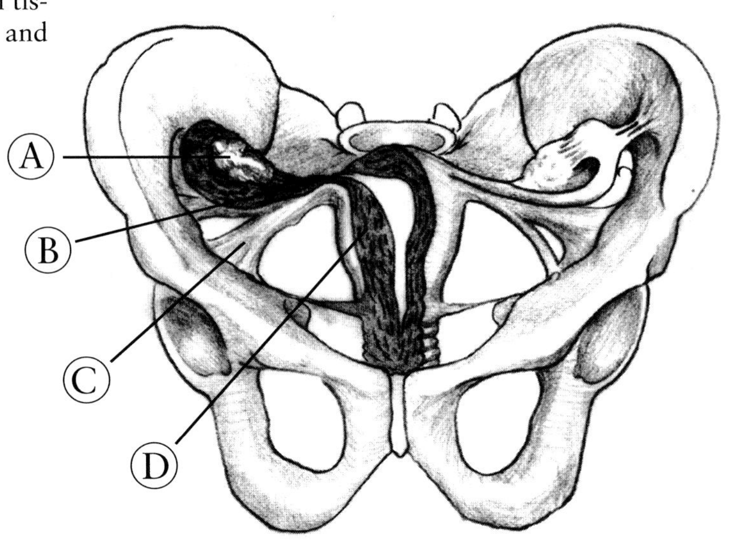

Figure 6-2
This illustration depicts the ovaries, fallopian tubes, uterus, and broad ligament in the pelvic girdle. These gynecological structures are suspended in the pelvic girdle by the broad ligament. When the pelvis subluxates the normal relationship is altered.
  (A) Ovary
  (B) Fallopian tube
  (C) Broad ligament
  (D) Uterus

The Sacrum

The sacrum is usually depicted as a solid bone, but I have found that even specimens 90-100 years old have viable discs in the sacrum between S1-S2 and S2-S3 (**See Figure 6-3**). The presence of a disc implies sacral motion because, from a physiological point of view, a fibro-cartilaginous disc requires motion for survival. These sacral discs are tied to, and bio-mechanically related to, the sacro-iliac joints and ligaments.

The sacrum and the sacroiliac joints are angled from top to bottom and from front to back (**See Figure 6-4**).The appearance of these structures on the variety of types of imaging and positions can be quite different. **See Figure 6-16** to see the different views in one study. To make the evaluation process more complex, the sacrum can be either parallel or nearly perpendicular to the ground (or anywhere in between) (**See Figure 6-15**).

The sacrum is an inverted pyramidal structure formed by the partial fusion of sacral vertebrae. It articulates with both innominates at the sacroiliac joints and the fifth lumbar vertebrae with the intervertebral disc and articular facets. It has a canal posterior to the bodies of the segments that is contiguous with the spinal canal. The distal end of the caudae equinae occupies the canal and the anterior and posterior foramen house the exiting sacral nerve roots.

The sacrum has five separate segments in a child and the partial fusion of S1 to S2 and S2 to S3 remains through life. S3, 4, and 5 can be fused by age 25. The presence of the sacral discs throughout life strongly suggests sacral motion. As previously mentioned, physiological function of intervertebral discs necessitates motion as a main mechanism of nutrition and waste elimination. This is likely to be the same for the avascular intrasacral discs.

The cortex of the sacrum is a contiguous and flexible wall. The sacral discs, as well as the intervertebral discs confer flexibility. There is only one mechanism for fluid and nutrient exchange for the intervertebral disc: imbibition (hydration) through the vertebral end plates via motion. This must also be true for sacral disc physiology and function. **See Figure 6-3**, a sacrum of an 86 year old individual. It is an obviously flexible structure, with healthy intrasacral discs.

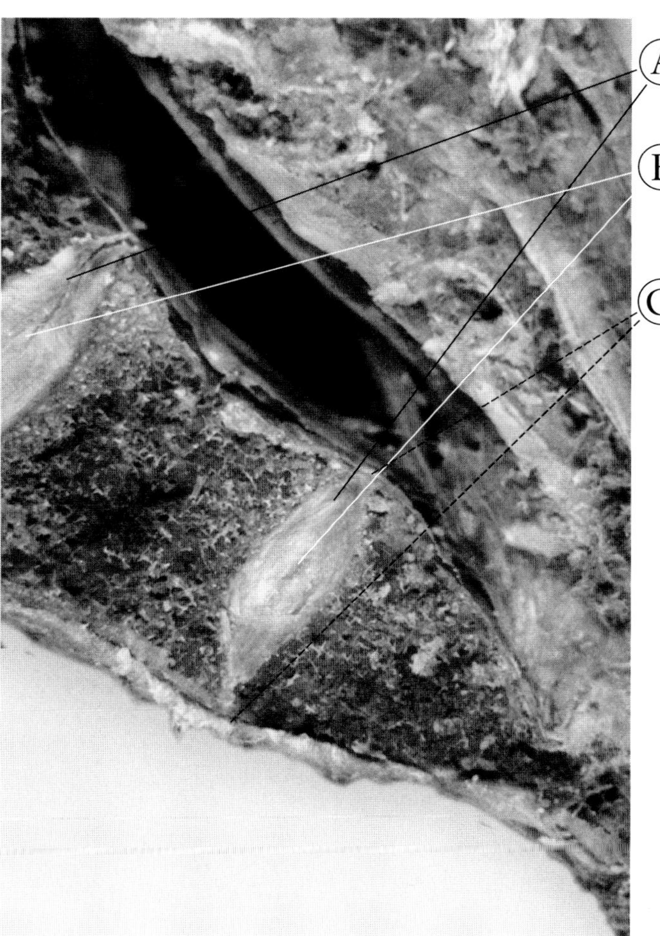

Figure 6-3
This is a view of the sacral discs of an 86 year old male.
The majority of elderly specimens had persistent sacral discs. The most persistent was the S1-2 disc. The S2-3 disc was less often observed. The S3-4 disc was occasionally seen, about 25%. This view was slightly off the mid-sagittal plane. Note the presence of annular rings and a nucleus pulposus. The sacral discs are oval in shape in the A to P and coronal planes (X-Y plane). Note the continuous cortical bone that must be radio dense. This is significant evidence of sacral motion front to back and side to side.
This is the anatomical explanation of the sacrum pumping the Cerebrospinal Fluid in the spinal canal. Sacral motion is likely to be connected to central nervous system physiology and function.
(A) Annulus fibrosus
(B) Nucleus pulposus
(C) Cortex of sacrum

The motion of the legs rotating from the acetabulum rocks the innominates with the anterior and posterior thigh musculature. The sacrotuberous and sacrospinous ligaments connecting to the sacrum from the innominate transfer movement alternating back and forward. The femur is an enormous lever. A handle on a wrench as long as the leg would snap a 3/4 quarter inch tightened bolt in a partial turn. The joints and ligaments that hold the pelvic girdle together must withstand tremendous rotational and shearing forces. Part of the strength and stability of the pelvis is its flexibility. The sacrum, forming the bottom of the spinal canal, must confer motion to the entire lower central nervous system, from the sacral nerve roots to the brainstem. Motion of the spinal cord is the major mechanism for capillary blood flow. A static spinal cord has reduced blood flow.

The sacral discs are evident to the 9th and 10th decades of life. In the limited study presented here there is evidence of intersacral subluxation. (See **Figures 6-36 through 6-41 on pages 202-203**). The S1-2 disc has a dorsal and ventral cortical bone covering. This will thicken with loss of integrity between the S1 and S2 segments and the disc will dehydrate. The S2 and S3 segments seem to have the same relationship.

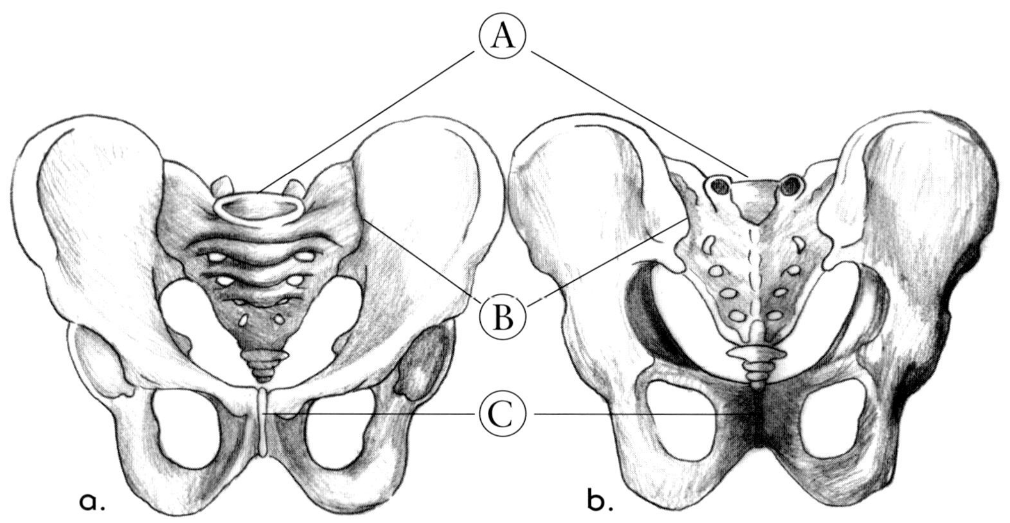

Figure 6-4

This shows the human pelvis from the (a) anterior and (b) posterior view. The three joints of the pelvis, the right and left sacroiliac joints, and the pubis symphysis can all be seen.
Note the sacrum is wider at the top (this is called the sacral base) narrower at the bottom (this the sacral apex). The sacrum is also wider in the anterior aspect than the posterior.
  (A) Sacrum
  (B) Sacroiliac joint
  (C) Pubis symphysis

The Sacroiliac Joints

Sacroiliac joints have two components: fibrous and cartilaginous (synovial). I have dissected more than 200 individuals' sacro-iliac joints, and have found extreme variation among specimens. The main differences are in the shape, contour, and size of the joint. The fibrous part is large in some specimens and small in others; the cartilaginous part shows the same variation, and there is no consistency in the ratios of one part to the other (**See Figures 6-5 and 6-6**). Such variation in a normal joint is unique among the bodies joints.

Other joints only show major variation from a "normal" configuration after injury or disease. The cartilage portion of the sacroiliac joint can be smooth and flat or extremely irregular and contoured. It can be in the same plane as the fibrous portion or at almost right angles at either medial or lateral orientation. This amount of variation of this significant joint complex can explain the wide range of responses to injury and recovery. Clinically it is common to find that the sacroiliac joint, once injured, never fully recovers.

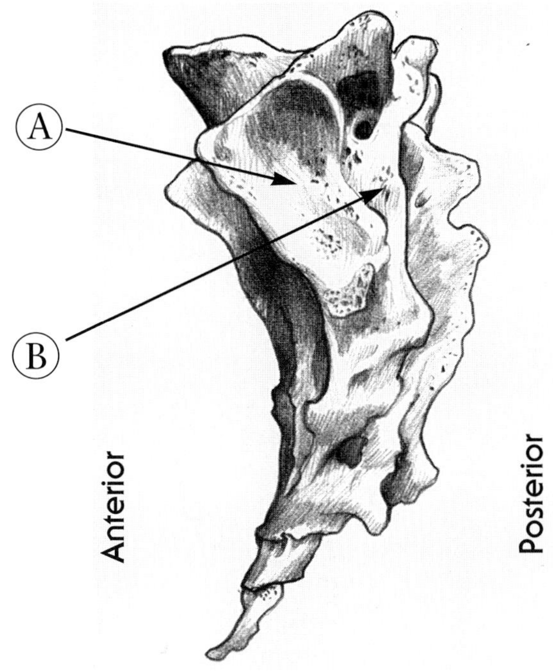

Figure 6-5
This illustration is a lateral view of the sacrum. The cartilage and synovial portion of the joint is generally anterior and inferior to the fibrous portion of the joint. These two components vary in size and contour between individuals. This is the most individually unique joint complex in the body. The sacro-iliac joint variations can explain the different responses to injury and recovery among individuals.
(A) The cartilage portion of the SI joint
(B) The fibrous portion of the joint

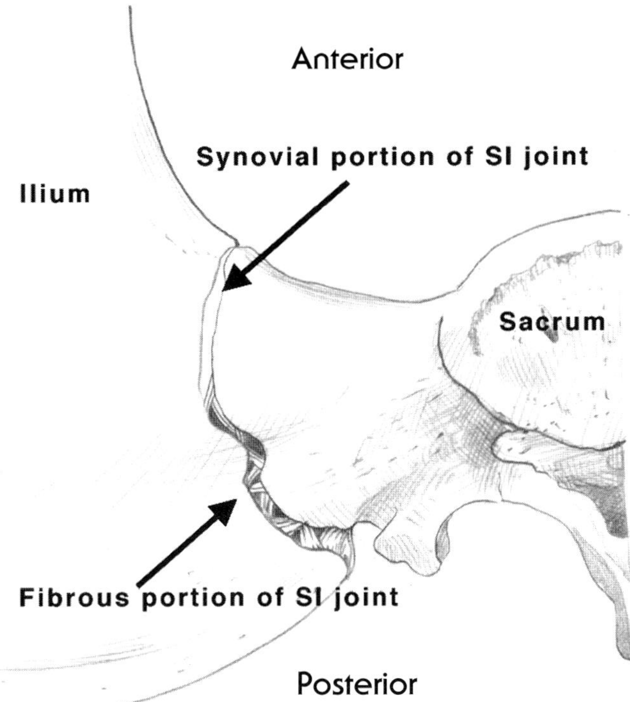

Figure 6-6
Sacroiliac Joint – Two Parts
The sacroiliac joint has a fibrous component, which is posterior and superior to the auricular surface. The auricular or cartilage component is anterior and inferior. There is cartilage on both surfaces and synovial fluid is a common finding. The auricular surfaces can be smooth or contoured; see **Figure 6-7**.

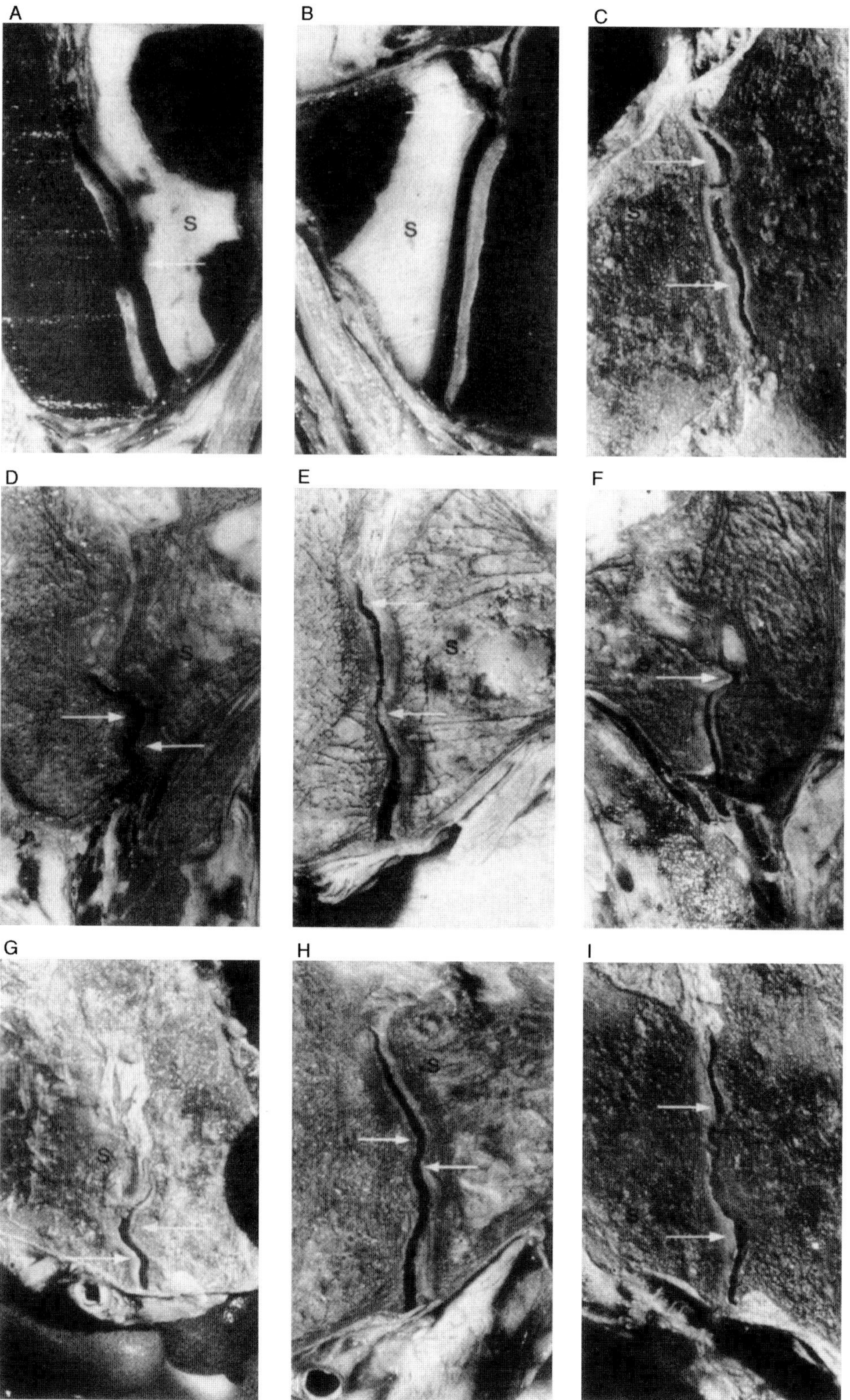

Figure 6-7

Frontal sections of the SI joints of enbalmed male specimens. S indicates the sacral side of the SI joint. **A** and **B** concern a 12-year-old boy. **C** to **I** concern male specimens older than 60 years. Arrows are directed at ridges and depressions. The ridges and depressions shown are covered by intact cartilage, which was checked by opening the joints afterwards.
With permission of Dr. A. Vleeming. Originally published in SPINE (European Ed.), 1990, 2: 130-132.

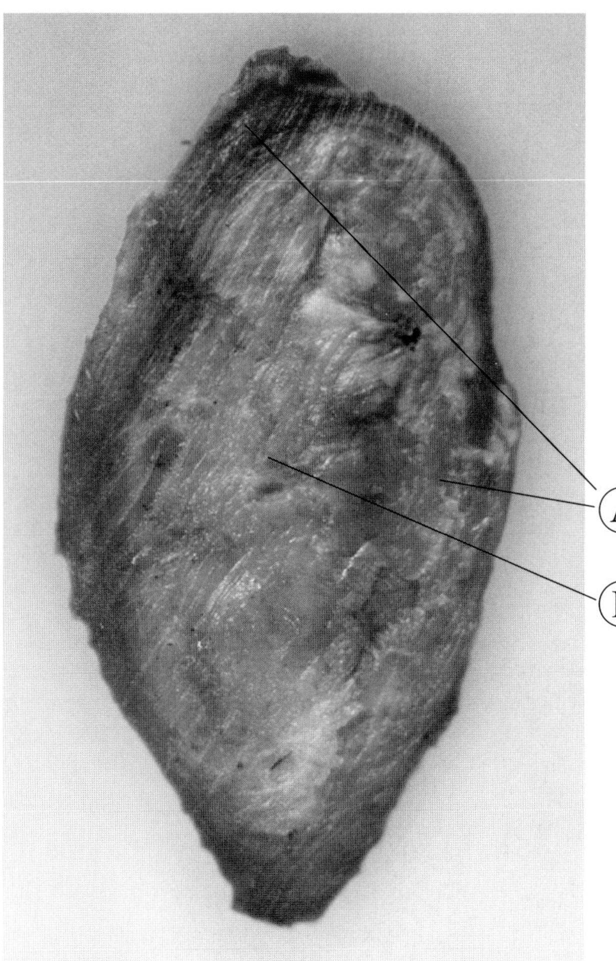

Figure 6-8
Because of the annular rings and a pulpy center, this illustrates a motion segment. Shearing or tearing of the intervertebral discs have been detailed in previous chapters. Similar disruption can occur to the pubis symphysis. Shearing of the vertebrae tear the disc; shearing of the pubic bones tear the pubic symphysis. The problem with the pubic symphysis over the IVD is having the transverse processes and spinous processes as lever arms to move the vertebrae. The pubic symphysis has the legs as levers for motion. This structure must withstand the significant mechanical advantage that the legs have as levers.
  (A) Annular ring
  (B) Nucleus pulposus

The Pubic Symphysis

The third joint of the pelvic girdle is the pubic symphysis, an avascular fibrocartilaginous disc. The end of each pubic ramus is covered by hyaline cartilage and the fibrocartilaginous pad in between has annular rings with a pulpy, spongy center. It is very similar to an intervertebral disc, even into advanced age. Extrapolation from intervertebral disc physiology would indicate that the pubic symphysis is supposed to move (**See Figure 6-8**) or else it cannot obtain sufficient nutrients.

The pubic symphysis, like any other movable joint, can subluxate and in different directions. Because of the complex ligamentous and muscular attachments that connect to the pubic rami, such subluxation can wreak physiological, proprioceptive, and painful havoc on the legs, thorax, and abdomen.

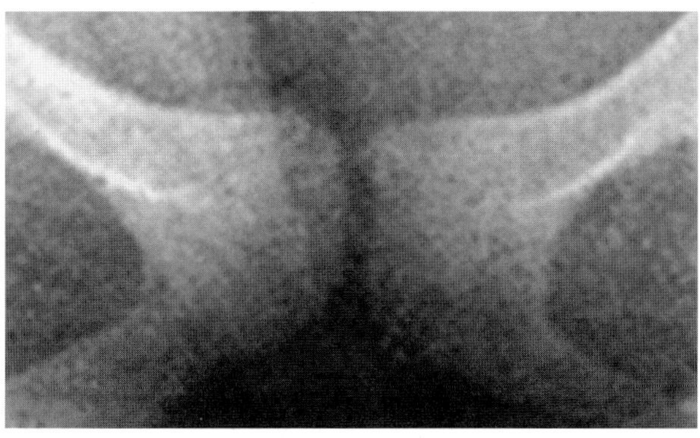

Figure 6-9
A-P pelvic X-ray with the right leg in adduction to 75 degrees. (Detail of Figure 6-11)
The pubis symphysis is showing movement with the left pubic bone superior to the right.

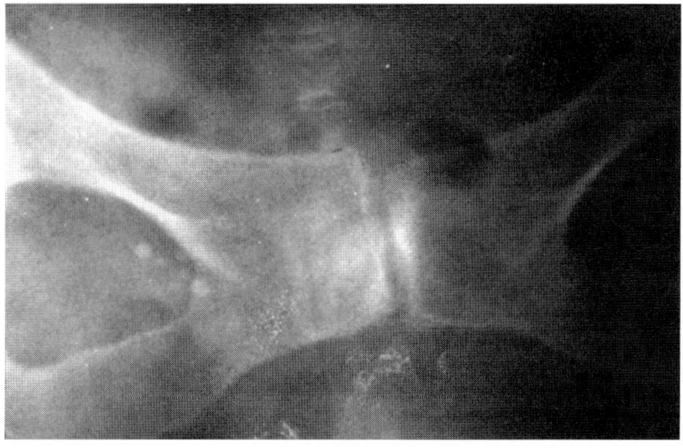

Figure 6-10
(Detail of Figure 6-12)
This subluxation of the pubis symphysis is chronic and sclerosis has occurred. This patient had a long history of groin, hip, and low back pain.

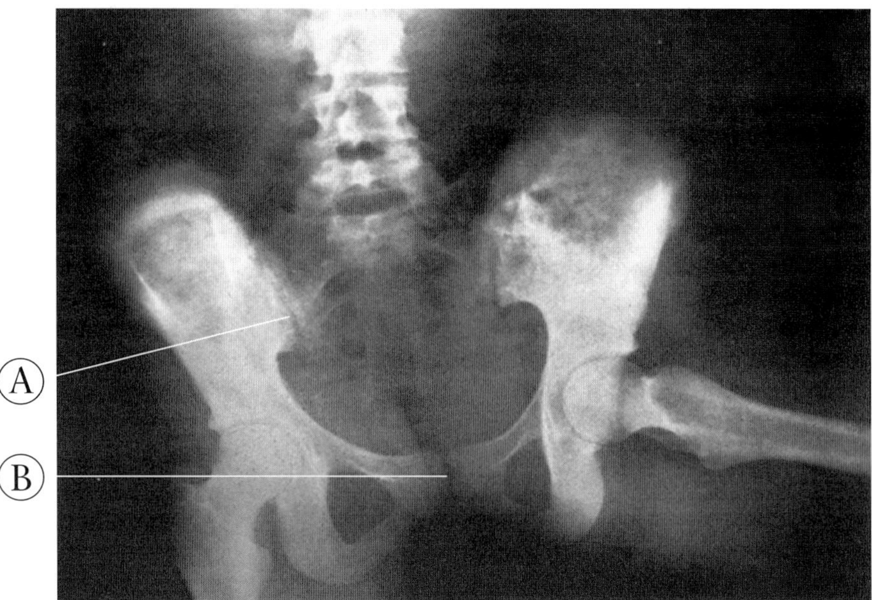

Figure 6-11
A-P pelvic X-ray with the right leg in adduction to 75 degrees.
(Used with permission from the Ilford publishing company.)
The sacroiliac joints can be seen to be asymmetrical with the left SI joint separating more than the right. The pubis symphysis is also showing movement with the left pubic bone superior to the right.
(A) Left sacroiliac joint
(B) Pubis symphysis

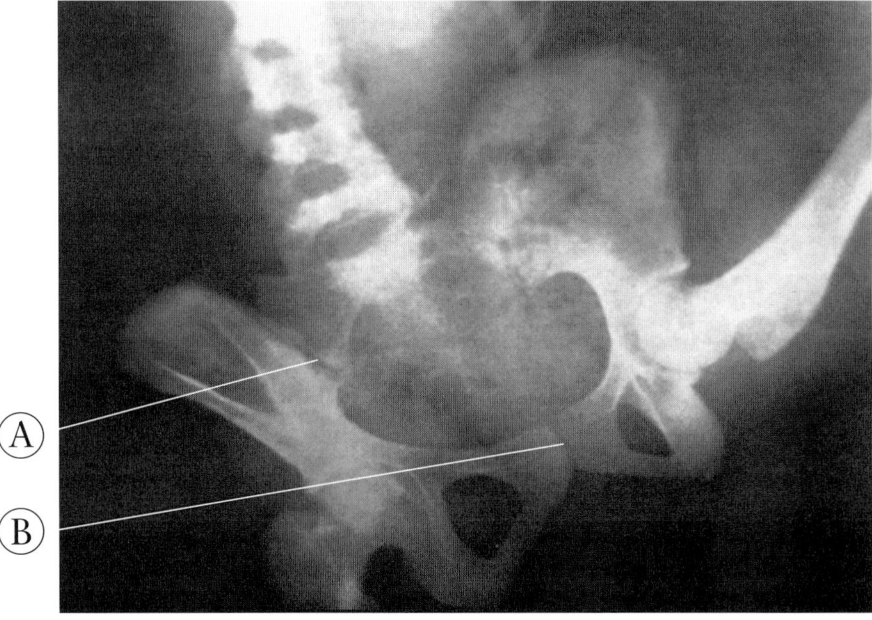

Figure 6-12
A-P pelvic X-ray with the right leg in adduction to 150 degrees.
(Used with permission from the Ilford publishing company.)
The gapping of the left SI joint is more pronounced than the previous picture. The pubis symphysis has continued to show mobility in this position.
(A) Left SI joint
(B) Pubis symphysis

Pelvic Motion

The joints of the pelvic girdle are the strongest in the body. In dynamic studies minor joint motion is seen (**See Figures 6-12 through 6-14**). The X-rays were taken weight bearing. The legs are the levers that move the pelvic joints, not lumbar motion. The last three pictures are positions of extreme motion. These are end range adduction and forward flexion of the hips and require athletic ability. The pelvic motion seen here is normal with leg motion. But the patterns of displacement seen here are commonly also seen in patients with both feet on the floor. The asymmetry of the SI joints and pubis symphysis seen with the patient in a neutral position is a sign of joint failure and a pathological condition. There are many of these "pain" patterns of the pelvic girdle.

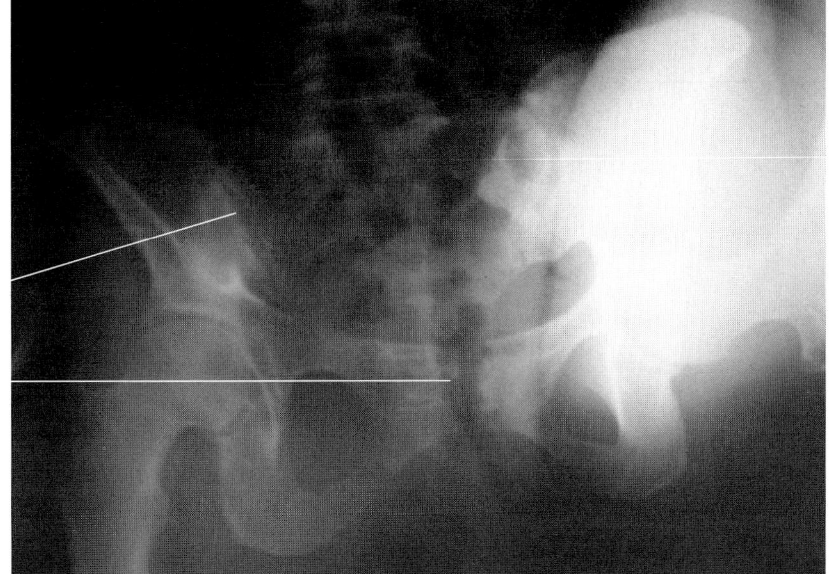

Figure 6-13

A-P pelvic X-ray with the right leg in hyperflexion.
The left SI joint has gapping similar to the previous X-rays. The pubis symphysis is showing some movement.
(A) Left SI joint
(B) Pubis symphysis

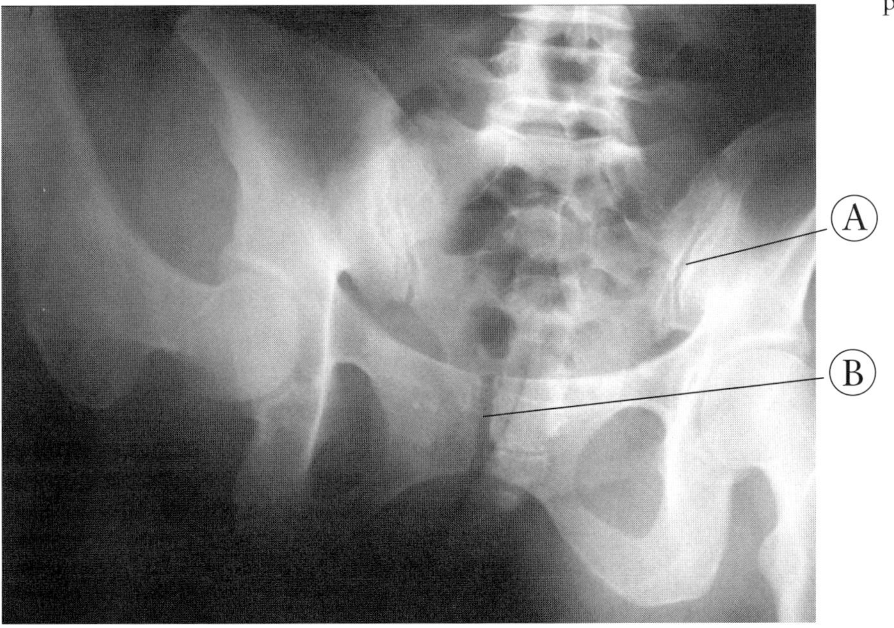

Figure 6-14

A-P pelvic X-ray with the left leg in hyperflexion.
The right SI joint is gapping and showing movement. The pubis symphysis is shifted so the right pubic bone is slightly superior.
(A) The right SI joint
(B) Pubis symphysis

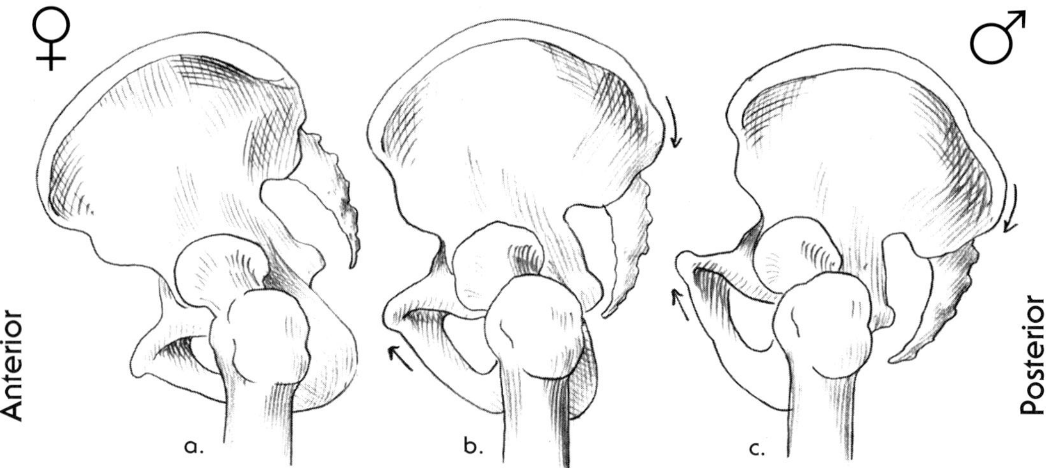

Figure 6-15

This illustrates the range of normal angles of pelvic tilt.
- (a) The anterior tilt is a typical female feature. The sacral base angle approaches zero or is perpendicular to the floor.
- (b) This is a neutral pelvic tilt. This is considered normal but a range of angles between (a) and (c) is commonly found.
- (c) This is a posterior tilt of the pelvis. The sacral base angle can be as high as 45 degrees. This is a typical male tilt. A central X-ray with A to P direction will give different appearances through each of (a), (b), and (c). The appearance on X-ray will change again with comparisons of recumbent and standing or seated views of the same individual.

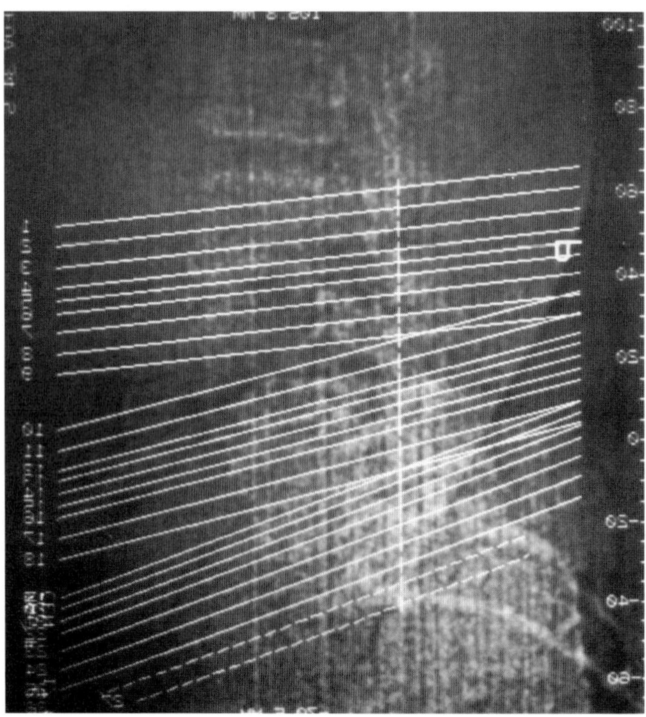

Figure 6-16

This lateral X-ray of the lumbar spine and pelvis have the planes of view of the CAT scan superimposed on it. Note the three different angles of views for the scans. Alignment and symmetry are important to evaluate, but the variety of angles of views can make this task more difficult.

Pelvic Tilt and Imaging

The normal pelvic tilt while standing can vary 45 degrees between the extremes of the anterior and posterior positions (See **Figure 6-15**). The A-P X-ray can show a sacral base almost perpendicular to the central ray of the X-ray or one nearly parallel. The X-ray is really just a shadow picture. This complicates evaluation and diagnosis. This also gives a different appearance on imaging. **Figure 6-16** shows the slices of axial or cross-section pictures in advanced images (MRI or CT Scan). The tilt of the pelvis can change the picture of the pelvic joints. The irregular contours and angles of the sacroiliac joints make easy evaluation impossible. The standing or weight-bearing A-P X-ray can have a different tilt than a recumbent X-ray of the same person. The seated A-P X-rays of the pelvis change the angle yet again. In **Figures 6-17** and **6-18**, the A-P X-rays of an anterior tilt and posterior tilt are shown. The diagnosis is the same for both individuals, but the appearance is different.

Figure 6-17
This is an A-P X-ray of an anterior tilted pelvis with a superior subluxation of the left innominate.
Note the relative alignment of the pubic symphysis; this is because the pubic rami are parallel to the central ray.
 (A) Right innominate
 (B) Right SI joint
 (C) Left innominate
 (D) Left SI joint
 (E) Pubis symphysis

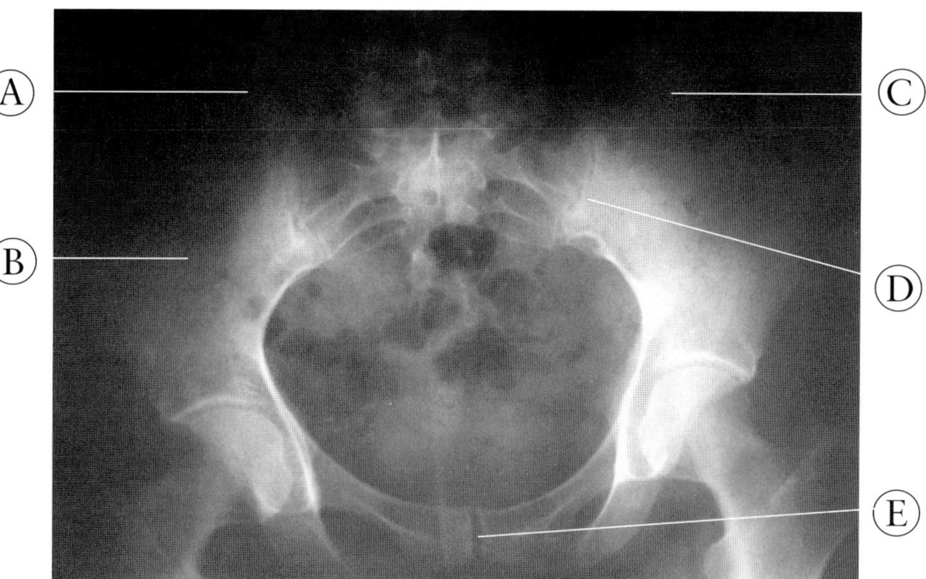

Figure 6-18
This A-P X-ray of a posterior tilted pelvis has a superior left innominate; note the asymmetry of the SI joints and the misalignment of the pubic symphysis. This appearance is possible because the pubic rami are perpendicular to the central ray.
 (A) Right innominate
 (B) Right SI joint
 (C) Left innominate
 (D) Left SI joint
 (E) Pubic symphysis

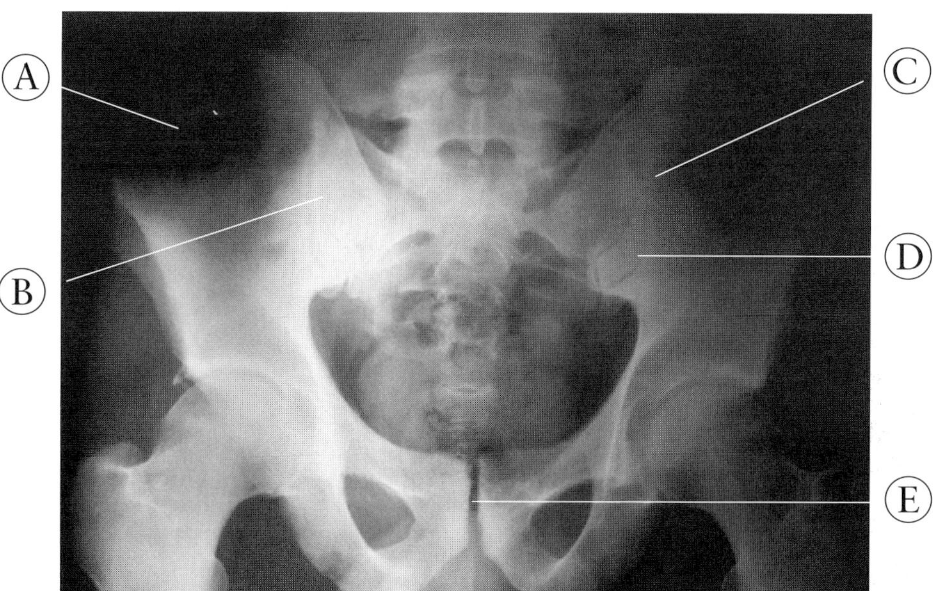

The Lumbosacral Relationship

The occurrence of even significant osteoarthritis in the lumbar spine can be a silent condition. An injury to the pelvis uncovers chronic degeneration and significant subluxa-tions. Remarkable activity levels can be enjoyed with massive joint dysfunction of the lumbar spine. The recent onset of pain can be injury to the pelvic joints (**See Figures 6-19 and 6-20**).

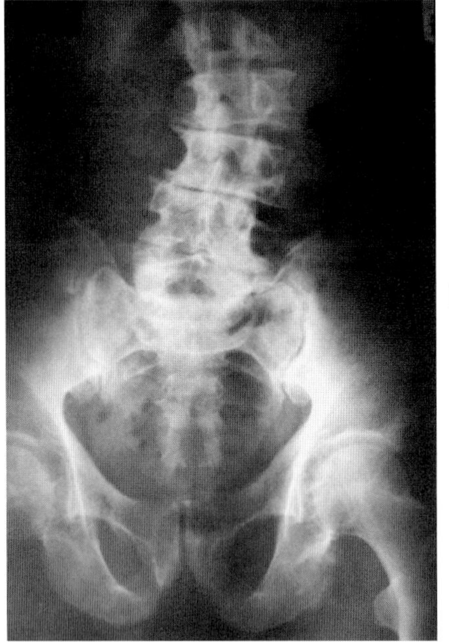

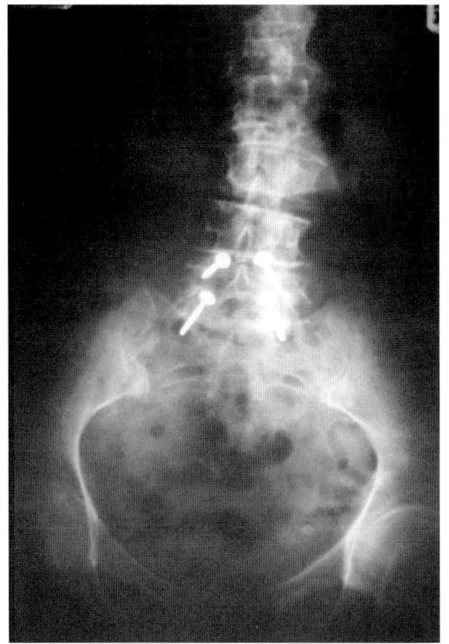

Figure 6-19
PELVIC TILT AND X-RAY APPEARANCE
A complete posterior rotation (right PI with ipsilateral superior pubis)

(a) Has a posterior tilt. The superior pubic rami are seen because they are generally perpendicular to central ray. Subject was an accomplished athlete for decades, and was still working out when film was taken.
(b) Has an anterior tilt and the pubic rami are generally parallel to the central ray. Note: in both cases spinal segments were not tender. The patients claimed very physically active lives and denied "years of pain." Both had the same complaint of right leg pain - rt. SI joint down the back of the leg with recent single event onset. Note the spinal damage and the denial of pain and restriction of activity.

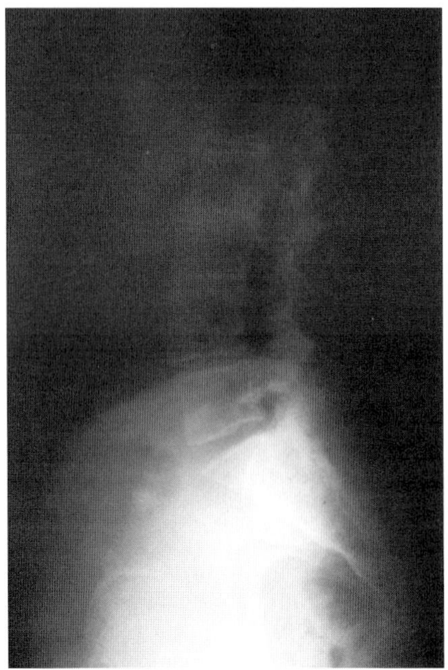

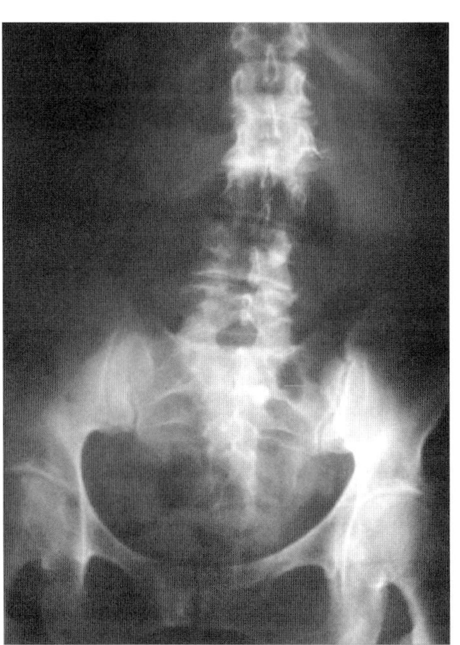

Figure 6-20
PELVIC SHEARING - non physiologic subluxations - VIII
Pelvic shearing in the presence of chronic degenerative osteoarthritis of the lumbar spine

These are A-P and lateral views of the lumbar spine and pelvis of a 72 year old woman who denies any history of back pain prior to a recent garden related event. Note fusion of L2-3 and other changes of the lumbar spine. Subject is a skilled (and regular) ballroom dancer.

PHYSIOLOGICAL SUBLUXATIONS

Figure 6-21 shows an axial plane MRI scan of an individual who complains of right hip and leg pain. The scan is taken with the R indicating the patient's right and the L indicating the patient's left. The top is anterior while the bottom is posterior, with the ilium (or innominates) and sacrum appearing in cross-section (like a slice of bread). This is a perfect example of how subluxations of the pelvic girdle can manifest themselves on MRI. Notice the left ilium is more posterior than the right one; also the sacrum is narrower on the left than it is on the right. This would indicate sacral lateral flexion or tipping to the left, with the apex of the sacrum angled to the right. This pattern is within the physiological limits of the ligaments. It is characterized by limited motion caused by muscle guarding, pain, and reduced symmetry of gait.

This is an example of a subluxation complex of the pelvic girdle. It results in a recognizable pain pattern, and should be viewed as a disease entity stressing the central nervous system, the peripheral nerves and the joints causing proprioceptive guarding of some or all of the muscles attached to the pelvic girdle.

It is important to know that pelvic subluxation can be viewed on advanced imaging. Advanced imaging usually focuses on the lumbar spine, and it is only in the last few panels in the study that part of the pelvic girdle can be seen. It is crucial to pay close attention to those details of the advanced imaging when patients present with pelvic and abdominal complaints, thigh cramps, or pain and tenderness.

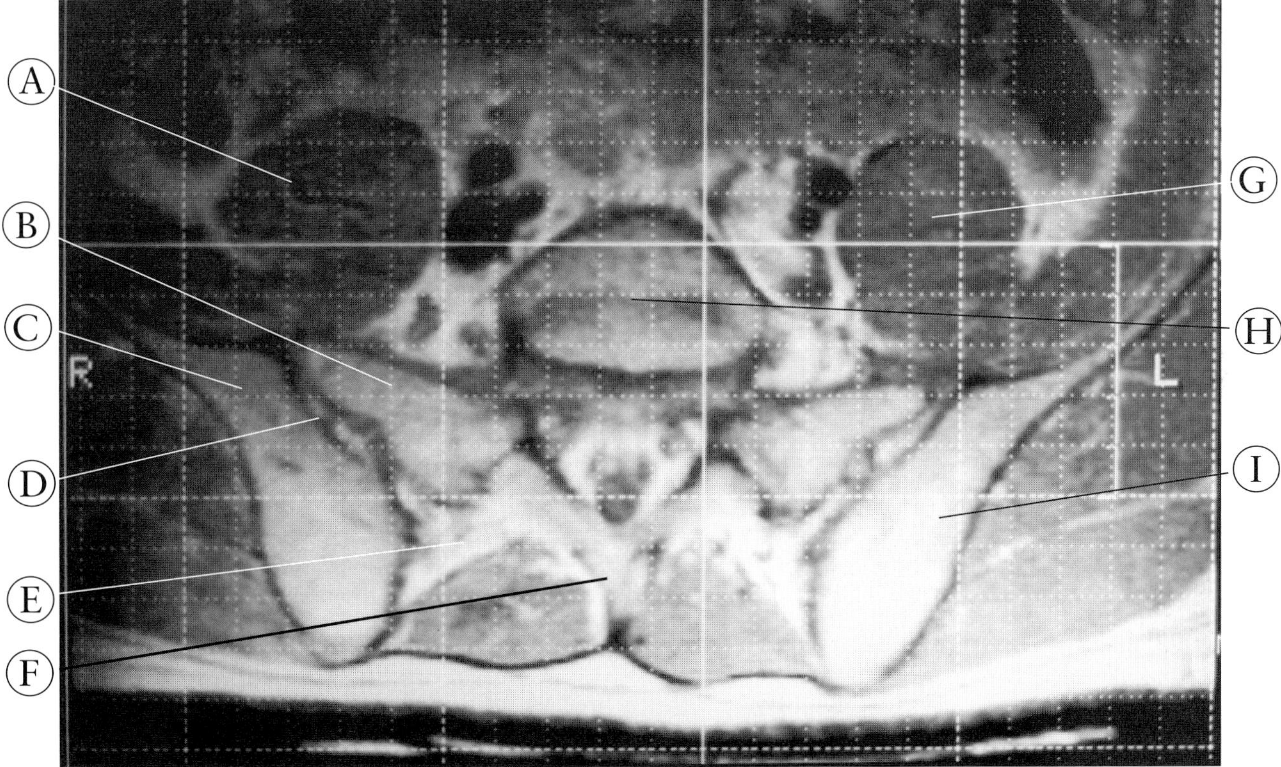

Figure 6-21

This an MRI axial view of the pelvis. The subluxation of the sacrum is seen at the right sacroiliac joint with the right sacral ala anterior of the ilium. Using the grid to evaluate, the sacrum appears rotated or the ilium has moved posteriorly. Also note the difference in the diameter of the right and left psoas, indicating spasm of the right psoas.

(A) Right psoas	(D) Synovial portion of SI joint	(G) Left psoas
(B) Right sacral ala	(E) Fibrous portion of SI joint	(H) Base of sacrum
(C) Right ilium	(F) S1 spinous	(I) Left ilium

Note the common explanation by radiologists of this subluxation complex is: "poor patient positioning." The X-ray technicians say that the patient is flat on their back with arms at the side aligned with the grid as best as possible, "the twists and misalignments are in the patient."

Flexion/Extension Rotation

Flexion/extension (PI/AS) rotation of an innominate around the femoral head is a common pelvic subluxation pattern. The posterior position of the innominate is a normal flexion motion of the hip. The anterior position is an extension of the hip. These subluxation patterns are physiological subluxations. If the degree of rotation is extreme, the pubic symphysis also subluxates as a result. Palpation and X-ray of the pubic symphysis reveals one ramus superior to the other.

NON-PHYSIOLOGICAL SUBLUXATIONS

Evidence from both dissection of cadavers and diagnosis and treatment of patients with pelvic trauma indicates that the innominates can subluxate, independently of one another, in the planes Y and Z. (The Cartesian coordinate system). This condition requires a significant amount of ligament failure or injury. It is not so well known, however, that substantial subluxation or rotation of the innominate can involve the pubic symphysis as well as at the sacroiliac joint. The analysis of the relative positions of the pubic rami at the symphysis is the key to understanding many pelvic subluxation patterns. Variability in pelvic structure among individuals is surprisingly great, and can complicate diagnosis.

In the Y axis, one innominate can translate unilaterally relative to the opposite side, primarily the +SY. (In physics the letter "S" is the symbol for distance or translation). In the Z axis, either +SZ or -SZ can occur. Both cause shearing at the sacroiliac joint and disruption of the pubic symphysis. These patterns of joint disruption exceed the physiological limits of the joints. They can be described as non-physiological subluxations. These injuries will not likely recover to a preinjury condition. The recovery to a functional, but limited, status will take many months to a few years.

Diagnosis of pelvic subluxation is further complicated by individual differences in the sacroiliac joint complexes. Wide variation occurs in the angles and curvatures of the joint complex itself. In some individuals the sacroiliac contact is flat, while in others it may exhibit ridged contours or deep sloping surfaces. The result is that, particularly in X-rays, the same subluxation may look very different among individuals. Conversely, different subluxations may mimic one another, as noted in the example above. **See Figures 6-17 and 6-18.** These two individuals have the same diagnosis: a superior subluxation of the left innominate. The different pelvic tilts leave a completely different X-ray appearance. **Figure 6-17** is a female with an anterior pelvic tilt and **Figure 6-18** is a male with a posterior pelvic tilt (**See Figure 6-15**).

Due to their variety, sacroiliac joints do not lend easily to any form of two-dimensional representation because, in the anatomical position, they are oriented obliquely in all three planes. To make matters even more confusing, the degree of obliqueness shows as much variation as the configuration of the joint surfaces. So, for the purpose of the following discussion, I will use supine and prone recumbent positions as my reference.

Anterior To Posterior Pelvic Shearing

The +Z Or -Z Innominate

The sacroiliac joints narrow from superior to inferior, and from posterior to anterior, so that one innominate can translate in the Z axis relative to the other. See **Figure 6-22**, a depiction of a shearing of one innominate forward relative to the other which involves all three joints with rotation of the sacrum. On X-ray of the anterior pelvis, the subluxation appears to be an inferior translation of the pubic rami. In a neutral or posterior pelvis, the subluxation can be hard to see, although the pubic bone can appear larger on one side. (Translation away from the X-ray film should increase the shadow effect and project a larger image.) This could also be rotation of the pubic rami.

Superior to Inferior Pelvic Shearing

The +Y Or -Y Innominate

Displacement of the innominate in the +Y plane is usually caused by a significant trauma such as falling on one ischium or one foot with the knee extended. This displacement of one innominate relative to the other is, as the B illustration in **Figure 6-23** shows, translation of the whole innominate in the positive Y axis. This results in one innominate being superior to the other. However, the same subluxation can appear to be different in standing AP X-rays, with different pelvic tilts. For instance, the +Y subluxation in an anterior pelvic tilt is not likely to be seen. A physical exam of the pubic symphysis and the other joints and landmarks is the key to analyzing this condition. A superior pubic symphysis is surrounded by ridged,

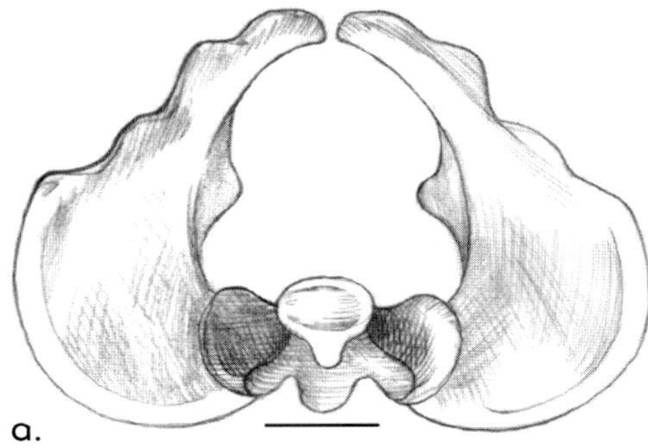
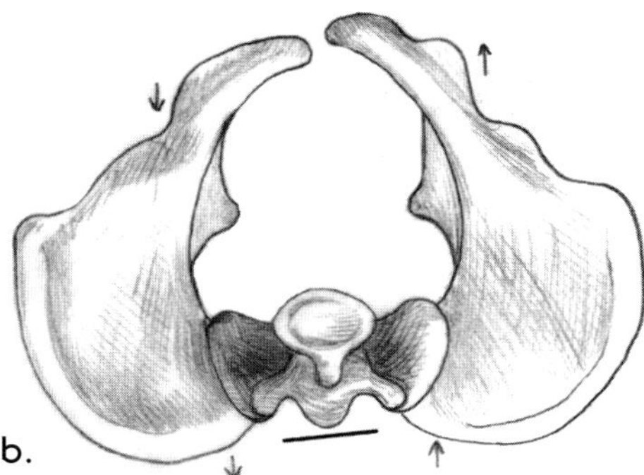

Figure 6-22

PELVIC SHEARING - non physiologic subluxations

This is an illustration of a theoretical view from above looking down on the whole pelvic girdle, not just a slice.
In (a) the three joints of the pelvis are seen, the right and left sacroiliac joints and the pubic symphysis are aligned.
In (b) the right pubic rami is anterior or ventral to the left and the sacrum is rotated. The shearing of the pelvis will have the appearance of positive and negative Z plane translations of one innominate relative to the other in the axial view. This type of injury involves sacral rotation as the right innominate shifts forward or anterior to the left. It is difficult to describe the axis of rotation in the varying pelvic tilts. Pubic symphysis shearing, tearing, and SI joint ligament damage are very likely in this type of injury.

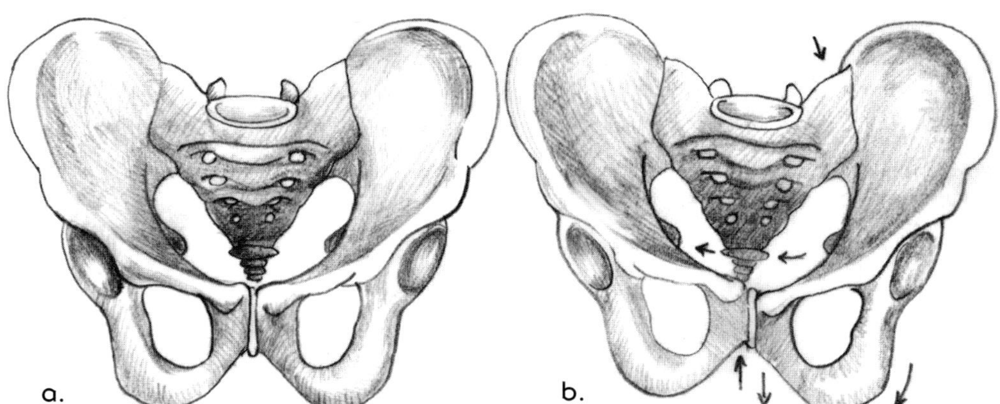

Figure 6-23

PELVIC SHEARING - non physiologic subluxations

(a) is an A to P view of a normal pelvis and (b) is the A-P appearance of a positive Y translation of the innominate on the left relative to the other. (Note the sacrum is tipped and the sacral apex is to the left of the pubic symphysis and the space between the ischial spine and the sacral border.) Also note the subluxation of the pubis symphysis, with the pubic rami on the left being elevated relative to other. I do not feel this an incidental finding. The psoas, iliacus, and all the muscles attaching to the ischium and pubis will be adversely affected.
This type of injury involves sacral shifting with the ala elevating with the superior innominate. This involves pubic symphysis and SI joint injury and intrinsic ligament damage because of the non physiologic displacement of the segments. Possible tearing of the pubis symphysis takes place. Axial imaging views will show the right iliac crest before the left in sequentially inferior views. Rotational displacement can be concomitant with Y or Z plane displacement. Combinations of these subluxation patterns in all planes can be present in one individual.

splinting musculature. The pubis can be tender or not, and palpation can refer pain to the SI joint. Comparison palpation and contact of the ischial tuberosities should indicate that one of the innominates is displaced in the positive Y direction.

Figure 6-24 shows an axial section of a CT scan at the level of S2. This is an advanced diagnostic image of a chronic subluxation of the pelvis. The asymmetry, joint sclerosis, and rotation are all signs pelvic girdle distortion subsequent to trauma. In this case the patient had fallen off of a loading dock 15 years earlier. **Figure. 6-25** is an MRI of the S2 level with the sacrum anterior to both illi. The left is worse than the right. This patient had been hit in a crosswalk by an automobile and suffered a gradual onset of left lower leg paralysis and foot drop. The left innominate was superior to the right. Subluxation of the pelvis can be a significant health factor adversely affecting many systems.

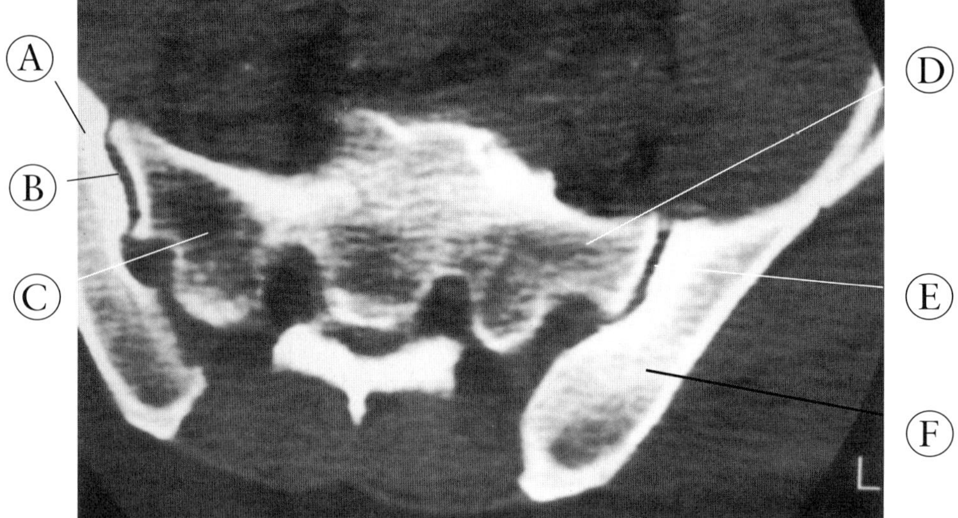

Figure 6-24

This CAT scan of the S2 level shows a subluxation complex of both SI joints. Note the difference in width between the right and left sides of the sacrum. This indicates that the sacrum is tipped. The left side is narrower and therefore a lower level of the sacrum, making the left sacral ala higher and the apex angled towards the left. The left ilium is posterior, larger, and at a different angle than the right innominate. The left SI joint is subluxated with the sacrum anterior to the ilium.

(A) Right ilium	(C) Right side of the sacrum	(E) Left SI joint
(B) Right SI joint	(D) Left side of the sacrum	(F) Left ilium

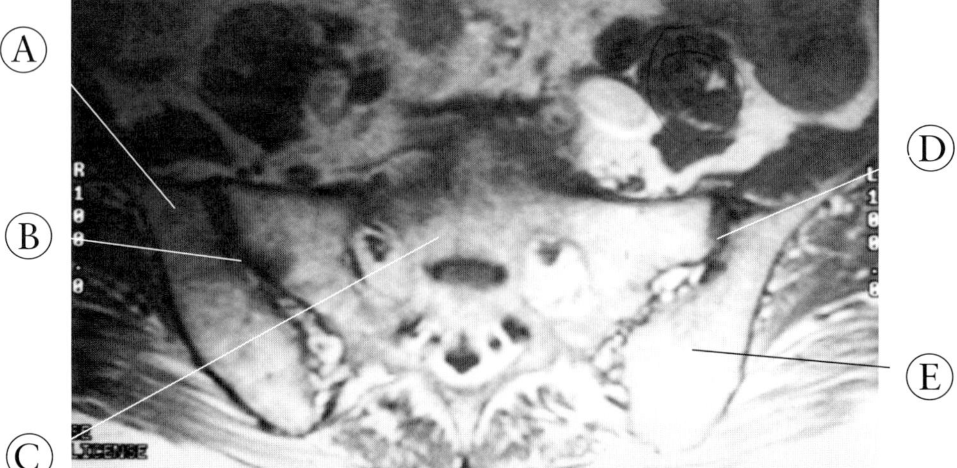

Figure 6-25

This is an MRI of a subluxated pelvis. The left innominate is posterior to the sacrum, the sacrum is rotated, the right side of the sacrum is anterior to the right ilium, and the illi are asymmetrical. This is the appearance of significant pelvic distortion resulting in neurological deficit, altered gait, and muscle atrophy.

(A) Right ilium	(C) Sacrum	(E) Left ilium
(B) Right SI joint	(D) Left SI joint	

Posterior Rotation of the Right Innominate Relative to the Left
A to P X-ray in the supine (recumbent) position.

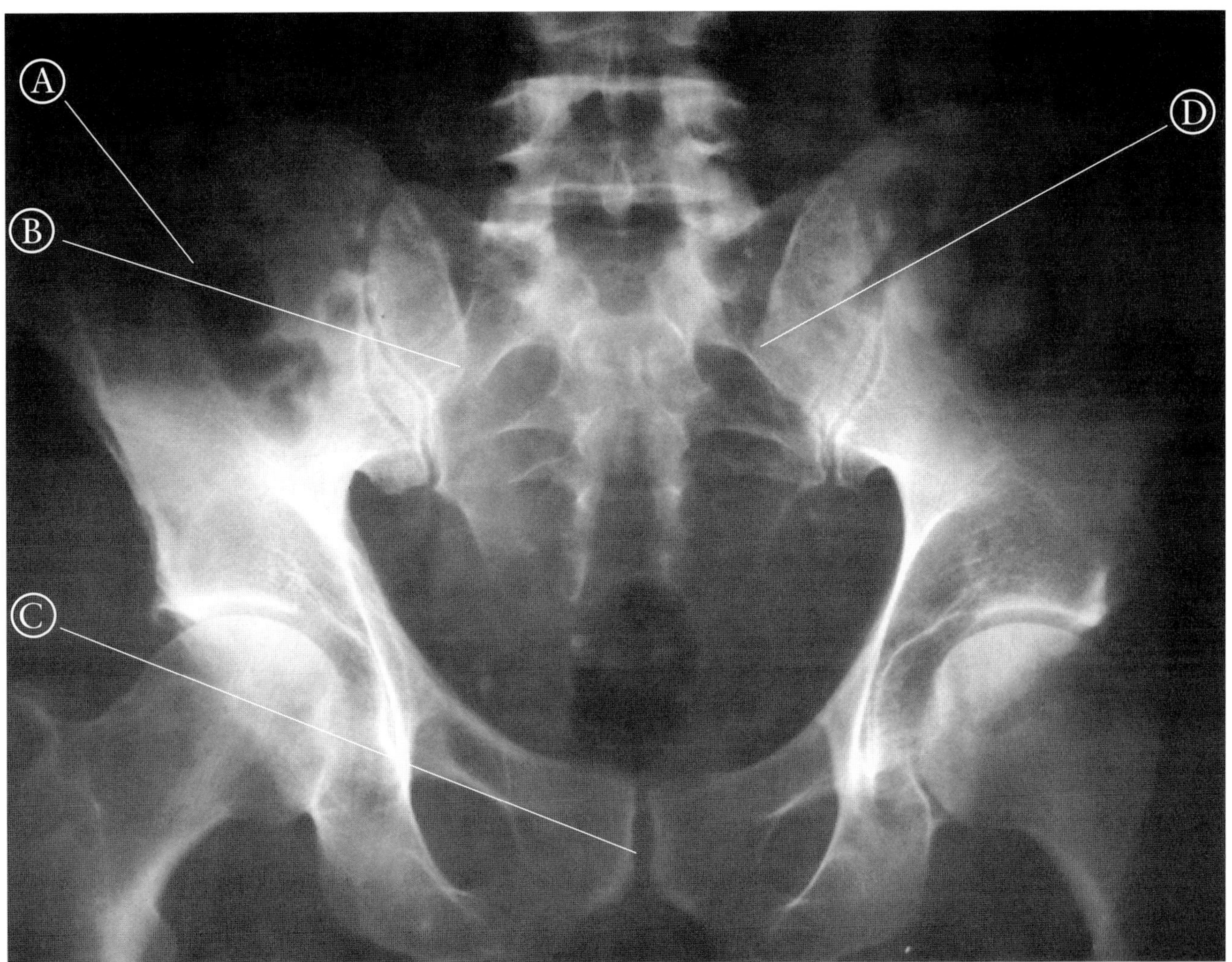

Figure 6-26

POSTERIOR OR FLEXION ROTATION OF ONE INNOMINATE
(a complete rotation of the right innominate or a right PI subluxation)

This is a recumbent view of a posterior pelvic tilt with a complete posterior rotation of the right innominate. The right posterior superior iliac spine (PSIS) is inferior to the left. Note elevation of right pubic rami. Correction of subluxation resulted in immediate relief and ability to walk.

(A) Right innominate
(B) Right posterior superior iliac spine
(C) Subluxated pubic symphysis
(D) Left PSIS

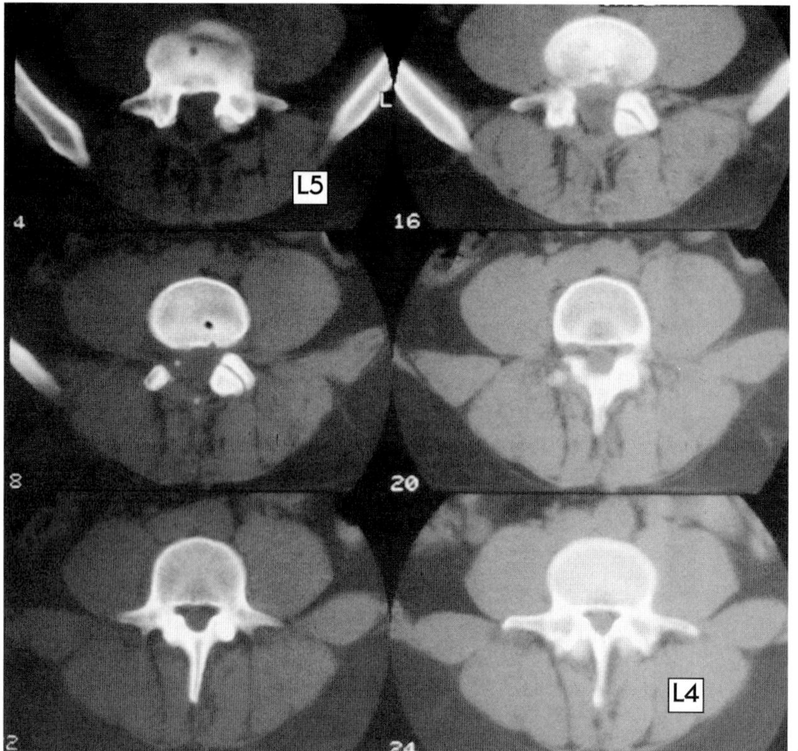

CAT Scan: Axial view

Figure 6-27
ROTATIONAL SUBLUXATIONS -
physiologic subluxations
Positive and negative rotations on the X axis.
This 12 panel series shows right innominate posterior rotation relative to the left and or left anterior rotation. Note the sacral rotation, a subluxation, that accompanies this condition because of the oblique orientation of the sacroiliac joints. Also note the right side is on the reading left, and the top left panel is the most inferior view and bottom right the most superior. Some frames have been labeled to help indicate level of image.
    (A)Posterior right ilium
Left   (B)Left ilium

a.

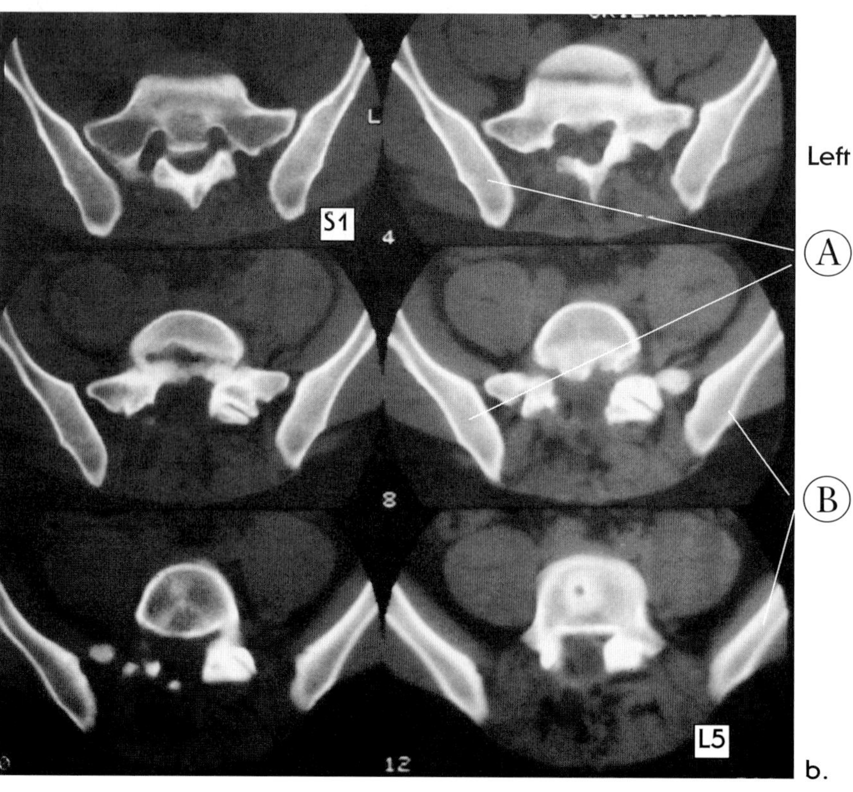

b.

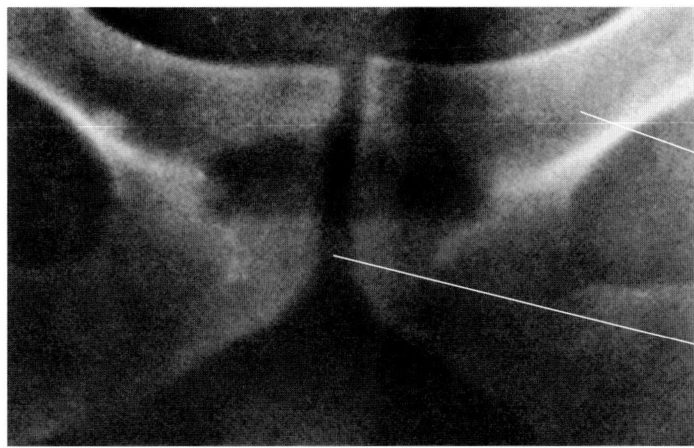

Pelvic Shearing:
Non-physiological subluxations

Figure 6-28
Subluxation of pubis symphysis
(A) Left pubic body
(B) Pubic symphysis

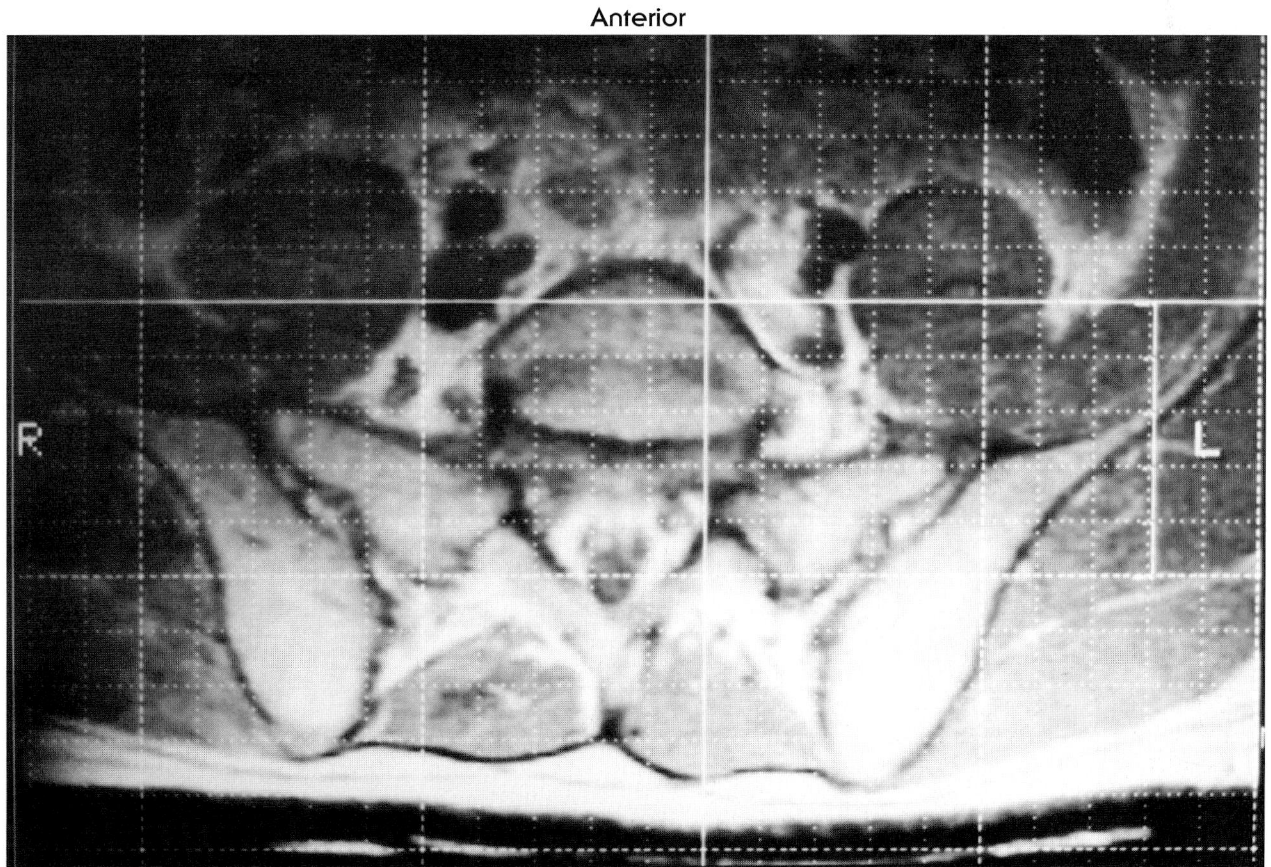

Figure 6-29
MRI and X-ray appearance of combinations of shearing and rotation
In the MRI the right innominate is anterior (+Z) to the left but is posterior to the sacrum indicating a rotation (rt PI) combination of subluxations. In the X-ray, the left innominate is superior (+Y) to the right side.

Pelvic Shearing: non-physiological subluxation of pelvis

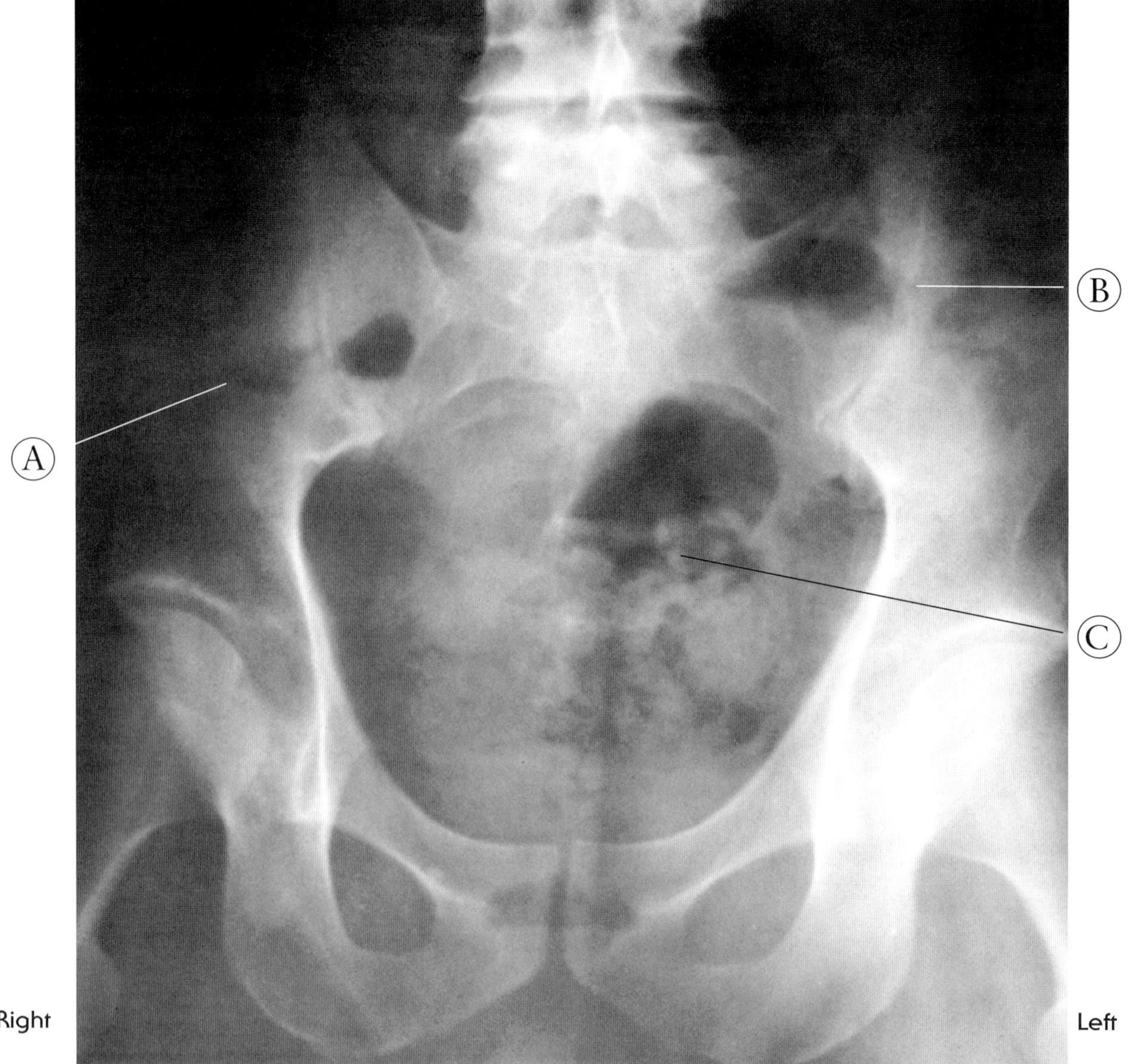

Figure 6-30
Standing A-P pelvic X-ray of a subluxated pelvis

This is an example of pelvic shearing, a non-physiological subluxation that must include ligament damage. The left innominate has superior (a +Y displacement) subluxation, but in the standing position appears lower. The acetabulum has moved up but the foot still has to be on the ground, angling and tipping the pelvis.

Note the sacrum is in the left side of the pelvic rim.

  (A) Right innominate
  (B) Left innominate
  (C) Sacrum

Superior subluxation of left innominate

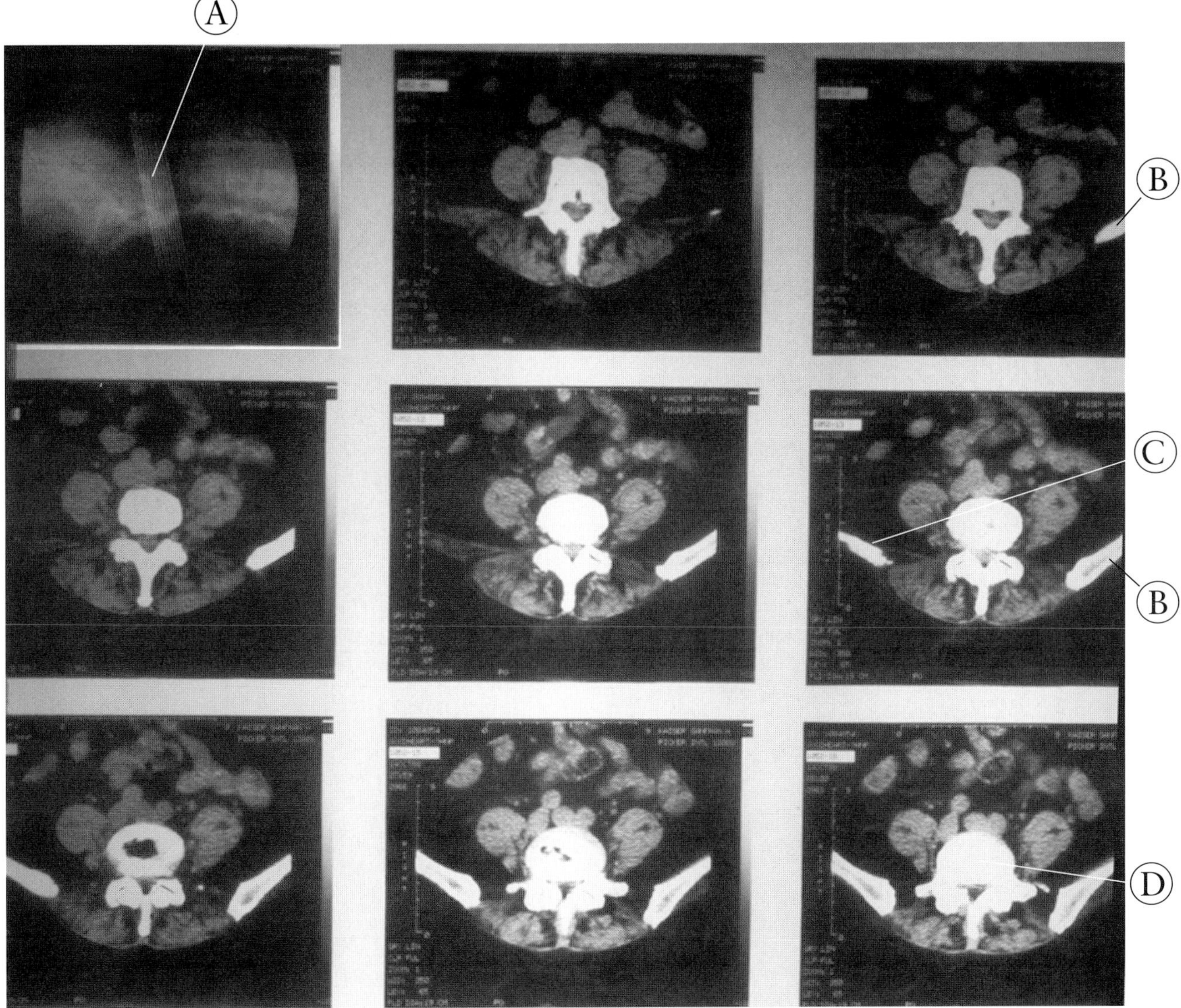

Figure 6-31
PELVIC SHEARING - non physiologic subluxations - V

This CT scan shows the top of the left iliac crest in the upper right panel. The second far right panel shows the top of the right iliac crest. This indicates a 15mm difference in height. A superior or +Y subluxation of the left innominate is present. Symptoms included severe left buttock, hip, and leg pain. The patient was referred to an orthopedic surgeon who recommended surgery of the lumbar spine.

(A) Planes of orientation of the scan shown with supine lateral lumbar X-ray
(B) Left iliac crest
(C) Right iliac crest
(D) L5

Superior subluxation of right innominate

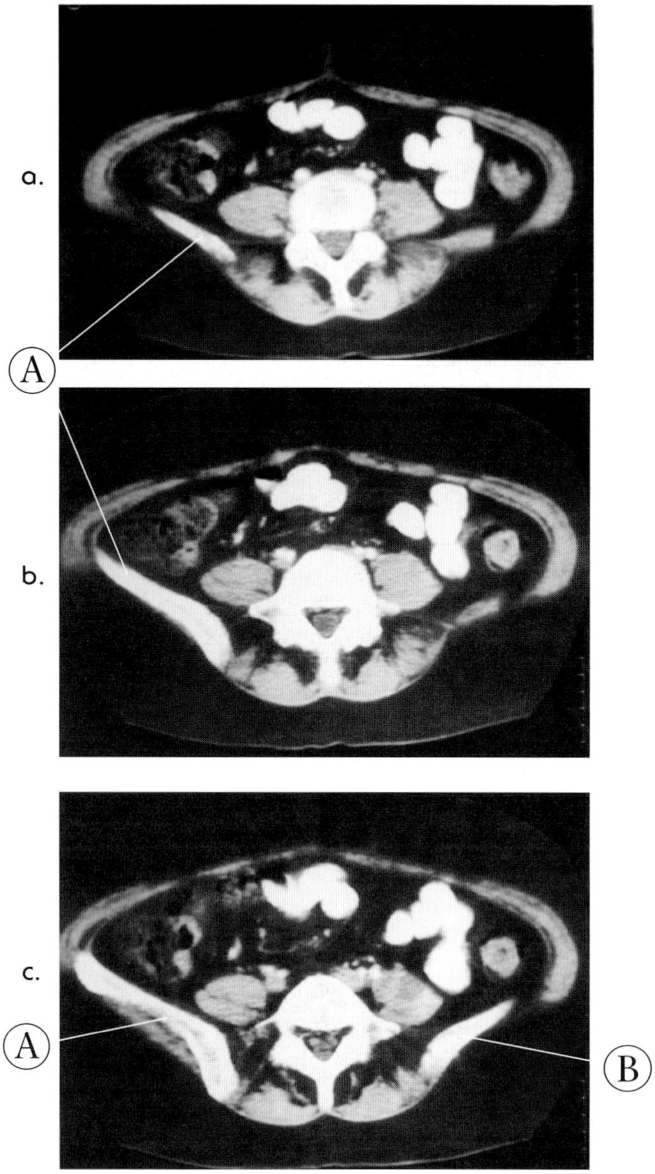

Figure 6-32

PELVIC SHEARING - non physiologic subluxation - IX
This is a CT scan of top of pelvis with right innominate +Y or superior subluxation.
The patient walks with a gait and has abnormalities that are improved with the correction of +Y right innominate translation.
  (A) Right innominate
  (B) Left innominate

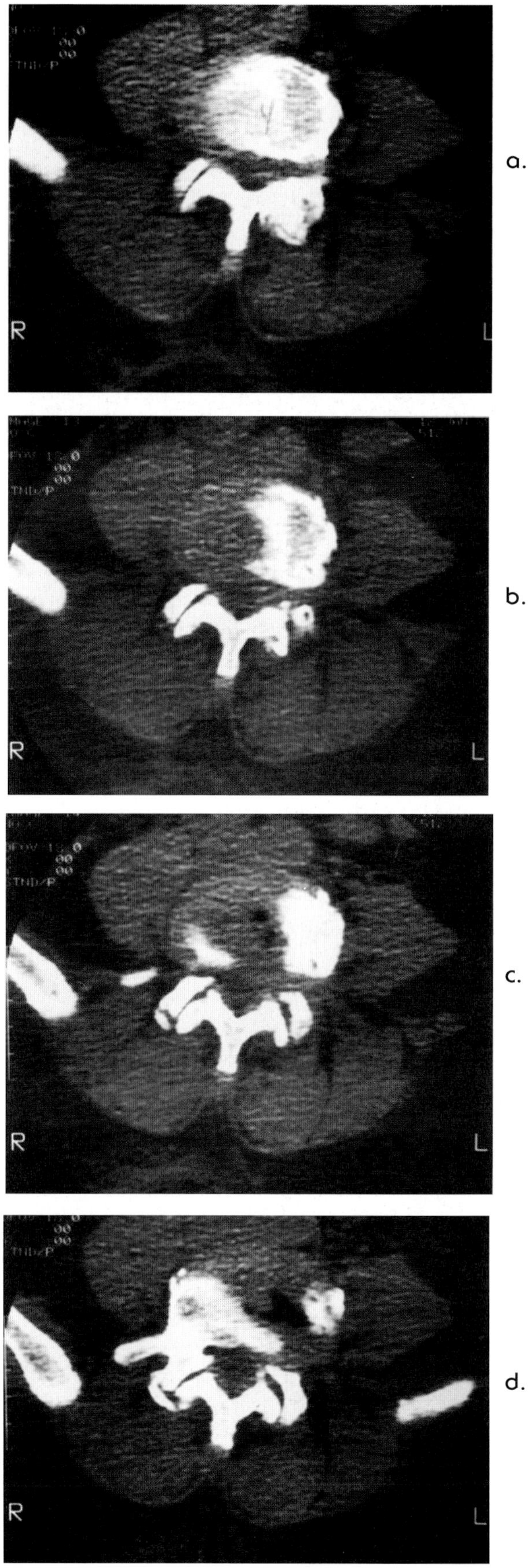

Figure 6-33

PELVIC SHEARING - non physiologic subluxation - X
Right innominate has +Y translation. Note left rotation and lateral flexion of L4&5 due to superior elevation of right side of sacral ala. Note black spaces in discs in panels two and four of discs L4-5 and L5-S1. Patient walked with cane and had obvious gait abnormality.

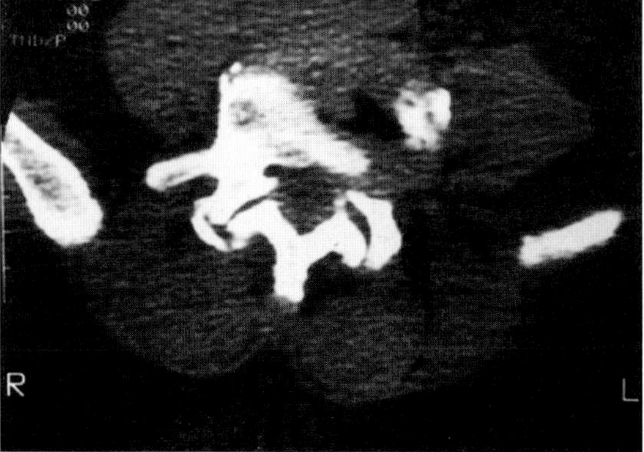

The Geriatric Pelvis

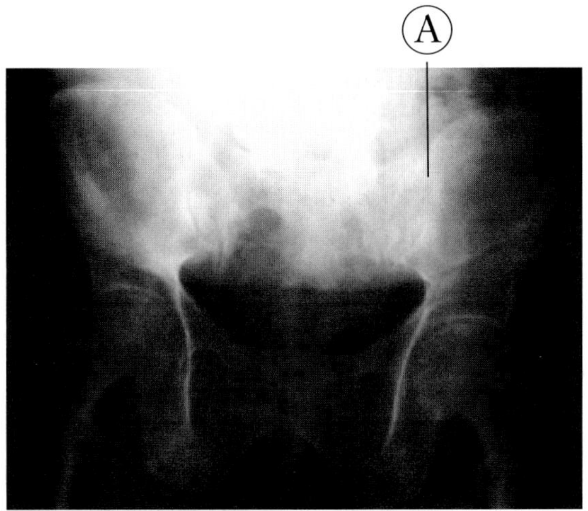

Figure 6-34

Multiple injuries have rendered this 84 year old man unable to walk. Note the asymmetry of the sacroiliac joints and the misalignment of the pubic symphysis. This is an example of superior (+Y) and anterior (+Z) shearing of the left innominate. The muscles of the hip, thighs, abdomen, and back were all rigid and painful. The patient was flexed at the hip as well as in knees and needed assistance to move. Correction of the pelvic subluxations allowed this individual to walk unaided.

(A) Left sacroiliac joint

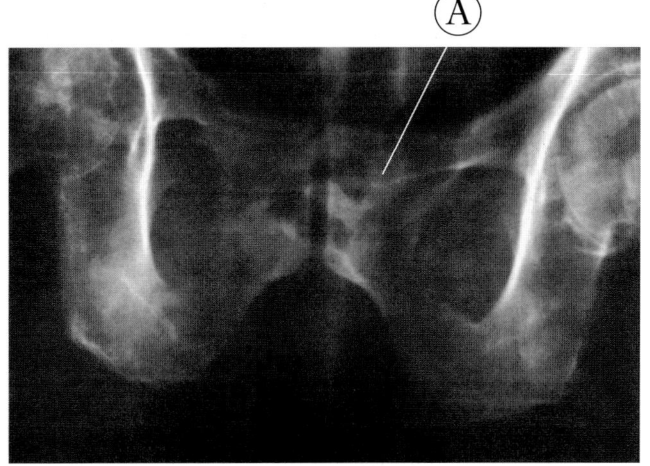

Figure 6-34 A
Detail from same study as Figure 6-34

Note shift of the left pubic bone upward relative to the right. This can result in spasms of the psoas, rectus abdominus, and thigh muscles.

(A) Left pubic bone

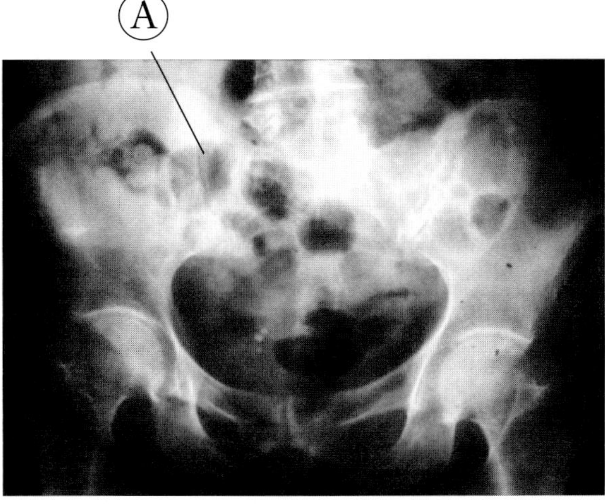

Figure 6-35

This 82 year old has a history of many falls, requires a walker, and moves slowly in a flexed forward position. Note the asymmetry of the sacroiliac joints and pubic symphysis. This is an example of a superior (+Y) and anterior (+Z) right innominate with a significant left innominate posterior rotation.

(A) Right sacroiliac joint

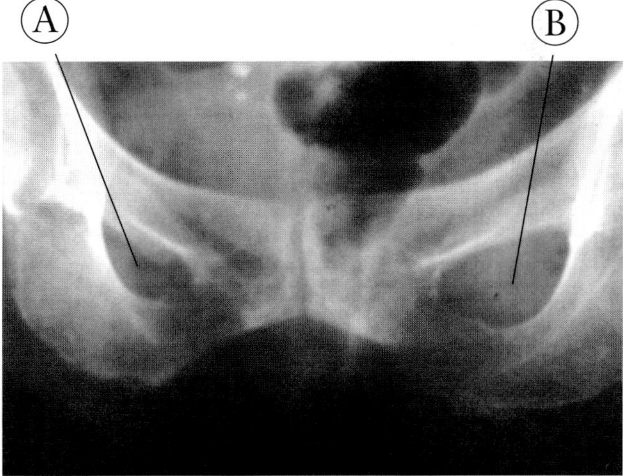

Figure 6-35 A
Detail from same study as Figure 6-35

Note the significant difference in the shape of the obturator foramen and the height of the pubic bones. This indicates rotation has taken place between the two innominates.

(A) Right obturator foramen
(B) Left obturator foramen

Intrasacral Subluxations

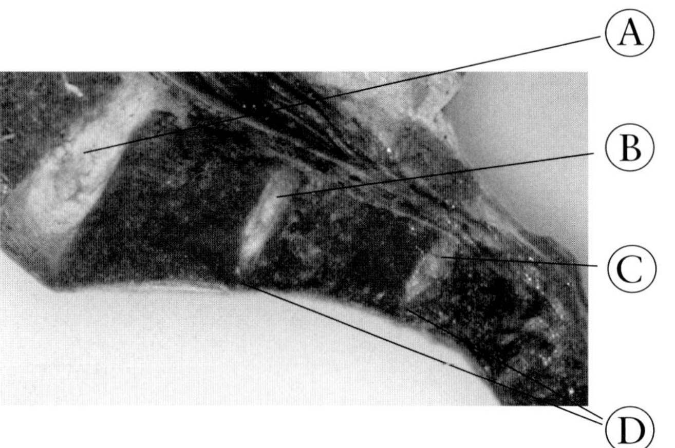

Figure 6-36
Most individuals have sacral discs. This would indicate sacral motion is normal.
Note the L5-S1, S1-2, and S2-3 discs are all present with the beginning signs of degeneration. The annular walls are darker and the cortical borders of the sacral discs are thickened.
  (A) L5-S1 disc
  (B) S1-2 disc
  (C) S2-3 disc
  (D) Cortex of sacrum

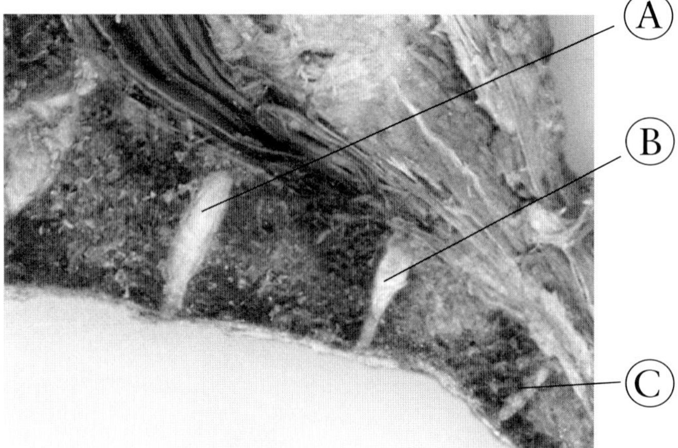

Figure 6-37
Shown are sacral discs in an elderly specimen. Note the discs between the segments of S1 and S2, S2 and S3, and S3 and S4. The avascular structures confer motion and need motion to persist late into life.
Note the loss of anterior disc height at the S2-3 disc and the angling of S3.
  (A) S1-2 disc
  (B) S2-3 disc
  (C) S3-4 disc

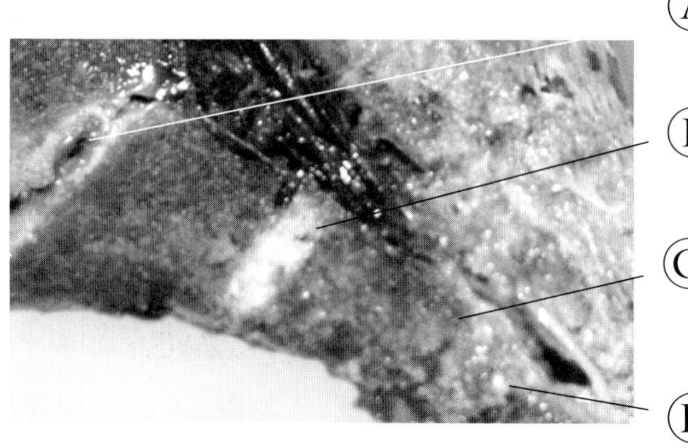

Figure 6-38
A sacral disc with degenerative joints above and below. The L5-S1 is sheared and degenerating because of the subluxation of L5 posteriorly.
Note the appearance of S3 being slightly anterior to S2 suggesting an intrasacral subluxation.
  (A) L5-S1 disc
  (B) S1-S2 disc
  (C) Site of S2-S3 fusion
  (D) S3

Intrasacral Subluxations

Figure 6-39

This shows a sacral disc with end stage degeneration above and below. The L5-S1 joint has sheared and fused. L5 is posterior to the sacrum. The S1-2 disc is dehydrated and the cortical bone has thickened. S3 is angled in ventral direction and the S2-3 disc is gone.

(A) L5
(B) S1
(C) S1-2 disc
(D) S2
(E) S3

Figure 6-40

This a picture of a sacral disc with a healthy L5-S1 joint and a fused S2-3 joint. The L5-S1 disc is slightly wedged anteriorly. The S1-2 disc is dehydrated and reduced in substance with a thickening of the cortical bone. S2 is angled in a dorsal direction.

(A) L5-S1 disc
(B) S1
(C) Thickened cortex
(D) S2

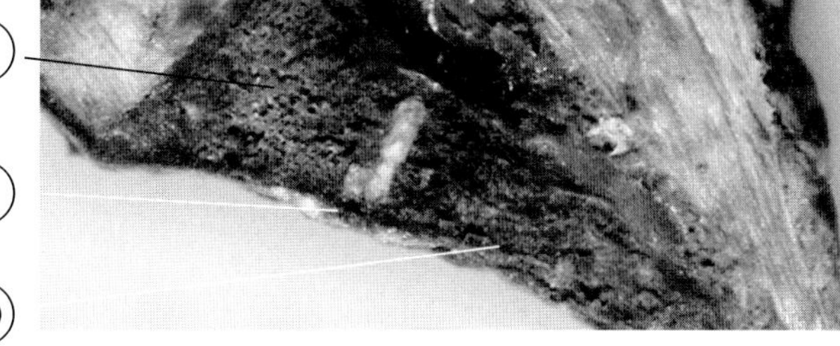

Figure 6-41

This specimen has a significant subluxation of S1 anterior to L5 with fusion. The S1-2 disc has barely persisted and the cortical bone has thickened.

(A) L5
(B) L5- S1 disc
(C) S1
(D) S1-2 disc
(E) Thickened cortex

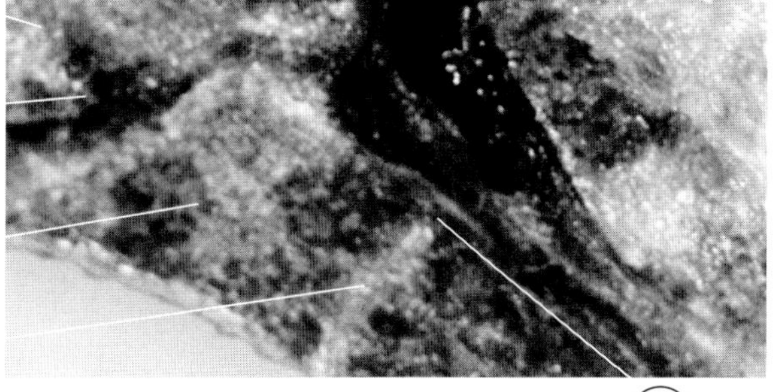

GLOSSARY

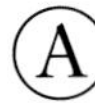

A

abdominal oblique muscles: internal and external

The external oblique originate at the lower eight ribs and insert at the iliac crest and linea alba (midline aponeurosis). Contraction of both compresses the abdomen. Contraction of one side alone laterally bends and rotates the vertebral column.

Innervated at the branches of thoracic nerves T7-T12 and iliohypogastric nerve.

The internal oblique originate at the iliac crest, inguinal ligament, and the thoracolumbar fascia, and insert at the cartilage of the last three or four ribs and linea alba. Contraction acts as external oblique. Innervated at the branches of thoracic nerves T8-T12, iliohypogastric nerve, and ilioinguinal nerves. A disruption in the pelvic girdle integrity will cause these muscles to partially or fully contract causing a disruption in the spinal curves by the massive muscle guarding.

absolute motion

A localized movement that affects the entire vertebral column. A movement in the cervical region globally affects the rest of the spine.

acetabulum

A deep, cup-shaped depression on the anterolateral surface of the pelvis, formed internally by the os pubis, superiorly by the ilium, posteroinferiorly by the ischium, and anteroinferiorly by the pubis. The head of the femur articulates here.

adaptive response

An adaptive response to subluxation is muscle guarding and a concomitant shortening of muscles and ligaments over time. An adaptive response, either anticipated or observed, is reason for care.

A to P

Anterior to posterior direction in taking and viewing X-rays.

adhesions

A joining of parts normally free to move independently to each other. This occurs as part of the inflammatory response to injury or irritation due to subluxations or other factors. The adhesions form by the edema's components coagulating in-between the tissues.

A.L.L.

Anterior longitudinal ligament

altered weight bearing

In the vertebral curve, normal weight bearing at each joint is balanced between three points, two facets and one body. Altering the weight bearing capacity of one or more points will alter the shape of the joint, alter the motion of the joint, and alter the surrounding tissue.

annulus fibrosus

The outer concentric layers of fibrocartilage which contain the nucleus pulposus in the intervertebral disc. Tearing or herniation of the annulus fibrosus changes the hydraulic capacity of the segments and can be concomitant with subluxation.

anterior

At or near the front of the body; ventral

anterior longitudinal ligament

A broad ligament that extends from the occipital bone to the sacrum. It supports the vertebral column and unites the vertebrae anteriorly.

anterior spinal artery

Supplies blood to the major substance of the spinal cord. Subluxation can block the anterior spinal artery and will cause the spinal cord to become hypoxic.

anterolisthesis

Anterior displacement of a vertebra with loss of joint integrity.

antero/posterior

Directed from the front toward the back.

apex

1. The outermost point of a convexity.
2. The apex of the sacrum is at the bottom where it joins with the coccyx.

arachnoid

The inside covering of the thecal wall. The presence of a subdural space indicates a pathology.

arthritis

Inflammation of a joint. The most common arthritic inflammatory condition of the spine is characterized by subluxation.

articulation

A joint. Indicates motion between two or more bones. Tissues associated with articulation depend on motion for their health.

atlantoaxial

Pertaining to the joint or space between the atlas and axis, the first two cervical vertebrae.

atlas

The first cervical vertebra, C1, having a two-point weight bearing system, lacking a body, and articulating superiorly with the occipital condyles of the occipital bone, which permits nodding of the head. The atlas articulates differently with C2, the axis, at the inferior articular facets.

autonomic nervous system

A division of the nervous system comprised of a series of reflex areas that control involuntary motor functions and innervate the heart, glands, viscera, and smooth muscle.

avascular

Lacking a direct supply of blood; oxygen, carbon dioxide, nutrients, and waste all diffuse through connective tissue via motion.

axial

1. Pertaining to the axis, C2.

2. Pertaining to the axial plane of the Cartesian coordinate system, the Y plane.

3. Pertaining to the axial skeleton, consisting of the bones of the skull, hyoid, ribs, sternum, and vertebral column.

axial loading

A mechanism of injury to the cervical spine in which an axially directed load exerts a longitudinally compressive force that results in a fracture of a mid-cervical vertebral body. This compression can be from the top-down or from the bottom-up.

axis

The second cervical vertebra, C2, is the first three-point weight bearing system in the vertebral column. The dens of the axis projects through the atlas, C1, and makes a pivot on which the head and atlas rotate, permitting side-to-side rotation of the head. The axis articulates superiorly with the atlas at the two superior articular facets and inferiorly with C3 at the two inferior articular facets and the body of the vertebra via the intervertebral disc.

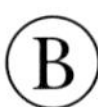

brain stem

The portion of the brain immediately superior to the spinal cord, made up of the medulla oblongata, pons, and midbrain. The brain stem is contiguous with the spinal cord and subject to forces initiated in the vertebral column. The blood supply to the brain stem is dependent on the integrity of the vertebral artery.

buckling

Deformation of an architectural structure due to rapid acceleration or deceleration of only part of the structure. This would be a good replacement term for "whiplash."

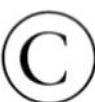

calcified

Crystallized and hardened tissues caused by the infiltration of tricalcium phosphate, calcium carbonate, and magnesium salts. They are deposited in the framework formed by the collagenous fibers of the matrix of a tissue. This can be a normal response to stress or a response to abnormal stress.

calcification

The process of deposition of mineral salts within a tissue or structure.

canal stenosis

The narrowing of the spinal canal.

1. A congenital condition, a narrower canal than normal, can be a silent condition until injury occurs.

2. A developed or acquired spinal canal stenosis is a result of subluxation of vertebrae and the subsequent widening endplates.

capillaries

A tiny, thin-walled blood vessel that connects arterioles and venules through which materials are exchanged between blood and tissue cells. The capillaries form a network or plexus in almost all the body's tissues. Blood flow is linked to the motion of the tissue, which act as a pump.

capsule

Joint capsule. The membrane that encloses a joint to form a closed cavity. It is primarily collagen fibers with a synovial membrane covering the inside and it is embedded with nerve endings of various types. Distress of this structure can result in reflex guarding of the muscle and tendon complexes that are involved.

cartilage

A specialized connective tissues composed of fibers and homogenous matrix containing various cells including chondrocytes that lie in spaces or lacunae in the matrix. The matrix can be white or gray, usually semiopaque, consisting chiefly of proteoglycans and collagen fibers, and is produced by cells called chondrocytes.

The matrix is avascular (without blood supply) and relies on movement to maintain its health and integrity. Hyaline cartilage is smooth in appearance and is found at the articulating facets of the vertebrae. Fibrocartilage is fibrous in appearance due to interlacing fibrous tissue strands in the matrix. It is found as transitional material from bone to the intervertebral disc material as well as the pubis symphysis.

Cartesian coordinate system

A three-dimensional coordinate system in which the coordinates of a point are its distances from three intersecting perpendicular straight lines or planes. These are described as the X, Y and Z axes or planes. It is used to describe position in human anatomy.

caudae equinae

Nerve rootlets of the spinal nerves that arise off the lower portion of the spinal cord in the lower thoracic and upper lumbar regions. It is the Latin for horse's tail, which it looks like. These hair-like fibers form the lumbar, sacral and coccygeal nerve roots.

cavitation

The formation of a cavity in the intervertebral disc by pathological processes. The degeneration of tissues of the disc can be initiated by shearing, loss of movement, and hyperloading which interrupts the nutrient pump.

central nervous system

The brain and spinal cord. The part of the nervous system that is contained in the skull and vertebral column.

cerebellum

The portion of the brain lying posterior to the medulla and pons, concerned with coordination of movement. Damage can cause ataxia (lack of muscle coordination), disturbance of gait, and severe dizziness. The position of the cerebellum in the occiput can be changed with vertebral column changes. The blood supply is vertebral artery dependent.

cerebrospinal fluid

This plasma like fluid continuously circulates through the ventricles of the brain and spinal canal surrounding the spinal cord in the subarachnoid space. The motion of the vertebral column and sacrum is the supposed mechanism of circulation.

cervical

Of or pertaining to the neck.

cervical curve

An essential architectural feature of the human spine. Changes in the shape of the cervical spine result in central nervous system deformation and joint pathology. The cervical curve is lordotic or the convex side of the curve is ventral.

cervicogenic

Symptoms produced from problems in the neck, i.e., cervicogenic headaches, unilateral cervicogenic deafness.

chronic

Long-term or frequently recurring.

chronic inflammation

A long-term, localized protective response to tissue injury designed to destroy, dilute, or wall off an infecting agent or injured tissue. Characterized by redness, pain, heat, swelling, and reduced or loss of function. Loss of joint integrity generates an inflammatory response.

clavicle

The collarbone. The medial end of the clavicle, the sternal extremity, is rounded and articulates with the sternum. The broad, flat, lateral end, the acromial extremity, articulates with the acromion of the scapula. These articulations are primarily ligaments and capsules and form the only bony articulation of the pectoral girdle to the chest.

clivus

The anterior portion of the occipital bone. It forms the front part of the foramen magnum. The dens of the axis attaches to the clivus.

coccyx

The most inferior portion of the spine, attached to bottom of the sacrum. It is the fusion of the three or four coccygeal vertebrae and is triangular in shape. The sacrococcygeal ligament is contiguous with the sacrotuberous ligaments.

compression fracture

A fracture due to impact loading in which the bone has been crushed. Seen in the vertebral bodies of osteopenic patients.

conductivity

The ability of a tissue to conduct a current or nerve impulse.

congenital stenosis

A narrowing of an opening or passage due to inherited variations.

contracture

1. A state of deformation and shortening of a soft tissue, such as a muscle or tendon, so that it cannot passively attain its normal length.

2. A state of diminished or loss of compliance of a normally pliant tissue. A shortening with a decrease range of motion, a common feature of chronic subluxation.

conus medularis

The inferior end of the spinal cord. It is tapered or cone-shaped and ends at the level of the intervertebral disc between the first and second lumbar vertebrae in the adult.

coronal

1. The frontal plane. It divides the body into anterior (front) and posterior (back) portions.

2. The X-Y plane in the Cartesian coordinate system.

cortex

1. The dense bone that forms the external surface of a bone called cortical bone.

2. The outer part of an organ.

cortical bone

The dense outer wall of a bone.

costotransverse

Pertaining to the ribs and transverse processes of the vertebrae. The transverse process is posterior to the rib and articulates with the neck of the rib.

costo-vertebral

Of or pertaining to a rib and a vertebrae. The typical costo-vertebral joint (T2-T10) is a three joint complex made up of the head of the rib, superior and inferior demifacets, and the intervertebral disc.

CNS

Central nervous system.

cross section

1. A section formed by a plane cutting through an object, usually at right angles to an axis.

2. Usually the X-Z plane of the Cartesian coordinate system.

cranium/cranial

The cranium can be defined as the bones of the skull that protects the brain and the organs of sight, hearing, and balance, including the frontal, parietal, temporal, occipital, sphenoid, and ethmoid bones. Cranial can be defined as a subdivision of the superior body cavity formed by the cranial bones and containing the brain.

degeneration

The process of the loss of normal function of the cells of a tissue. A pathological process of a progressive nature.

degenerative joint disease

A chronic joint condition characterized by a loss of normal integrity, space or height, articular cartilage, and motion. The process causes bone hypertrophy, and new bone in the margins of the joint, particularly the weight-bearing joints. The most common pathological feature of this condition is subluxation and resulting loss of joint space.

dehydration

The loss of water from any tissue or from the body.

demifacet

A thoracic vertebral body structure that articulates with the heads of the ribs.

dens

A toothlike process projecting upward from the body of the second cervical vertebra that articulates with the interior of the anterior arch of the atlas. It acts as a pivot around which the atlas rotates. It is also called the odontoid process.

dentate ligament

A narrow fibrous band situated on each side of the spinal cord throughout its entire length and separating the anterior from the posterior roots of the spinal nerves. The inner border is continuous with the pia mater. The outer serrated border is fixed at intervals to the dura mater.

The dentate ligament is used to support the spinal cord in the cerebrospinal fluid. Synonym: denticulate.

desiccated

Dried, lacking water, easily crumbled.

deviation

1. A variation from normal.

2. Displacement of one of the body's masses relative to the others. When at rest, it is no longer aligned with one or more coordinate system planes.

disc

The intervertebral disc.

D.J.D.

Degenerative joint disease.

dorsal

Relative to or situated on the posterior or back surface; opposite of ventral. Synonym: thoracic.

dura

The dura mater. The outer wall of the thecal sac.

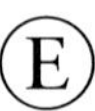

eburnation

A radiodensity feature on X-ray that is a product of degeneration of the cartilage at the articulating surface of a bone. This is also called sclerosis and is part of the process of changing the shape and density of articular bone. This is a common feature of degenerative changes in an articulation.

endplate

The fibrocartilage that defines the disc from above and below, separating it from the adjacent bony cortex of the vertebral body. There are endplates on the superior and inferior surfaces of each vertebral body.

epidural adhesion

An adhesion between the vertebral canal wall and the dura mater in the epidural space. This can be due to subluxation and the resulting chronic inflammation, a feature of degenerative joint disease and mechanical distress. It can also be seen as a result infectious insult or post operative finding.

epidural space

The outermost space covering the brain and spinal cord, located on or over the dura mater and inside a mostly bony encasement.

erector spinae

This is the largest muscular mass of the back and consists of three groupings: iliocostalis, longissimus, and spinalis. They originate on the sacrum and iliac crests and ascend the spine and rib cage to the neck and in some cases the skull. These groups, in turn, consist of a series of interlapping muscles. The iliocostalis group is laterally placed, the longissimus group is intermediate in placement, and the spinalis group is medially placed. The proprioceptive links are to the sacroiliac joints and the position of the ilium relative to the ribs and vertebrae.

esophagus

A muscular collapsible tube that lies behind the trachea, that connects the phyarnx to the stomach. The posterior wall of the esophagus is adhered to the anterior surface of the cervical spine. It is 23 to 25 cm long and begins at the end of the laryngopharynx, passes through the diaphragm through the esophageal hiatus, and terminates in the superior portion of the stomach. It is innervated by among others, the vagus nerve, recurrent laryngeal nerves and the cervical sympathetic chain.

extension

The unfolding of a joint so that the two articulated segments are moved apart, thereby increasing the joint angle approaching 180 degrees. Relating to the vertebral canal, when the head and or spine is tipped backward the canal length is shortened. Bending backwards.

extremity

1. An arm or leg.

2. A distal or terminal portion.

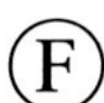

facet

The paired, posterior zygopophyseal joints of the spine. They are gliding, diarthrodial articulations. The facets are weight bearing, covered with cartilage, and surrounded by synovial capsules. These capsules are imbedded with proprioceptors. The angle of orientation and shape varies throughout the spine, in the cervical region by an anteroposterior position, in the thoracic region by an anteromedial position, and in the lumbar region by a lateral position. There are the superior articulating facets at the superior end of the vertebra and the inferior articulating facet at the inferior end of the vertebra.

facetal capsule

Ligamentous type enclosures of the gliding articulations of the vertebral column. They have a synovial lining on the inside. The capsules are innervated with proprioceptors that will respond to altered positions (subluxations). Threshold irritation can cause reflex splinting and constant noxious neurological stimuli.

fascia

The ubiquitous connective tissue throughout all regions of the body. Fascia is pervasive and interconnects all the body tissues.

femur

The leg or thigh bone. Its proximal end articulates with the acetabulum of the hipbone.

fibrocartilage

Cartilage that contains collagen fibers of various combinations in the matrix. The fibers are angled, in bundles, imbedded in a matrix with small spaces containing chondrocytes. The spine has various types in the intervertebral discs, the pubis symphysis, and at the attachments of tendons and ligaments to bone.

fibrous

Containing or composed of fibers, usually dense and interconnecting tissues.

filum terminale

The thread-like attachment of the conus medularis to the bottom of the thecal sac. It is contiguous with, and an extension of, the pia mater.

flexion

In the spine, it can refer to forward bending, head moving towards knees. Flexion elongates the spinal canal and spinal cord. Bending or having two parts move closer together as in the extremities.

foramen

A passage through which nerves or blood vessels pass. Usually found in bones, but can consist of a combination of tissues.

foramen magnum

The large opening in the base of the occipital bone that connects the cranial cavity and the spinal canal. The spinal cord/brain stem passes through this opening.

fusion

1. The normal process for bone formation.
2. The end stage of the degenerative process of joint pathology, i.e., the total loss of joint space and uniting of two bones.

glycoprotein

A macromolecule that is a combination of protein and sugar. Glycoproteins are a major component of the nucleus pulposus of the intervertebral disc.

gravitational load

The force applied by the mass of the body on the joints and tissues due to gravity. The load increases inferiorly.

guarding

A description of a functional aspect of muscle tissue, a muscle spasm, i.e., to protect a distressed joint complex. This is a neurological reflex.

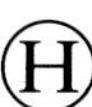

herniation

In referring to the human intervertebral disc, a rupture of an intervertebral disc so that the nucleus pulposus protrudes outside the annulus fibrosus. Contact and pressure on nervous tissue is possible. Trauma and other excessive forces on the disc can result in a loss of annulus fibrosus integrity allowing nucleus pulposus migration.

hydration

Combining or causing to combine with water.

hydraulic

Operated by a fluid under pressure, e.g., an intervertebral disc. A hydraulic system transmits force.

hydrophilic

Having an affinity for water. The nucleus pulposus of the intervertebral disc is hydrophilic due to glycoproteins and other components.

hyoid bone

A single U-shaped bone that is a component of the axial skeleton but does not articulate with any other bone. It is located in the neck between the mandible and larynx. It supports the tongue and provides attachment for some of its muscles and for muscles of the neck and pharynx.

hyperkyphosis
The condition of the kyphotic curve of the thoracic spine having a greater than normal curve.

hyperload
The loss of normal three point weight bearing can result in all the weight being supported by one point or joint leading to excessive loading. This will cause an alteration of the tissue, bone and ligament, to accommodate this change in weight bearing.

hypertonic
An adjective of hypertonia. A condition of muscle and tendon tension that is significantly greater than normal resting muscle tone. It can be directly related to noxious proprioceptive input from the joint distress, subluxation. Hypertonic muscles at rest should be a neurological finding. It leads to loss of joint space and reduced articular excursion. It is a common feature of arthritic degeneration.

hypertrophy
An increase in thickness or size of an organ or tissue. This usually occurs as an adaptive response to increased stress or demand on a tissue or organ.

hypokyphosis
The condition of the kyphotic curve of the thoracic spine having a lesser than normal curve.

hypolordotic
The condition of the lordotic curve of the cervical and lumbar spine having less than the normal curve.

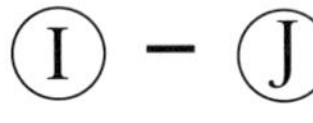

iliacus muscle
The iliacus originates at the iliac fossa and base of the sacrum and inserts with the tendon of the psoas major at the lesser trochanter of the femur. Action is to flex and rotate the thigh laterally, and it also flexes the vertebral column. Innervation is the femoral nerve. Proprioceptive links are to the sacroiliac joint and the pubis symphysis.

ilium
The ilium is the superior and largest of the three original bones of the innominate. Its superior border, the iliac crest, ends anteriorly in the anterior superior iliac spine. Posteriorly, the iliac crest ends in the posterior superior iliac spine. The posterior inferior iliac spine is just inferior to it. The spines serve as points of attachment for the abdominal wall and erector spinae musculature. Inferior to the posterior inferior iliac spine is the greater sciatic notch. The internal surface of the ilium seen from the medial side is the iliac fossa, a concavity where the iliacus muscle attaches. Posterior to this fossa is the iliac tuberosity, a point of attachment for the sacroiliac ligament, and the auricular surface, which articulates with the sacrum to form the sacroiliac joint.

imbibition
The flow or absorption of fluid through or into a tissue. Osmotic pressure or the pumping action of motion are the most common mechanism of imbibition.

inferior
Lower in place or position, anatomically, i.e., closer to the feet.

inferior articular facet
See facet.

inflammation
The protective reaction of tissues to all forms of injury and irritation. It is a neurological response involving vascular changes characterized by heat, redness, swelling, pain, and loss of function.

innominate
The hip bone. In early life it is three bones, the ilium, ischium and pubis. The three bones fuse as the individual reaches adolescence.

intercostal
Between the ribs.

interspinous ligament
Thin, almost membrane like ligaments that connect spinous processes with fibers running anterosuperiorly from the apex of the spinous process below toward the root of the spinous process above. They are embedded with proprioceptors and other nerve structures.

intervertebral disc
The thick, fibrous, avascular pad between the vertebrae. Composed of a nucleus pulposus (center) and an annulus fibrosus (outer wall). It is largely composed of water and therefore a hydraulic system and it transmits force to the vertebral body. It is, therefore, not a shock absorber but allows a flexible vertebral column (this is essential to spinal cord vascular function).

intervertebral foramen
Openings that are along the lateral border of the intervertebral canal. They are formed anteriorly by the intervertebral disc, the lower portion of the vertebral body above, and the upper portion of the vertebral body below; posteriorly by the posterior zygapophyseal joint and ligamentum flavum; and superiorly and inferiorly by the a vertebral pedicle. The spinal nerve roots and vascular components of the spinal column pass through these openings.

intrathecal
Inside the thecal sac or the subarachnoid space, between the arachnoid mater and the pia mater.

intrathecal adhesions
An adhesion between the arachnoid mater and pia mater. This is a product of inflammation and will cause an interruption of normal thecal and spinal cord dynamics or

motion. It can also impede the flow of cerebrospinal fluid and entrap neurological and vascular structures.

ischial tuberosity
The inferior aspect of the ischium and innominate, the point of contact in the sitting position. Origin of the sacrotuberous ligament, inferior gemellus, quadratus femoris, semimembranosus, semitendinosus and biceps femoris muscles.

ischium
The inferior and posterior of the three bones that make up the innominate. It contains an ischial spine, a lesser sciatic notch below the spine, and an ischial tuberosity. The ischium has a ramus which joins with the pubis and together they form the obturator foramen.

I.V.D.
Intervertebral disc.

I.V.F.
Intervertebral foramen.

kyphosis
Pertaining to a kyphotic curve.

kyphotic curve
A normal architectural feature of the human vertebral column in the thoracic and sacral regions. It is characterized by the concavity of the curve facing the ventral or anterior surface. Alteration of the kyphotic curve changes the shape of the central nervous system and other associated tissues.

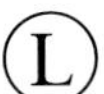

lamina
In the vertebra, it is a paired structure on either side that unites posteriorly to form the spinous process. The lamina forms the roof of the posterior vertebral arch.

laminectomized
The surgical removal of the lamina or posterior bony arches of one or more vertebrae in order to expose the neural elements of the spinal cord.

larynx
The voice box. It is a short passageway that connects the pharynx with the trachea. It lies in the midline of the neck anterior to the fourth through sixth cervical vertebrae, C4-C6.

lateral
On the side. Opposite of medial.

lateral flexion
A flexion to either side.

lateralisthesis
A displacement lateral to normal position.

ligament
The fibrous connective tissue joining two or more bones, cartilages, or other structures together. A ligament gives stability, usually to a joint, preventing excessive motion in certain directions. It is embedded with proprioceptors and other nerve structures. The loss of ligament integrity (subluxation) initiates degenerative arthritis.

ligamentum flavum
The yellow elastic tissue attached to and extending between the ventral portions of the laminae between the vertebrae. They close the spaces between the vertebral arches in the spinal canal.

lordosis
Pertaining to a lordotic curve.

lordotic curve
A normal architectural feature of the human vertebral column in the cervical and lumbar regions. It is the angle formed by perpendicular lines drawn from the superior endplate of L1 and the inferior endplate of L5. Alteration of these curves changes the shape of the central nervous system and other tissues.

lumbar
Pertaining to the lower region of the spine, between the thorax and the pelvis. Usually vertebrae, L1-L5.

lumbar curve
An essential architectural feature of the human spine. Changes in the shape of the lumbar region of the spine result in central nervous system deformation and joint pathology. The lumbar curve is lordotic or the convex side of the curve is facing the ventral or anterior surface.

lumbosacral aponeurosis
The thick fascia connecting the musculature of the lower thoracic and lumbar region with the sacrum, iliac crests, and abdominal wall muscles. Synonym: thoracolumbar fascia.

luxation
A complete dislocation of an articulation.

magnetic resonance imaging
An imaging technique that uses radio waves and an intense magnetic field to produce accurate images of the inside of the body. These image show soft tissue contrast without bony artifact. There is also excellent imaging of the water content and condition of the intervertebral discs.

mandible
The lower jawbone.

marginal osteophytes
A horizontal bone extension of the vertebral endplate. It is the response of the body to a shearing of the intervertebral disc usually as a result of trauma. This ossification process is a response to stress due to altered architecture.

mastication
Chewing.

mastoid process

The posterior, lateral projection of the temporal bone inferior to the external auditory meatus. This is the origin of the occipitalis and digastric muscles and insertion of sternocleidomastoid, splenius capitis, and longissimus capitis muscles.

medial

Near the midline of the body.

medullary bone

The marrow part of bone, occupying space within the cortex of a bone.

meningeal

Pertaining to the meninges.

meninges

The supportive and enclosing tissues of the central nervous system; the dura mater, the arachnoid, and the pia mater and other structures. They protect and impart motion to the central nervous system.

midsagittal

A vertical plane at the midline that divides the body into left and right portions.

military neck

Loss of the cervical curve. It is a straightening rather than a reversal.

MRI

Magnetic resonance imaging.

myelopathy

The pathological condition of the spinal cord or nervous tissues usually caused by later stages of degenerative joint processes. These changes to the spinal cord produce signs and symptoms of cord dysfunction.

necrosis/necrotic

The death of a cell or group of cells comprising a tissue or tissues as a result of injury or disease.

nerve root

The bundles of nerve fibers that arise from the spinal cord join together as a nerve root. These bundles are paired and are the dorsal and ventral nerve roots. The nerve roots combine to form the spinal nerve.

nerve rootlets

Hair-like fibers extending from the spinal cord. They converge laterally and gather into a nerve fiber and root.

neuron

A nerve cell which has a cell body, dendrites, and an axon.

neutral position

Normal anatomical position; the body is erect and facing observer, arms hanging at the sides.

neurovascular bundle

A bundle of nerves and blood vessels that both innervate and supply blood to a region or tissue.

non marginal osteophytes

An osteophyte forming on the vertebral body not at the endplate. This ossification process is a response to stress due to altered architecture.

nucleus pulposus

The glycoprotein, hydrophilic, center of the intervertebral disc. It is a hydrodynamic structure that has a greater fluid content than the rest of the disc and resists compression.

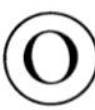

osmotic

The pressure that develops when two solutions of different concentrations are separated by a permeable membrane.

ossification

Formation of or conversion into bone.

osteoarthritis

A progressive joint disorder involving deterioration of the articular structures usually due to trauma and loss of normal joint integrity. The neurological response to the altered joint mechanics is muscle guarding, inflammation, reduced joint space, cartilage erosion, and increased bone formation in the subchondral regions. This condition changes the shape and function of the joint and can be described as degenerative joint disease. This condition can occur as a result of the pathogenesis of subluxation.

osteophyte

A projection or outgrowth of bone; a bone spur. The tissue attaching or inserting into bone can be under mechanical distress causing its calcification and forming the outgrowth.

osteoporosis

A bone disorder characterized by decreased density of normally mineralized bone resulting in bone fragility. Causes of osteoporosis are post-menopause, disuse, diet, chronic illness, and endocrine abnormalities.

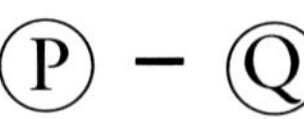

parasagittal

A vertical line that does not pass through the midline and that divides the body or organs into unequal left and right portions.

para spinal phyte

Ossification of the soft tissue structures that surround the vertebral body. This ossification process is a response to stress due to altered architecture.

parasthesia

A condition of altered sensation.

pedicle

One of the paired bony processes projecting posteriorly from the body of a vertebra, which connect with the lamina on either side. These structures assist in transferring weight bearing to the facets.

pelvis/pelvic girdle

The three bone, three joint complex that provides the weight-bearing and muscular anchoring of the trunk and lower extremities while protecting the lower abdominal viscera. It consists of the two innominate bones that articulate posteriorly with the sacrum and anteriorly at the pubis symphysis. The pelvis articulates with the femurs at the acetabuli to form the hip joints. A major portion of the body's muscle mass arises from the pelvis. Distortion of the pelvic girdle (subluxation) will initiate guarding responses of the muscles and organs attached.

pelvic shearing

A non-physiologic displacement of the innominates relative to each other in the Y and/or Z planes. Significant ligament injury occurs in both the sacroiliac joints and the pubis symphysis.

pharynx

The throat. This is a region posterior to the nasal cavity, oral cavity, and larynx, and is just anterior and attached to the cervical vertebrae.

pia mater

The inner membrane of the thecal sac. It invests or covers the spinal cord and roots into cord matrix. The pia mater supports and shapes the spinal cord. It is attached to the arachnoid mater via the dentate ligaments and other structures.

P.L.L.

Posterior longitudinal ligament.

pons

The part of central nervous system above the medulla and anterior to the cerebellum. It connects the spinal cord with the brain and parts of the brain with each other. The longitudinal fibers of the pons belong to the motor and sensory tracts that connect the spinal cord or medulla with the upper part of the brain stem.

posterior

Rear, back, or dorsal surfaces of the body.

posterior impression

An anatomical feature of the intervertebral disc. The indented posterior surface helps to give shape to the spinal canal.

posterior longitudinal ligament

The ligament that runs on the posterior surfaces of the vertebral bodies. It extends from the axis down through the entire length of the vertebral column. It widens at the vertebral margins to reinforce the intervertebral discs. It covers the anterior surface of the spinal canal.

posterior superior iliac spine

Uppermost and rearmost surface of the ilium. *See,* ilium

proprioception

The neurological perception of position and change of position of the body and its parts. Proprioception is transmitted through nerve sensors, most of which are in muscles, tendons and joint tissues.

proprioceptive reflex

An automatic response of muscle and tendon initiated by stimuli that arise from joint distress. The reflex mechanism itself is mediated by sensory afferent stimulation of motor neurons of the involved musculature. Since there is a direct connection at the spinal cord level with no higher motor neuron involvement, its a reflex. This occurs in spinal cord lesion victims below the lesion as do the standard neurological reflexes.

protrusion

In the intervertebral disc, a migration of the nucleus pulposus beyond the boundary of the annulus fibrosus. This occurs in all directions around the perimeter of the disc.

pseudo-joint

A false joint is formed where two bones contact each other when they should be apart. Common in degenerative changes of the spine. The most common occurrence in the spine is the spinous processes in the lumbar region.

PSIS

The posterior superior iliac spine.

psoas major

The psoas major originates at the transverse processes and bodies of the lumbar vertebrae and inserts at the lesser trochanter of the femur. The action flexes and rotates the thigh laterally and also flexes the vertebral column. Innervated at the lumbar nerves L2-L3. It has proprioceptive links to the sacroiliac joints and pubis symphysis. The lumbar nerve roots exit the spine into the psoas and the lumbar plexus is in the belly and tendons of the muscle. The psoas attaches to the diaphragm and anterior longitudinal ligament.

pubic body

The medial portion of the pubic bone. Each side joins with the fibrocartilaginous disc called the pubis symphysis.

pubis symphysis

The pubis symphysis has annular rings and a spongy center, is avascular, and motion is a major component of its physiology. This joint can tear and subluxate and suffer major stability problems. Misalignment of this joint automatically misalign one or both sacroiliac joints. Proprioceptive links are to the psoas, iliacus, all the hip muscles, medial and anterior muscles of the thigh and the abdominal and erector groups.

rectus abdominus

The rectus abdominus originates at the pubic crest and pubis symphysis and inserts at the cartilage of the fifth to seventh ribs and the xiphoid process. Its action is to compress the abdomen, and flex the vertebral column. Innervation is from the branches of thoracic nerves T7-T12. Proprioceptive innervation is between pubic bone and lower rib cage. Unilateral or bilateral rectus abdominus splinting can be a sign of pubis symphysis subluxation.

recumbent position

The body position of lying down on a horizontal surface.

retro

Abbreviation for retrolisthesis.

retrolisthesis

Any posterior displacement of a vertebra in relation to the one below it causing stress and probable tearing of the annulus fibrosus and nucleus pulposus. Also, the altered biomechanics and loss of normal motion resulting from a retrolisthesis is the etiology of almost all degenerative or arthritic changes to the disc, vertebral body, facet, and other associated tissues.

retropulsion

The process of being pushed posteriorly. This usually describes a vertebral body fracture and refers to fragments that have moved back into the spinal canal.

rib

One of the bones that forms the outer skeleton of the thorax. The twelve pairs of ribs form the rib cage. The rib articulates with one of the twelve thoracic vertebrae at the transverse process and with one or two of the vertebral bodies . The anterior end is attached to a section of cartilage joined to the sternum. The first seven pairs, the true ribs, are connected directly to the sternum by their costal cartilages. The next three pairs, the false ribs, are attached indirectly to the sternum. Each is connected by its cartilage to the rib above it. The last two pairs, the floating ribs, end freely in the muscles of the anterior body wall.

rootlets

Nerve rootlets.

rotation

The movment around an axis. One of the primary motions in physics. The unit of measurement is usually in degrees.

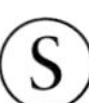

sacral ala

The wing-like projections evolving from the transverse processes of S1. They form part of the sacral base and the lateral edges form part of the sacroiliac joint.

sacral apex

The inferior aspect of the sacrum, articulating with the superior portion of the coccyx.

sacral base

The superior aspect of the sacrum, articulating with the inferior portion of L5 and laterally with innominates.

sacral disc

The disc between sacral segments. As the sacrum ages, it begins to fuse, becoming for all practical purposes, a single but flexible bone. When these bones, S1-S5, articulate, the intersacral discs remain in place and act just the same as the intervertebral discs of the other vertebrae. The cortex of the sacrum is contiguous but this must be a flexible structure. Physiological function of intrasacral discs necessitates motion as the only mechanism of nutrition and waste elimination. The sacral discs do what the intervertebral discs do: confer flexibility. There is only one mechanism for fluid and nutrient exchange for the intervertebral disc and that is imbibition through motion. This must also be true for sacral disc physiology and function.

sacroiliac joint

The paired articulations between the sacrum and the iliac bone in the pelvis. These two joint complexes are different in each individual. Some of the factors are the size of the joint, size of each portion, shape of each portion, and orientation of each portion to each other. These factors could explain the different responses to the same treatment with the same diagnosis.

sacroiliac ligament (anterior and posterior)

Anterior: This ligament is contiguous with periosteum of ilium and sacrum. This is one of the structures involved with S.I. joint injuries, sustaining a sprain with either physiological or non-physiological subluxations.

Posterior: This ligament is contiguous with and attached to the lumbosacral fascia from above and the medial attachment of the gluteus maximus muscle from below. It connects the sacrum and the ilium behind and forms the chief connection between these bones.

sacrospinous ligament

The ligament from the lateral edge of the sacrum to the spine of the ischium. This ligament along with the sacrotuberous ligament is primarily responsible for conferring motion to the sacrum. As the leg swings forward for heel strike, the innominate nutates with the ilium moving posterior and the ischial tuberosity moving forward and via the sacrotuberous and sacrospinous ligaments, moves the ipsilateral side of the sacrum forward.

sacrotuberous ligament

The ligament from the lateral edge of the sacrum to the ischial tuberosity. Fibers of the sacrotuberous can be contiguous with the tendon of the biceps femoris. Unilateral shortening of the ligament can rotate and or angle the sacrum between the ilium creating a contralateral stretching and irritation to various structures, this could be a factor in a number of syndromes. The sacrotuberous ligament, along with the sacrospinous ligament, confer motion to the sacrum with motion of the leg.

sacrum

The sacrum is a triangular shaped bone formed by the partial fusion of sacral vertebrae. It articulates laterally with the innominates, superiorly with L5, and inferiorly with the coccyx. The sacrum is five separate segments in the child and S1-S5 are fused by age 25 to form, for all practical purposes, a single but flexible bone.

sagittal

A vertical plane that divides the body into left and right portions. This is the Y-Z plane in the Cartesian coordinate system.

Schmoral's node

An invagination in the endplate of a vertebral body that is surrounded by repaired compact bone. It is formed by a prolapse of the nucleus pulposus into the vertebral body through the endplate and into the medullary bone. On a lateral X-ray a Schmoral's node is seen as a radiolucency in the upper or lower margin of the body of the affected vertebra surrounded by compact bone.

sclerosis

In bone, the increase in density of an area, usually, in cortical bone in the region of an articulation. This gives an increased white appearence on X-ray and is associated with degenerative changes of a joint or an adaptive response to increased stress on part of a bone. In general, sclerosis is hardening or thickening of a tissue or organ, usually by an increase in fibrous tissue.

segment

1. Another term for a vertebrae in the context of the vertebral column.
2. A portion of a larger body or structure.

shearing

A type of deforming force applied in the axial plane to the spine resulting in angular deformation. Involves numerous ligament, joint, muscle and nervous tissue structures besides the vertebrae.

SI joint

Sacroiliac joint

sinuvertebral artery

A small branch or arterial twig off the vertebral artery that enters the intervertebral foramen. It supplies blood to the thecal sac and spinal cord. Loss of lordotic curve and subluxation of numerous cervical vertebrae can cause translation of the cord, thecal sac, and nerve roots into the anterior wall of the spinal canal and the intervertebral foramen. Chronically compressed sinuvertebral artery could cause negative sympathetic syndrome.

soft tissue

The non osseous tissue of the body, including intervertebral discs, tendons, muscle, connective tissues, nerves, vascular structures and ligaments.

spasm

Involuntary musculature contraction. It can be due to proprioceptive sensory bombardment, peripheral nerve entrapment or central nervous distress, all of which can be due to subluxation.

spinal canal

A continuous channel running longitudinally through the vertebral column. The anterior wall is formed by the posterior surfaces of the vertebral bodies and intervertebral discs and by the posterior longitudinal ligament. The posterior wall is formed by the vertebral laminae, the ligamentum flava and the intervertebral foramina. Canal length (flexion increases 5-7 cm the length over extension) and shape (side bending and rotation create a concave-convex formation of the lateral surfaces of the canal) are affected by the shape or posture of the spinal column. The anatomic relationship with the spinal cord and caudae equinae determine the shape of the lower central nervous system. A kyphosis of the cervical spine is a flexion deformity that affects the entire length of the canal, spinal cord, brain stem and nerve roots.

spondylolithesis

The anterior displacement of a vertebra in relation to the lower vertebra. Usually associated with a break or fracture of the posterior elements of a vertebrae.

spondylosis

One of the descriptive terms used to indicate degenerative changes of both the disc and the zygapophyseal joints of the spine. Spondylosis is a feature of osteoarthritis and includes narrowing of both the disc space and the neural foramina, as well as the presence of osteophytes. The most common etiology is subluxation.

spinal column

The spinal column includes the all the tissues of the vertebral column, meninges, and spinal cord.

spinal cord

The lower part of the central nervous system inside in the vertebral column. It begins as a continuation of the medulla oblongata at the inferior part of the brain stem and extends from the foramen magnum of the occipital bone to a tapered end at the junction of L1-L2. It consists of nerve cells and bundles of nerves connecting all parts of the body to the brain. The spinal cord changes it shape with the changing shape of the spinal canal and meninges. The spinal cord can increase in length 3-5 cm going from full extension to flexion. With flexion and spinal cord lengthening, the dentate ligaments stretch and narrow, pulling the edges of the cord with them. Acting together, they pull the from the right and the left and increase the coronal diameter. The anterior to posterior diameter decreases, making the cord appear oval on axial view. Pia mater invests the spinal cord with roots into the cord matrix. The subarachnoid space is the CSF filled space between the pia mater covering of the spinal cord and the inside of the thecal sac covered with the arachnoid mater.

spinal laminar junction

A radiographic line. The vertebral lamina unite posteriorly to form the spinous process. At the point of junction there is a white line which is the posterior wall of the vertebral canal.

spinous process

That part of a vertebra that projects posteriorly from the arch, producing a lever arm for introduction of motion by attaching muscle groups.

spurring

An osteophyte, or bony lip, on or near the articular margin of a bone. Vertebral endplate spurs are all disc related, posterior as well as anterior and lateral.

stairstepping

In a radiograph, stairstepping has the appearance of stairs due to repeated subluxations from vertebra to vertebra, resulting in a sequential loss of alignment in a series of vertebrae.

stenosis

A closing or narrowing of an opening or passage, such as the spinal canal, can be congenital or acquired. It is a common finding with chronic subluxation with involved segments.

sternum

The breastbone. It is located in the median line of the anterior chest wall and measures about 15 cm in length. The sternum consists of three basic portions: the superior manubrium, the medial body, and the inferior xiphoid process. The manubrium articulates with the medial or proximal ends of the clavicles as well as the first and second ribs. The body articulates directly or indirectly with the second through tenth ribs, via the costal cartilages. The xiphoid process provides the insertion point for the rectus abdominus and transversus abdominus muscles.

subarachnoid adhesions

An adhesion occurring between the arachnoid and pia mater. *See* intrathecal adhesions.

subarachnoid space

The space between the arachnoid and pia mater. It contains circulating cerebrospinal fluid and large blood vessels. Obliteration of the anterior subarachnoid space seen in advanced imaging by the spinal cord taken in the supine position can be a sign of central nervous system tethering and distress. Loss of space due to fibrous adhesions or stenosis is considered pathological and relate to severe neurological conditions.

subdural space

Theoretical or potential space between the dura mater and arachnoid mater. It looks and acts like a single tissue, hence the term, theca. These two layers of tissue are normally adhered together.

subluxation

Loss of joint alignment and integrity. This describes an injury to the joint structures such as the ligaments, discs, joint capsules, supporting tendons, and fascia. Subluxation is the most common etiology of osteoarthritis and is characterized by immobilization, inflammation, pain and muscle spasms.

superior

Situated above or towards the upper part of the body or head; opposite of inferior.

superior articular facet

See facet.

supine

The position of the body when on the back facing upwards.

sympathetic chain

Long nerve complexes on each side of the vertebral column from the base of the skull to the coccyx. It is the extravertebral portion of the central nervous system containing part of the autonomic nervous system.

sympathetic nervous system

One of the two subdivisions of the autonomic nervous system, having cell bodies of preganglionic neurons in the lateral gray columns of the thoracic segment and first two or three lumbar segments of the spinal cord. It is primarily concerned with processes involving the expenditure of energy. Paravertebral ganglia as well as spinal nerve roots have been observed to be adversely affected by chronic degenerative processes of the vertebral column.

synovial joint

A joint in which there is a space between the articulating bones. A synovial joint is freely movable and is classified as a diarthroses. They are surrounded by a capsule and held together by ligaments. Disruption of normal relationships (subluxation) causes inflammation, muscle guarding and limited range of motion leading to arthritic changes if allowed to become chronic.

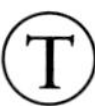

tendon/tendinous

The extension of a muscle's tissue that forms a dense fibrous cord or band which attaches it to a bone. Muscle contraction pulls on the tendon, which moves the bone. The tendons are embedded with proprioceptors and other neurological structures.

tethered cord syndrome

A collection of signs, symptoms and complaints that are the result of central nervous system distress from chronic elongation of the neural canal in the vertebral column. Characterized by translation of the spinal cord into the anterior canal wall obliterating the patency of the anterior spinal artery. Also known as filum terminale syndrome or cord traction syndrome.

theca/thecal

The theca or thecal sac refers to part of the meninges, the dura mater and the arachnoid mater.

thoracic

Pertaining to the thoracic region of the spine, T1-T12.

thoracic curve

An essential architectural feature of the human spine. Changes in the shape of the thoracic region of the spine result in central nervous system deformation and joint pathology. The thoracic curve is kyphotic or the concave side of the curve is ventral.

thoracolumbar fascia

A thick, broad tissue anchoring the erector spinae, abdominal muscles, and latissimus dorsi. It connects the lower thoracic area, lumbar spine, sacrum, and iliac crests.

thorax

The chest; the thoacic spine and rib cage.

three-point weight bearing

The three-point weight bearing system in the vertebral column is based on weight distributed between three points, the body of the vertebra and the two articular facets. This system works for each joint in the vertebral column from C2 to S1. Disruption of the three-point weight bearing system alters the dynamics of the joint and associated tissues and leads to osteoarthritis. *See* altered weight bearing.

trabecula

1. The inner or medulary bone has a latice like construction called trabecular bone.

2. The trabecula of the arachnoid are delicate fibrous threads connecting the inner surface of the arachnoid to the pia mater.

trachea

The windpipe. It is a tubular passageway for air, it is located anterior to the esophagus.

tractioned

Stretching or elongating a tissue, e.g., spinal cord from deformation of spinal column.

transverse abdominus

The transverse abdominus originates at the iliac crest, inguinal ligament, lumbar fascia, and cartilages of the last six ribs and inserts at the xyphoid process, linea alba, and pubis. Action is to aid in lateral flexion and rotation of the trunk. Innervation is from the branches of the thoracic nerves T8-T12, the iliohypogastric and ilioinguinal nerves. It is proprioceptily linked to the sacroiliac joints, pubis symphysis, and the lower ribs.

transverse processes

The bony wings projecting from the sides of the vertebra at the junction of the pedicle and the lamina. They serve as levers for the action of splenius cervicis, iliocostalis, longissimus, scalenes, quadratus lumborum, intertranversarii muscles, and other muscles.

trochanter

Refers to the greater trochanter of the femur. The bony protuberance that projects from below, and lateral to, the neck of the femur. The gluteus medius, gluteus minimus, piriformis, obturator internus, superior gemellus, and inferior gemellus insert at the greater trochanter.

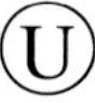

urogenital

The region of the pelvic floor below the pubis symphysis, bounded by the pubis symphysis and the ischial tuberosities and containing the genital and urinary structures.

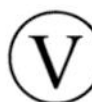

vascular

Pertaining to or containing many blood vessels.

vasoconstriction

A neurologically mediated decrease in the size of the lumen of a blood vessel caused by the contraction of the smooth muscle in the wall of the vessel.

ventral

Pertaining to the anterior or front side of the body; opposite of dorsal.

vertebral artery

This vessel is a branch of the subclavian artery, it supplies the cervical spinal cord and lower and posterior cranial structures. It enters the foramen in the sixth cervical vertebra and ascends through the foramina in the transverse processes of all the vertebrae above this. It passes through the atlas, beneath the posterior occipitoatlantal ligament, pierces the dura mater and arachnoid, and enters the skull through the foramen magnum.

vertebral canal

See spinal canal.

vertebral column

The flexible column of the axial skeleton composed of vertebrae separated by intervertebral discs and facets, and bound together by ligaments. One of the three systems of spinal tissues. *See* spinal column.

visceral

Pertaining to the viscera; a collective term for the internal organs.

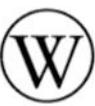

whiplash

A term for an injury in which one part of the spine is unexpectedly and violently forced or "whipped" in one direction then suddenly in the opposite direction.

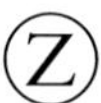

zygapophyseal joint

Of or pertaining to the lateral and posterior articulating joints of the spine. *See* facet.

REFERENCES

Adams, C. B. T., Logue, V., Studies in cervical spondylotic myelopathy (1. Movement of the cervical roots, dura and cord, and their relation to the course of the Extrathecal roots). *Brain*, 1971, 94:557-658.

Adams, M. A., Hutton, W. C., The Effect of Posture on the Fluid Content of Lumbar Intervertebral Discs, *Spine,* 1983, 6:665-671.

Adams, M.A., Hutton, W.C., The Effect of Posture on the Role of the Apophysial Joints in Resisting Intervertebral Compressive Forces, *Journal of Bone and Joint Surgery*, 1980, 3:358-362.

Ader, R., Cohen, N., Felton, D., "Psychoneuroimmunology: Interactions between the Nervous System and the Immune System", *The Lancet,* 1995, v. 345, 99-103.

Ahmed, M., Bjurholm, A., Kreicbergs, A., Schultzberg, M., Neuropeptide Y, Tyrosine Hydroxylase and Vasoactive Intestinal Polypeptide-Immunoreactive Nerve Fibers in the Vertebral Bodies, Discs, Dura Mater, and Spinal Ligaments of Rat Lumbar Spine, *Spine,* 1993, 2:268-273.

Allison, R. D., Pain in the Chest Wall Simulating Heart Disease, *British Medical Journal*, 1950, Feb:332-334

Al-Mefty, O., Harkey, H. L., Marawi, I., Haines, D. E., Peeler, D. F., Wilner, H. I., Smith R. R., Holaday, H. R., Haining, J. L., Russell, W. F., Harrison, B., Middleton, T. H., Experimental Chronic Compressive Cervical Myelopathy, *Journal of Neurosurgery,* 1993, 79:550-561.

Avramov, A. I.,Cavanaugh, J. M., Ozaktay, C. A., Getchell, T. V., King, A. I., The Effects of Controlled Mechanical Loading on Group-II, and IV Afferent Units from the Lumbar Facet Joint and Surrounding Tissue, *Journal of Bone & Joint Surgery*,1992, 10/v. 74-A, 1464-1471.

Basbaum, A. I., Levine, J. D., The Contribution of the Nervous System to Inflammation and Inflammatory Disease, *Canadian Journal of Physiological Pharmacology*, 1991, 69:647-651.

Behar, A. J., Feldman, S., Pathogenesis of Adhesive Arachnoiditis, An Experimental Study, *Journal of Neuropathology and Experimental Neurology*, 1957, 16:261-268.

Bernhardt, M., Bridwell, K. H., Segmental Analysis of the Sagittal Plane Alignment of the Normal Thoracic and Lumbar Spines and Thoracolumbar Junction, *Spine,* 1989, 7:717-721.

Bernick, S., Walker, J. M., Paule, W. J., Age Changes to the Anulus Fibrosus in Human Intervertebral Discs, *Spine,* 1991, 5:520-524.

Blau, J. N., Rushworth, G., Observations on the Blood Vessels of the Spinal Cord and Their Responses to Motor Activity, *Brain,* 1958, Vol. 81:354-363.

Boden, S. D., Davis, D. O., Dina, T. S., Patronas, N. J., Wiesel, S. W., Abnormal Magnetic-Resonance Scans of the Lumbar Spine in Asymptomatic Subjects, *The Journal of Bone and Joint Surgery,* 1990, 3:403-408.

Bogduk, N., The Innervation of the Vertebral Column, *The Australian Journal of Physiotherapy*, 1985, 3:89-94.

Bogduk, N., Lambert, G. A., Duckworth, J. W., The Anatomy and Physiology of the Vertebral Nerve in Relation to Cervical Migraine, *Cephalalgia,* 1981, 1:11-24.

Bogduk, N., Macintosh, J. E., The Applied Anatomy of the thoracolumbar Fascia, *Spine,* 1984, 2:164-170

Bogduk, N., Windsor, M., Inglis, A., The Innervation of the Cervical Intervertebral Discs, *Spine,* 1988, 1:2-8.

Bowen, V., Cassidy, J. D., Macroscopic and Microscopic Anatomy of the Sacroiliac Joint from Embryonic Life Until the Eighth Decade, *Spine,* 1981, 6:620-627.

Brain, L., Some Unsolved Problems of Cervical Spondylosis, *British Medical Journal,* 1963, 23:771-777.

Brain, W. R., Northfield, D., Wilkinson, M., The Neurological Manifestations of Cervical Spondylosis, *Brain,* 1952, 75:187-225.

Breig, A., *Adverse Mechanical Tension in the Central Nervous System*, Alquist and Wiksell, 1978.

Breig, A., Overstretching of and Circumscribed Pathological Tension in the Spinal Cord- A Basic Cause of Symptoms in Cord Disorders, *Journal of Biomechanics*,1970, 3:7-9.

Breig, A., Marions, O., Biomechanics of the lumbosacral nerve roots, *Acta Radiologica,* 1962, 1:1141-1160.

Breig, A., Renard, M., Stefanko, S., Renard, C., Anatomic Basis of Medical and Surgical Technique, Healing of the Severed Spinal Cord by Biomechanical Relaxation and Surgical Immobilization. *Anatomia Clinica*,1982, 4:167-181.

Breig, A., Turnbull, I., Hassler, O., Effects of Mechanical Stresses on the Spinal Cord in Cervical Spondylosis, A Study on Fresh Cadaver Material, *Journal of Neurosurgery,* 1966, 25:45-56.

Brickley-Parsons, D., Glimcher, M. J., Is the Chemistry of Collagen in Intervertebral Discs an Expression of Wolff's Law?, *Spine,* 1984, 2:148-163.

Brower, A.C., *Arthritis in Black and White*, W.B. Saunders Co., Philadelphia, 1988.

Brunner, C., Kissling, R., Jacob, H. A. C., The Effects of Morphology and Histopathologic Findings on the Mobility of the Sacroiliac Joint, *Spine,* 1991, 9:1111-1117.

Bullough, P.G., Boachie-Adjer, O. *Atlas of Spinal Diseases,* J.P. Lippincott, 1988.

Cavanaugh, J. M., El-Bohy, A., Hardy, W. N., Getchell, T. V., Getchell, M. L., King, A. I., Sensory Innervation of Soft Tissues of the Lumbar Spine in the Rat, *Journal of Orthopaedic Research,* 1989, 7:378-388.

Condon, B. R., Hadley, D. "Quantification of Cord Deformation and Dynamics During Flexion and Extension of the Cervical Spine using MR Imaging, *Journal of Computer Assisted Tomography,* 1988,12:947-955

Crock, H. V., Yamagishi, M., Crock, M. C., *The Conus Medullaris and Cauda Equina in Man, An Atlas of the Arteries and Veins,* Springer- Verlag Wien New York, 1986

Culver, G.J., Pirson, H.S., Preventive Effect of Aortic Pulsations on Osteophyte Formation in the Thoracic Spine, *American Journal of Radiology and Radiation Therapy,* 1960, 5:932-940.

De La Porte, C., Siegfried, J., Lumbosacral Spinal Fibrosis (Spinal Arachnoiditis), *Spine,* 1983, 6:593-603

Di Chiro, G., Fischer, R. L., Contrast Radiology Of the Spinal Cord, *Archives of Neurology,* 1964, 2:125-143.

Dijkstra, P. F., Vleeming, A., Stoeckart, R., Complex Motion Tomography of the Sacroiliac Joint An Anatomical and Roentgenological Study, *Interdisciplinary World Conference on Low Back Pain and Its Relation to the Sacroiliac Joint,* 1992, San Diego, Ca.

Dillon, W.P., Norman, D., Newton, T. H., Bolla, K., Mark, A., Intradural Spinal Cord Lesions: Gd-DTPA-Enhanced Mr Imaging, *Radiology,* 1989, 1:229-238

Donaldson, I., Gibson, R., Spinal Cord Atrophy Associated with Arachnoiditis as Demonstrated by Computed Tomography, *Neuroradiology,* 1982, 24:101-105.

Dolan, E.J., McBroom, R.J., Taguchi, T., Macnab, I., The Effect of Spinal Distraction on Regional Spinal Cord Blood Flow in Cats, *Journal of Neurosugery,* 1980, 53:756-764

Dooley, J.F., McBroom, R.J., Taguchi, T., Macnab, I.,Nerve Root Infiltration in the Diagnosis of Radicular Pain, *Spine,* 1988, 1:7983

Ducker, T.B., Kindt,G. W., Kempe, L. G., Pathological Findings in Acute Experimental Spinal Cord Trauma, *Journal of Neurosurgery,* 1971, Dec.:700-708.

Egund, N., Olsson, T. H., Schmid, H., Selvik, G., Movements in the Sacroiliac Joints Demonstrated With Roentgen Stereophotogrammetry, *Acta Radiologica Diagnosis,* 1978, 19(5):833-846.

El-Bohy, A., Cavanaugh, J. M., Getchell, M. L., Bulas, T., Getchell, T. V., King, A. I., Localization of Substance P and Neurofilament Immunoreactive Fibers in the Lumbar Facet Joint Capsule and Supraspinous Ligament of the Rabbit, *Brain Research,* 1988, 460:379-382.

Elliott, H.C., Cross-sectional Diameters and Areas of the Human Spinal Cord, *Anatomical Record,* 1945, Vol.93,287-293.

Eng, K., Rangayyan, R. M., Bray, R. C., Frank, C. B., Anscomb, L., Veale, P., Quantitative Analysis of the Fine Vascular Anatomy of Articular Ligaments, *IEEE Transactions on Biomedical Engineering,* 1992, 3:296-305.

Evans, W., Jobe,W., Seibert, C., A Cross-Sectional Prevalence Study of Lumbar Disc Degeneration in a Working Population, *Spine,* 1989, 1:60-64.

Frank, C., Woo, S. L-Y., Amiel, D., Harwood, F., Gomez, M., Akeson, W., Medial Collateral Ligament Healing, *The American Journal of Sports Medicine,* 1983, 6:379-389.

Frank, E., " HLA-DR Expression on Arachnoid Cells, A Role in the Fibrotic Inflammation Surrounding Nerve Roots in Spondylotic Cervical Myelopathy," *Spine,* 1995, 19/v. 20, 2093-2096.

Friberg, S., Anatomical Studies on Lumbar Disc Degeneration, *Acta Orthop. Scand.,* 1948, 17:224-230.

Fujita, Y., M.D., Yamamoto, H., M.D. "An Experimental Study on Spinal Cord Traction Effect," *Spine,* 1989, Vol. 14, 7:698-705.

Fujiwara, K., Yonenobu, K., Hiroshima, K., Ebara, S., Yamashita, K., Ono, K., Morphometry of the Cervical Spinal Cord and its Relation to Pathology in Cases with Compression Myelopathy, *Spine,* 1988, 13/11:1212-1218.

Fukuyama, S., Nakamura, T., Ikeda, T., Katsumasa, T., The Effect of Mechanical Stress on Hypertrophy of the Lumbar Ligamentum Flavum, *Journal of Spinal Disorders,* 1995, 2-126-130.

Giles, L. G. F., *Anatomical Basis of Low Back Pain,* Williams and Wilkens,1989, Baltimore.

Giles, L. G. F., Harvey, A, R., Immunohistochemical Demonstration of Nociceptors in the Capsule and Synovial Folds of Human Zygapophyseal Joints, *British Journal of Rheumatolgy,* 1987, 26:362-364.

Ghosh, P., *The Biology of the Intervertebral Disc,* CRC Press, 1988.

Godwin-Austen, R. B., The Mechanoreceptors of the Costo-Vertebral Joints, *Journal of Physiology,* 1969, 202:737-753.

Gordon, S.J., Yang, K.H., Mayer P. J., Mace, A. H., Kish, V. L., Radin, E. L., Mechanism of Disc Rupture, A Preliminary Report, *Spine,* 1991, 4:450-456.

Gronblad, M., Korkala, O., Konttinen, Y. T., Nederstrom, A., Hukkanen, M., Tolvanen, E., Polak, J. M., Silver Impregnation and Immunohistochemical Study of Nerves in Lumbar Facet Joint Plical Tissue, *Spine,* 1991, 1:34-38.

Hadley, L., M.D. *Anatomico-Roentgenographic Studies of the Spine,* Charles C. Thomas, 1981.

Haher, T. R., Felmy, W., Baruch, H., Delvin, V., Welin, D., O'Brien, M., Ahmad, J., Valenza, J., Parish, S., The Contribution of the Three Columns of the spine to Rotational Stability, A Biomechanical Model, *Spine,* 1989, 7:663-669.

Halata, Z., Ruffini Corpuscle - A Stretch Receptor in the Connective Tissue of the Skin and Locomotion Apparatus, *Progress in Brain Research,* 74:221-229.

Hampton, D., Laros, G., McCarron, R., Franks, D., Healing Potential of the Anulus Fibrosus, *Spine,* 1989, 4:398-401.

Harrison, D. D., Janik, T. J., Troyanovich, S. T., Holland, B., Comparisons of Lordotic Cervical Spine Curvatures to a Theoretical Ideal Model of the Static Sagittal Cervical Spine, *Spine,* 1996, 6:667-675.

Hasegawa, T., An, H.S., Haughton, V.M., Nowicki, B.H., Lumbar Foraminal Stenosis: Critical Heights of the Intervertebral Discs and Foramina, *The Journal of Bone and Joint Surgery,* 1995, 1/v. 77-A, 32-38.

Hassler, O., Blood Supply to Human Spinal Cord, *Archives of Neurology,* 1966, 15:302-307.

Hoff, J. T., Wilson, C. B., The Pathophysiological of Cervical Spondylotic Radiculopathy and Myelopathy, *Clinical Neurosurgery,* 1977, 24:474-487.

Hoffman, G.S., Spinal Arachnoiditis, What is the Clinical Spectrum ? I., *Spine,* 1983, 5:538-540.

Hoffman, H.J., Hendrick, E.B., Humphreys, R.P., The Tethered Spinal Cord: Its Protean Manifestations, Diagnosis and Surgical Correction, *Child's Brain,* 1976, 2:145-155

Hoffman, H. H., Kuntz, A., Vertebral Nerve Plexus, Components Anatomical Relationships, and Surgical Implications, *A.M.A. Archives of Surgery,* 1957, 74:430-437.

Horwitz, T., Degenerative Lesions in the Cervical Portion of the Spine, *Archives of Internal Medicine,* 1942/1178-1191

Hoy, K., Hansen, E.S., He, S.Z., Soballe, K.. Henriksen, T.B., Kjolseth, D., Hjortdal, V., Bunger, C., Reginal Blood Flow, Plasma Volume, and Vascular Permeability in the Spinal Cord, The Dural Sac, and Lumbar Nerve Roots, *Spine,* 1994, 24/19 2804-2811.

Hoyland, J.A., Freemont, A. J., Denton, J., Thomas, A. M. C., McMillian, J. J., Jayson, M. I. V., Retained Surgical Swab Debris in Post-laminactomy Arachnoiditis and Peridural Fibrosis, *The Journal of Bone and Joint Surgery,* 1988, 4:659-662.

Hughes, J. T., *Pathology of the Spinal Cord,* Year Book Medical Publishers, Chicago, 1966, Pg.114-125.

Jayson, M. I. V., The Inflamtory Component of Mechanical Back Problems, *British Journal of Radiology,* 1986, 25:210-213.

Jayson, M. I. V., Keegan, A., Million, R.,Tomlinson, J., A Fibrinolytic Defect in Chronic Back Pain Syndromes, *The Lancet,* 1984, Nov.:1186-1187.

Jarzem, P. F., Quance, D. R., Doyle, D. J., Begin, L. R., Kostuik, J. P., Spinal Cord Tissue Pressure During Spinal Cord Distraction in Dogs, *Spine,* 1992, 85:S227-S234.

Jiang, H., Raso, J. V., Moreau, M. J., Russell, G., Hill, D. L., Bagnall, K. M., Quantitative Morphology of the Lateral Ligaments of the Spine, Assessment of their Importance in Maintaining Lateral Stability, *Spine,* 1994, 23:2676-2682.

Jiang, H., Russell, G., Raso, J., Moreau, M. J., Hill, D. L., Bagnall, K. M., The Nature and Distribution of the Innervation of Human Supraspinal and Interspinal Ligaments, *Spine,* 1995, 8:869-876.

Kaigle, A. M., Magnusson, M., Pope, M. H., Broman, H., Hansson, T., In Vivo Measurement of Intervertebral Creep: A Preliminary Report, *Clinical Biomechanics,* 1992, 7:59-62

Keller, T. S., Holm, S. H., Hansson, T. H.,Spengler, D. M., The Dependence of Intervertebral Disc Mechanical Properties on Physiologic Conditions, *Spine,* 1990, 8:751-760.

Kobrine, A. I., Doyle, T. F., Martins, A. N., Local Spinal Cord Blood Flow in Experimental Traumatic Myelopathy, *Journal of Neurosurgery,* 1975, 42:144-149.

Konttinen, Y. T., Gronblad, M., Antti-Poika, I., Seitsalo, S., Hukkanen, M., Polak, J. M., Neuroimmunohistochemical Analysis of Peridiscal Nociceptive Neural Elements, *Spine,* 1990, 5:383-386.

Korkala, O., Gronblad, M., Liesi, P., Karaharju, E., Immunohistochemical Demonstration of Nociceptors in the Ligamentous Structures of the Lumbar Spine., *Spine,* 1985, 2:156-157

Kunert, W., Functional Disorders of Internal Organs Due to Vertebral Lesions, *Ciba Symposium,* 1965, 13:85-96

Lawson, T. L., Foley, W. D., Carrera, G. F., Berland, L. L., The Sacroiliac Joints: Anatomic, Plain Roentgenographic, and Computed Tomography Analysis, *Journal of Computer Assisted Tomography,* 1982, 2:307-314.

Levine, J. D., Dardick, S. J., Basbaum, A. I., Scipio, E., Reflex Neurogenic Inflammation, 1. Contribution of the Peripheral Nervous System to Spatially Remote Inflammation Reponses That Follow Injury, *The Journal of Neuroscience,* 1985, 5:1380-1386.

Levine, J. D., Moskowitz, M. A., Basbaum, A. I., The Contribution of Neurogenic Inflammation in Experimental Arthritis, *The Journal of Immunology,* 1985, 2:843s-847s.

Lew, P. C., Morrow, C. J., Lew, A. M., The Effect of Neck and Leg Flexion and Their Sequence on the Lumbar Spinal Cord, *Spine,* 1994, 21:2421-2425.

Louis, R. Spinal Stability as Defined by the Three-Column Spine Concept, *Anatomica Clinica,* 1985, 7:33-42.

Lundborg, G., Rydevik, B., Effects of Stretching the Tibial Nerve of the Rabbit, A Preliminary Study of the Intraneural Circulation and the Barrier Function of the Perineurium, *The Journal of Bone and Joint Surgery,* 1973, 55/ 2:390-401.

Macdonald, R. L., Findlay, J. M., Tator, C. H., Microcystic Spinal Cord Degeneration Causing Posttraumatic Myelopathy, *Journal of Neurosurgery,* 1988, 68:466-471.

Macnab, I., The Traction Spur, An Indication of Segmental Instability, *Journal of Bone and Joint Surgery,* 1971, 4:663-670.

Marcus, M. L., Heistad, D. D., Ehrhardt, J. C., Abboud F. M., Regulation of Total and Regional Spinal Cord Blood Flow, *Circulation Research,* 1977, 1:128-134.

Markolf, K. L., Morris, J. M., The Structural Components of the Intervertebral Disc, *The Journal of Bone and Joint Surgery,* 1974, 4:675-687.

Marzluff, J. M., Hungerford, G. D., Kempe, L. G., Rawe, S. E., Trevor, R., Perot, P. L., Thoracic Myelopathy Caused by Osteophytes of the Articular Processes, Thoracic Spondylosis, *Journal of Neurosurgery,* 1979, 50:779-783

Mclain, R. F., Mechanoreceptor Endings in Human Cervical Facet Joints, *Spine,* 1994, 19/5:495-500.

Miller, J. A. A., Schmatz, C., Schultz, A. B., Lumbar Disc Degeneration: Correlation with Age, Sex, and Spine Level in 600 Autopsy Specimens, *Spine,* 1988, 2:173-178

Morton, S. A., Localized Hypertrophic Changes in the Cervical Spine With Compression of the Spinal Cord or its Roots, *The Journal of Bone and Joint Surgery,*1936, 4:893-898

Nathan, H., Compression of the Sympathetic Trunk by Osteophytes of the Vertebral Column in the Abdomen: An Anatomical Study with Pathology and Clinical Considerations. *Surgery,* 1968, 4:609-625.

Nowicki, B. H., Haughton, V. M., Ligaments of the Lumbar Neural Foramina: A Sectional Anatomic Study, *Clinical Anatomy,* 1992, 5:126-135.

Okada, Y., Ikata, T., Katoh, S., Yamada, H., Morphologic Analysis of the Cervical Spinal Cord, Dural Tube, and Spinal Canal by Magnetic Resonance Imaging in Normal Adults and Patients with Cervical Spondylotic Myelopathy, *Spine,* 1994, 19/20:2331-2335.

Owen, J. H., Naito, M., Bridwell, K., Relationship Among Levels of Distraction, Evoked Potentials, Spinal Cord Ischemia and Integrity, and Clinical Status in Animals. *Spine,* 1990,15:846-81.

Owen, J. H., Naito, M., Bridwell, K., Oakley, D., Relationship Between Duration of Spinal Cord Ischemia and Postoperative Neurologic Defects in Animals. *Spine,* 1990, 15:846-851.

Osti, O. L., Vernon-Roberts, B., Fraser, R. D., Anulus Tears and Intervertebral Disc Degeneration, An Experimental Study Using an Animal Model, *Spine,* 1990, 8:v. 15 762-767.

Pal, G. B., Routal, R. V., A Study of Weight Transmission Through the Cervical and Upper Thoracic Regions of the Vertebral Column in Man, *Journal of Anatomy,* 1986, 148:245-261.

Pal, G.P., Sherk, H.H., The Vertical Stability of the Cervical Spine, *Spine,* 1988, 5:447-449.

Palleske, H., Kivelitz, R., Loew, F., Experimental Investigation on the Control of Spinal Cord Circulation, *Acta Neurochirurgica,* 1970, 22:29-41.

Pang, D., Wilberger, J.E., Tethered Cord Syndrome in Adults, *Journal of Neurosurgery,* 1982, 57:32-47

Parke, W. W., Watanbe, R., The Intrinsic Vasculature of the Lumbosacral Spinal Nerve Roots, *Spine,* 1985, 6: 508-515.

Parry, D. A. D., Barnes, G. R. G., Craig, A. S., A Comparison of the Size Distribution of Collagen Fibrils in Connective Tissues as a Function of Age and a Possible Relation Between Fibril Size Distribution and Mechanical Properties, *Proceedings of the Royal Society of London,* 1978, 203:305-321.

Patterson, M. M., Steinmetz, J. E., Long-lasting Alterations of Spinal Reflexes: A Potential Basis for Somatic Dysfunction, *Manual Medicine,* 1986, 2:38-42.

Pech, P., Daniels, D. L., Williams, A. L., Haughton, V. M., The Cervical Neural Foramina: Correlation of Microtomy and CT Anatomy, *Radiology,* 1985, 1:143-146.

Pedersen, H. E., Blunck, C. F. J., Gardner, E., The Anatomy of Lumbosacral Posterior Rami and Meningeal Branches of Spinal Nerves (Sinu-Vertebral Nerves), With an Experimental Study of Their Functions, *Journal of Bone and Joint Surgery,* 1956, 2:377-390.

Porter, R. W., Oakshot, G., Spinal Stenosis and Health Status, *Spine,* 1994, 8:901-903

Posner, I., White, A. A., Edwards, W. T., Hayes, W. C., A Biomechanical Analysis of the Clinical Stability of the Lumbar and lumbosacral Spine, 1982, *Spine,* 4:374-388.

Pountain, G. D., Keegan,A. L., Jayson, M. I. V., Impaired Fibrinolytic Activity in Defined Chronic Back Pain Syndromes, *Spine,* 1987, 2:83-85.

Ragnarsson T. S., Durward, Q. J., Nordgren, R. E., Spinal Cord Tethering After Traumatic Paraplegia with Late Neurological Deterioration, *Journal of Neurosurgery,* 1986, 64:397-401.

Reid, J. D., Effects of Flexion-Extension Movements of the Head and Spine Upon the Spinal Cord and Nerve Roots,*Journal of Neurology, Neurosurgery and Psychiatry,* 1960, 23:214-221.

Resnick, D., Osteophytes, Syndesmophytes and Other "Syghtes", *Postgraduate Radiology,* 1981, 1:217-231.

Resnick, D., Niwayama, G., Goergen, T. G., Degenerative Disease of the Sacroiliac Joint, Investigative *Radiology,* 1975, 10:608-621.

Rhalmi, S., Yahia, L, Newman, N., Isler, M., Immunohistochemical Study of Nerves in Lumbar Spine Ligaments, *Spine,* 1993, 2:264-267.

Ross. J. S., Masaryk, T. J., Modic, M. T., Delamater, R., Bohlman, H., Wilbur, G., Kaufman, B., MR Imaging of Lumbar Arachnoiditis, *American Journal of Radiology,* 1987, 149:1025-1031.

Rothman, R. H., Simeone, F. A., *The Spine,* W. B. Saunders Company, Philadelphia, 1982,

Sashin, D., A Critical Analysis of the Anatomy and the Pathologic Changes of the Sacro-iliac Joints, *Journal of Bone and Joint Surgery,* 1930, 12:891-910.

Sato, A., The Reflex Effects of Spinal Somatic Nerve Stimulation on Visceral Function, *Journal of Manipulation and Physical Therapy,* 1992, 15/1:57-61

Schmorl, G., Junghanns, H., *The Human Spine in Health and Disease,* Grune and Stratton, New York and London, 1971.

Schneider, S. J.,Rosenthal, A. D., Greenberg, B. M., Danto, J., A Preliminary Report on the Use of Laser-Doppler Flowmetry during Tethered Spinal Cord Release, *Neurosurgery,* 1993, 2:214-218,

Schwarzer, A. C., Aprill, C. N., Bogduk, N., The Sacroiliac Joint in Chronic Low Back Pain, *Spine,* 1995, 1/20, 31-37.

Schwarzer, A. C., Aprill, C. N., Derby, R., Fortin, J., Kine, G., Bogduk, N., The Prevalence and Clinical Features of Internal Disc Disruption in Patients With Chronic Low Back Pain, *Spine,* 1995,17:1878-1883.

Seti, M., Maeda, M., Effects of Electrical Stimulation of Motor and Cutaneous Nerves on Spinal Cord Blood Flow, *Spine,* 1993, 13:1798-1802.

Senter, H. J., Venes, J. L., Loss of Autoregulation and Posttraumatic Ischemia Following Experimental Spinal Cord Trauma, *Journal of Neurosurgery,* 1979, 50:198-206.

Shapiro, R., Batt, H.D., Unilateral Thoracic Spondylosis, *American Journal of Radiology and Radiation Therapy,*1960, 4:660-662.

Shaw, M.D.M., Russell, J.A., Grossart, K.W., The Changing Pattern of Spinal Arachnoiditis, Journal of Neurology, *Neurosurgery and Psychiatry,* 1978, 41:97-107.

Stephens, M. M., Evans, J. H., O'Brien, J. P., Lumbar Intervertebral Foramens, An in Vitro Study of their Shape in Relation to Intervertebral Disc Pathology, *Spine,* 1991, 5:525-529

Stewart, T. D., Pathologic Changes in Aging Sacroiliac Joints, A Study of Dissecting-room Skeletons, *Clinical Orthopaedics and Related Research,* 1984, 183:188-196.

Stilwell, D. L., Stanford, M. D., Structural Deformities of Vertebrae, Bone Adaptation and Modeling in Experimental Scoliosis and Kyphosis, *The Journal of Bone and Joint Surgery,* 1962, 4:611-633.

Sunderland S., Meningeal-Neural Relations in the Intervtebral Foramen, *Journal of Neurosurgery,* 1974, 40:756-763.

Sunderland, S., Bradley, K, C., Stress-Strain Phenomena in Human Spinal Nerve Roots, *Brain,* 1961, 84:120-124.

Tachibana, S., Kitahara, Y., Iida, H., Yada,K., Spinal Cord Intramedullary Pressure, *Spine,* 1994, 19:2174-2179.

Takahashi, K., Nomura, S., Tomita, K., Matsumoto, T., Effects of Peripheral Nerve Stimulation on the Blood Flow of the Spinal Cord and the Nerve Root, *Spine,* 1988,11-1273-1283.

Tetsworth, K. D., Ferguson, R. L., Arachnoiditis Ossificans of the Caudae Equina, *Spine,* 1986, 7:765-766

Tipton, C. M., Matthes, R. D., Maynard, J. A., Carey, R. A., The Influence of Activity on Ligaments and Tendons, *Medicine and Science in Sports,* 1975, 3:165-175.

Turnbull, I. M., Blood Supply of the Spinal Cord: Normal and Pathological Considerations, *Clinical Neurosurgery,* 1973, Vol. 20: 56-84

Turnbull, I. M., Microvasculature of the Human Spinal Cord, *Journal of Neurosugery,* 1971, 35:141-147.

Turnbull, I. M., Breig, A., Hassler, O., Blood Supply of Cervical Spinal Cord in Man, A Microangiographic Cadaver Study, *Journal of Neurosurgery,* 1966, 24:951-965.

Van Buskirk, C., Nerves in the Vertebral Canal, Their Relation to the Sympathetic Innervation of the Upper Extremities, *Archives of Surgery,* 427-432

Vernon-Roberts, B., Pirie, C. J., Degenerative Changes in the Intervertebral Discs of the Lumbar Spine and Their Sequelae, *Rheumatology and Rehabilitation,* 1977, 16:13-21.

Vleeming, A., Stoeckart, R., Snijders, C. J., A Description of the Integrated Function of the Lower Spine, A Clinical Anatomical and Biomechanical Approach, *A Lecture delivered at the 11th Annual Meeting of the American Association of Orthopaedic Medicine,* 1994, Orlando, Florida.

Vleeming, A., Stoeckart, R., Volkers, A. C. W., Snijders, C. J., Relation Between Form and Function in the Sacroiliac Joint, Part I: Clinical Anatomical Aspects, *Spine,* 1990, 2:130-132

Vleeming, A., Stoeckart, R., Volkers, A. C. W., Snijders, C. J., Relation Between Form and Function in the Sacroiliac Joint, Part II: Biomechanical Aspects, *Spine,* 1990, 2:133-135.

Vleeming, A., Van Wingerden, J. P., Snijders, C. J., Stoeckart, R., Stijnen, T., Load Application to the Sacrotuberous Ligament; Influences on Sacroiliac Joint Mechanics, *Clinical Biomechanics,* 1989, 4:204-209.

Volger, J. B., Brown, W. H., Helms, C. A., Genant, H. K., The Normal Sacroiliac Joint: A CT Study of Asymptomatic Patients, *Radiology,* 1984, 151:433-437.

Voutsinas, S. A., MacEwen, G. D., Sagittal Profiles of the Spine, *Clinical Orthopaedics and Related Research,* 1986, 210:235-242

Watanabe, R., Parke, W. W., Vascular and Neural Pathology of Lumbosacral Spinal Stenosis, *Journal of Neurosurgery,* 1986, 64:64-70.

Wicke, L., *Atlas of Radiologic Anatomy,* Urban & Schwarzenberg, Baltimore-Munich, 1982.

Xiuqing,C., Bo, S., Shizhen, Z., Nerves Accompanying the Vertebral Artery and their Clinical Relevance, *Spine,* 1988, 12:1360-1364.

Yabuki, S. & Kikuchi, S., Nerve Root Infiltration and Sympathic Block, An Experimental Study of Intraradicular Blood Flow, *Spine,* 1995, 8/v. 20:901-906.

Yahia, L. H., Newman, N., Rivard, C. H., Neurohistology of Lumbar Spine Ligaments, *Acta Orthopaedia Scandinavia,* 1988: 59(5):508-512

Yamada, S., Zinke, D.E., Sanders, D., Pathophysiology of "Tethered Cord Syndrome", *Journal of Neurosurgery,* 1981, 54:494-503.

Yamashita, T., Cavanagh, J. M., El-Bohy, A. A., Getchell, T. V., King, A. I., Mechanosensitive Afferent Units in the Lumbar Facet Joint, *The Journal of Bone and Joint Surgery,* 1990, 6:865-870.

Yu, S., Haughton, V. M., Sether, L. A., Wagner, M., Anulus Fibrosus in Bulging Intervertebral Disks, *Radiology,* 1988, 3:761-763.

Zagra, A., Lamartina, C., Pace, A., Balzarini, E., Zerbi, A., Scoles, P., Ajello, F., Mazzarella, G., Pillitteri, G., Posterior Spinal Fusion in Scoliosis: Computer-assisted Tomography and Biomechanics of the Fusion Mass, *Spine,* 1988, 2:155-161.

INDEX

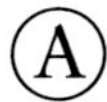

A

Abdominal
    complaints, 191
    oblique muscles
        internal, 179
        external, 179
    tissues, lining, cavity, 180
Absolute motion, 2, 3, 6 *see also*
        Global motion
Acetabulum, 180, 182, 198
Adaptive response, 88, 90
Adhesions
    epidural, 20
    fibrous, 81
    intrathecal, 14
    subarachnoid, 21, 22, 81
A.L.L. (Anterior longitudinal
        ligament), 10, 12, 26, 33,
        93, 103, 106, 153, 154,
        161, 171
Altered weight bearing, 2, 15, 17,
        23, 39, 45, 46, 51, 60, 62,
        69, 83, 117, 122, 124, 166
Annular rings (Annulus Fibrosus),
        12, 119, 120, 181, 185
Annulus fibrosus *see* Annular rings
Anterior longitudinal ligament
        see A.L.L.
Anterior spinal artery,18, 20, 81
Anterolisthesis, 11, 12, 40, 68, 88,
        94, 96, 100, 105, 148
A-P (Anterior to posterior), 7, 44,
        110
    alignment, 121
    direction, X-ray, 188
    displacement of vertebrae, 176
    subluxations of the lumbar
        spine, 131
    subluxation, lack of and DJD,
        137
    subluxation, sacrum, 147
    view of normal pelvis, 193
    X-ray in supine position, 195
Arachnoid
    mater, 2, 4, 5, 22
    trabeculae, 5, 22
Arthritis, 124

Articulation, 11
    posterior, 2
    rib-disc, 77
Atlanto-axial, 2
Autonomic nervous system, 78
Avascular
    fibrocartilaginous disc, 185
    intrasacral discs, 181
    structures, 12, 119, 202
Axial
    views, 7, 13, 20-22, 26, 77, 181,
        188, 191, 193, 194, 196
    skeleton, 77
Axial loading, 97

B

Brain stem, 2, 7, 21, 36, 37
Buckling, 23

C

Calcified
    A.L.L., 10 *see also* A.L.L.
    discs, 15, 109
    P.L.L., 10, 107 *see also* P.L.L.
Calcification
    A.L.L., 12, 106
    C4-5, C5-6, C6-7, 33
    L2, 154, 155
    L5 loss of disc height and, 151
    T5 fracture and, 108
    T6-7 to T11-12, 103
    T9-10 and T10-11, 107
    T11-12, 107
Canal stenosis, 9, 15, 16, 24-25,
        32, 37, 41, 43, 50, 53, 61,
        63, 67, 70, 122, 124, 157
Capillaries, spinal cord, 10, 182
Cartilage, 183
    deterioration, 12
    hyaline, 185
    SI joint, 183, 184
    vertebral column, 2
Cartesian coordinate system, 192
Caudae equinae, 2, 7, 19, 169, 175,
        181
Cavitation, 17, 41, 57, 99, 105,
        117, 131, 141, 144, 147,
        149, 155, 159, 161-163,
        165, 167, 173
Central nervous system *see* C.N.S.
Cerebellum, 3, 4, 24, 36, 37, 73

Cerebrospinal fluid, 181
Cervical curve, 14, 15, 17, 18, 22,
        25, 48, 79, 111
    lordotic cervical, 30, 32, 34,
        36, 38, 40, 42, 44
    loss of, 48
Cervicogenic, 23
Chronic
    inflammation, 20-22, 81
    lumbar subluxation, 117
    neurological distress, 83
    pelvis, subluxation, 194
    posterior stairstepping, 162
    spasm, the cause of some
        headaches, 23
Chronically degenerative, 12, 50,
        79, 122, 167, 189, 190
Clavicles, 26
Coccyx, 2, 5, 6
Compression fracture, 81, 88, 95,
        100, 105, 108, 114, 120,
        132, 133, 140, 148, 158,
        162, 163, 172-174
Conductivity, 21, 81
Congenital stenosis, 9, 30, 64
Conus medularis, 2, 7, 175
    and thoracic disc herniation, 80
Coronal, 119, 181
Cortex
    of sacrum, 181, 202, 203
Cortical bone, 181, 182, 202, 203
Costotransverse, 77, 79
Costo-vertebral, 77, 78, 79
CNS (Central nervous system)
    anatomy and physiology, 1-10
    and nutrient delivery, 7, 23, 25,
        181, 182
    effects of motion, 19, 182,
    proprioceptive input and, 180
    subluxation and, 13, 17, 21, 24,
        55, 191
Cranial
    flexion, 7
Cross section
    in advanced imaging, 188
    of lumbar disc, 119
    of sacrum, 191
Curve *see*
    cervical
    kyphotic
    lordotic
    lumbar
    thoracic

D

Degeneration, 1, 14, 16, 17, 24, 26, 30, 31, 33, 36, 40, 42, 49, 56, 58, 59, 71, 89, 95, 96, 97, 98, 100-102, 106
  beginning signs, 202
  chronic, 189, 190
  end stages, 22, 52, 164, 166, 203
  initiated by immobility, 10, 180
  of discs, 117, 118, 130, 133, 134, 142, 146, 151, 158, 177
  of facets, 51
  of sacrum, 145
  patterns, causes of, 23, 83, 122
  subluxation and, 50, 124, 150, 154, 167, 176
Degenerative joint disease *see* D.J.D.
Dehydration, 101, 117, 122, 182, 203
Demifacet, 77
Dens, 8, 49, 56
Dentate ligament, 4, 5, 7, 26
Dessicated, 12
Disc, 117, 118, 119, 181
  protrusion, 35, 80, 92, 120
D.J.D. (Degenerative joint disease), 12, 20, 37, 59, 78, 99, 104, 105, 170
Dorsal spinal artery, 4
Dura mater, 2, 4, 5, 20, 22

E

Eburnation, 34
End plate, 12, 37, 43, 58, 59, 65, 78, 86, 93-95, 97, 98, 106, 119, 124, 138, 139, 150, 152, 156, 157, 159-164, 166, 177
Epidural adhesions, 20, 21
Epidural space, 7
Erector spinae, 179, 180, 124, 177
Esophagus, 26
Extension
  flexion-extension, 3, 7, 25
  hip, 192
  lordotic curve, 5
  lumbar spine, 18
  spinal canal, 22
  thecal sac, 3, 7
Extremity, upper, 17, 18

F

Facet, 2, 3, 10-11, 20, 77, 117, 122
  altered weight bearing, 60
  articular, 117, 181
  degeneration, 51
  gapping, 55
  height loss, 45
  hypertrophy, 34, 62
  inferior articulating, 13
  jamming, 51, 59
  separation, 6
  sclerosis, 12, 59, 151
  superior articulating, 13
  uncoupling of, 122
  weight bearing, 31, 41
  zygopophyseal joints, 12
Facetal capsule, 122
Fascia, 124, 136, 147
Femur, 182
Fibrous, 183
  adhesions, 81
  portion of the SI joint, 183, 191
Filum terminale, 7
Flexion, 3, 6, 16, 17, 18, 19, 25, 43, 49, 73, 92
  cervical, 18, 19, 175
  cranial, 7
  deformity, 15, 19
  flexion/extension, 25, 192
  forward, 7, 15, 187
  lateral, 7, 191, 200
Foramen magnum, 6, 37, 56
Foramen
  jugular, 4
  intervertebral (IVF), 6, 7, 24, 81, 124
Fusion, 17, 42
  C5 and C6, 60
  C6-7 fused with C7, 65
  C6-7, 43
  cervical spine, 10
  L2-3, 190
  L3, 156, 164, 167
  L5-SI joint, 123, 148, 155, 161, 163, 203
  S2-S3, 202, 203
  S3, 4, and 5 fused by age 25, 181

G

Glycoprotein, 118
Gravitational load, 117
Guarding (spasmed), 11, 180, 191

H

Herniation, 87, 90
  multiple disc, 86
  posterior disc, 79, 80
  thoracic disc, 80
Hydration
  loss of, 14
  low, 86
  poor, 89
  (imbibition), vertebral end plates, 181
Hydraulic
  function interruption, 117
  system, closed, 120
Hyoid bone, 26
Hyperkyphosis
  due to compression fracture, 114
  from altered weight bearing, 15
  osteoporosis and, 80, 106, 108
  progressive spurring, 110
  thoracic spine, 80, 115
Hyperload, 12
Hypertonic, 179
Hypertrophy
  of A.L.L., 93, 97, 99, 103, 107, 109, 149, 153, 161
  of facets, 34, 62, 117
  vertebrae, 117
  unciate process, 24
Hypokyphotic, 19
Hypolordotic, 25
Hydrophilic disc, 118, 119, 121

I – J

Iliacus muscle, 179, 180, 193
Ilium, 179, 191, 194, 196
Imbibition, 86, 181
Inferior articulating facet, 13
Innominate, 179, 181, 182, 189, 191-201
Intercostal
  artery, 78
  nerve, 78, 79
  neurovascular bundles, 79
  vein, 78
Interspinous distance, 19, 34, 49

Intervertebral disc, 77, 181, 185, 119
Intervertebral foramen *see* I.V.F.
Intrasacral, 181, 182, 202, 203
Intrathecal, 14, 21, 22, 97, 101
Ischial tuberosities, 194
Ischium, 179, 193
I.V.F. (Intervertebral foramen), 6, 7, 19, 24, 81, 124

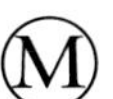 K

Kyphosis, 18, 19, 72, 81, 83
Kyphotic, 15
    cervical, 13, 52, 54, 56, 58, 60, 62, 64, 66, 68, 70, 72, 74, 79
    sacral, 1
    thoracic, 80, 81, 86, 88, 91, 96, 98, 106, 108, 177

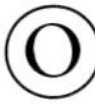 L

Lamina, 2, 6, 20, 22, 24, 26, 43, 77
Laminectomized, 3
Larynx, 26
Lateral flexion
    L4 and L5, 200
    sacral, 191
    spinal cord, 6, 7
Lateralisthesis, 79
Ligament *see*
    A.L.L. (Anterior longitudinal ligament)
    Dentate ligament
    P.L.L. (Posterior longitudinal ligament)
    SI (Sacroiliac) joint/ ligament
    Sacrospinous ligament
    Sacrotuberous ligament
Ligamentum flavum, 2, 20, 21, 22, 35, 74, 75
Lordotic curve, 23, 117, 121, 122, 124, 128, 134, 136, 140, 143, 144, 148, 151, 154, 160 *see also* cervical, lordotic
    loss of, 25, 48, 158, 164, 176
    reversal of, 168, 170, 172, 174
Lumbar curve, 14, 15, 111, 123, 138, 142
    normal, 130, 134
Lumbo-sacral aponeurosis, *see* Thoracolumbar fascia
Luxation, 11

 M

Magnetic resonance imaging *see* MRI
Mandible, 3, 26
Marginal osteophytes, 83, 107
Mastication, 26
Mastoid process, 23
Medullary bone, 119, 120
Meningeal, Meninges, 2, 5, 7, 22
Mid-sagittal, 11, 16
Military neck, 18, 46, 48, 50
MRI (magnetic resonance imaging)
    cervical, 17, 18, 19, 20, 21, 22, 24, 26, 41, 67, 72, 74
    lordotic, 176
    pelvic, 188, 191
    sacrum, 194, 197
    thoracic, 82, 112, 114
Myelopathy, 17

 N

Necrosis or necrotic, 58, 65
Nerve root, 6, 7, 20, 78
Nerve rootlets, 4, 7, 20, 22, 81
Neutral position, 4, 16, 19, 20, 73, 82, 92, 187
Neurons, 10, 20, 80, 81
Neuro-vascular bundle, 180
Non-marginal osteophytes, 83 *see also* Osteophyte
Nucleus pulposus, 12, 118, 119, 120, 140, 157, 181, 185

O

Osmotic, 121
Ossification, 97
Osteoarthritis, 12, 23, 117, 124, 189, 190
Osteophyte, 12, 18, 20, 24, 51, 74, 75, 81, 87, 102, 107, 117, 124, 176, 177 *see also* non-marginal osteophyte
Osteoporosis, 2, 15, 80, 106, 108

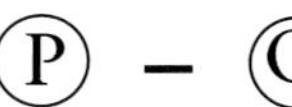 P — Q

Parasthesia, 18
Para spinal phyte , 97, 103, 110
Pedicles, 80, 117
Pelvis, 1, 77, 160, 163, 179, 180, 182, 188-194, 198, 200, 201 *see also* Pelvic girdle

Pelvic girdle, 179, 180-183, 185, 187, 189, 191, 193, 194, 195, 197, 199, 201, 203
Pharynx, 26
Pia mater, 5, 7, 20, 22
P.L.L. (Posterior longitudinal ligament), 8, 10, 12, 22, 79, 159
Pons, 1, 2, 7, 8, 24, 25, 49
Posterior impression, 119
Posterior longitudinal ligament *see* P.L.L
Posterior superior iliac spine *see* PSIS
Proprioceptive, 179, 185
    guarding, 122, 191
    noxious stimuli, 180
Pseudo-joint, 153
    atlas and C2, 71
    spinous process contact forming, 153, 161
PSIS (Posterior superior iliac spine), 195
Psoas, 180, 191, 193, 201
    major hip flexors, 179
    pubic bone, 185, 186, 187, 192, 201
Pubis symphysis, 179, 180, 185, 189-190, 192, 193, 195, 197, 201

R

Rectus abdominus, 201
Retrolisthesis, 11, 47, 79, 117, 154
    C3, 40, 55, 56, 72,
    C3 through C5, 32
    C5 to C4, 17, 48
    C5, 19, 21, 66
    C6, 24, 32, 59, 60, 63, 71
    L1, 174, 176
    L3, 172
    L4, 117, 159, 168
    L5, 142
    lumbar, stairstepped, 12, 38, 170
    mid-sagittal, 11
    T11, 99
Retropulsion, 114
Rib, 79
    articulation, 77, 79, 80
    cage, 1, 77
    spine relationship, 78
    thoracic spine, 82

Rootlets *see* Nerve rootlets
Rotation, 192, 193, 201
　　and joint sclerosis, 194
　　C1 to C2, 13
　　complete posterior, 190, 195, 201
　　lateral flexation and, 7, 200
　　lateralistheses and, 79
　　shearing and, 197
Rotational, 182, 193, 196
　　misalignments, 23

S

Sacral ala, 191, 194, 200
Sacral
　　apex, 136, 177, 182, 193
　　base, 159, 165, 182, 188
　　disc, 19, 149, 161, 177, 181,
　　　　202, 203
Sacroiliac joint *see* SI joint
Sacrospinous ligament, 182
Sacrotuberous ligament, 182
Sacrum, 2, 122-124, 129, 131, 136,
　　　　137, 139, 141, 142, 144-
　　　　147, 149, 151, 153, 155,
　　　　157, 159, 161, 163, 165,
　　　　167, 169, 171, 173, 175,
　　　　177, 179, 180-183, 191-
　　　　194, 197, 198, 202
Schmoral's node, 95, 96, 105, 138,
　　　　157
Sclerosis, 78, 185
　　compression fracture with, 132
　　end plates, 98
　　facet, 12, 24, 51, 59, 151
　　joint, 194
　　lower, 41
Segmental motion, 2, 37
Sheared, Shearing, 12, 47, 48, 63,
　　　　66-67, 69, 122-123, 182,
　　　　185, 190, 192, 193, 197-
　　　　203
Sinuvertebral artery, 13
SI (Sacroiliac) joint/ligament, 179,
　　　　182-187, 189, 190-194,
　　　　201
Soft tissue, 46, 83, 124
Spinal canal, 1-3, 6, 9, 12, 13, 21,
　　　　22, 24, 25, 37, 70, 117,
　　　　122, 124, 153, 171, 172,
　　　　173, 181, 182
Spinal column, 1, 2, 4, 6, 7, 10, 15

Spinal cord, 1, 2, 5-10, 13-26, 33,
　　　　41, 45, 47, 53, 56, 57, 59,
　　　　63, 67, 69, 70, 72-75, 77,
　　　　79-83, 97, 99, 103, 105,
　　　　109, 113-115, 182
Spinal laminar junction, 17
Spinous process
　　cervical, 6, 20, 26, 56, 71
　　lumbar, 117, 129, 149, 171
　　thoracic, 77
Spondylosis, 12, 83, 124
Spondylolisthesis, 123
Spurring, 12, 15, 17, 18, 80, 117,
　　　　122, 124
　　acquired, 57
　　and cervical curve reverse, 16
　　and vertebral body enlargement,
　　　　17, 124
　　cervical, 30, 36, 38, 41-43, 48,
　　　　51, 53, 57-60, 63, 65-67
　　congenital, 9, 64
　　impressions on spinal cord, 81
　　lumbar, 123, 151-155, 158-160,
　　　　162, 163-175
　　thoracic, 89, 92, 93, 94, 96, 98,
　　　　99, 102, 106, 108-110
Stairstepping, 12
　　cervical, 38
　　lumbar, 154, 160, 162, 170
Stenosis, 14, 15
　　of spinal canal, 25, 30, 32, 37,
　　　　41, 43, 45, 50, 51, 53, 54,
　　　　61, 63, 67, 70, 122, 157
Sternum, 26
Subarachnoid adhesions, 21, 22,
　　　　81, 97
Subarachnoid space, 5, 7, 22, 81
Subdural space, 4
Subluxation, 1, 11
　　adhesions, inflammation, 20-21
　　advanced degeneration, 17, 22
　　and circulation, 13
　　and tractioning, 22
　　and vertebral canal, 13
　　and weight bearing, 2
　　complexes, 12
　　differences, individuals, 14
　　pelvic and sacral, 179
Subluxation of
　　costovertebral joint, 78
　　occiput- C1, 40-41, 54-63
　　C1-C2, 13, 30-31, 36-43, 46-47,
　　　　54-63

C2-C3, 17, 30-31, 36-37, 40-41,
　　　　44-57, 62-63, 68-73
C3-C4, 16-19, 30-75
C4-C5, 16-19, 30-75
C5-C6, 16-19, 30-75
C6-C7, 16-19, 30-71, 74-75
C7- T1, 16, 19, 30-31, 40-41,
　　　　44-45, 48-53, 64-65, 70-71
T1-T2, 70-71, 80, 86-87,92-
　　　　93,106-109
T2-T3, 80, 86-93, 96-97, 100-
　　　　103, 106-107
T3-T4, 80, 88-89,92-93,102-103
T4-T5, 80, 88-93, 100-103,
　　　　108-109, 114-115
T5-T6, 80, 86-93, 100-101
T6-T7, 80, 86-87, 92-93, 96-99
T7-T8, 80, 86-87, 92-95, 98-101
T8-T9, 86-87, 92-93, 98-101
T9-T10, 80, 86-87, 90-95, 98-101
T10-T11, 80, 88-89, 92-95, 98-
　　　　99, 102-105
T11-T12, 80, 90-93, 98-99,
　　　　104-109
T12-L1, 130-131, 154-155, 174-
　　　　175
L1-L2, 122-123, 130-131, 134-
　　　　137, 148-157, 160-167,
　　　　170-177
L2-L3, 122-123, 128-129, 134-
　　　　135, 140-141, 146-155,
　　　　160-167, 170-177
L3-L4, 122-123, 128-131, 134-
　　　　135, 140-141, 146-177
L4-L5, 122-123, 128-135, 138-
　　　　145, 148-161, 164-173,
　　　　176-177
L5-L6, 134-136
L5-S1, 122-123, 128-133, 136-
　　　　139, 142-155, 158-165,
　　　　168-177
　　pubic symphysis, 179, 180, 182,
　　　　185-187, 189-190, 192-
　　　　193, 195, 197-198, 201
　　sacral segments, 202-203
　　sacroiliac joint, 189-201
Superior articulating facet, 13
Supine, 18, 19, 114, 177, 192, 195,
　　　　199
Sympathetic chain, 78, 79
　　"Storm", 13
Sympathetic nervous system *see*
　　　　Sympathetic chain
Synovial, 77, 183, 191

T

Tendon or tendinous, 23, 124
Tethering, 19, 82
    adhesions, 20, 21, 81
    and anterior weight bearing, 83
    and conductivity, 21, 81
    cord cervical, 18, 20, 49, 63, 70
    disc herniation and, 79
    thoracic, 22, 112
Theca or thecal, 2-8, 22, 103
Thoracic, 77
    A-P, 3
    tethering *see* Tethering
Thoracic curve, 15, 88, 90, 94, 96, 98
Thoracic spine
    adhesions, 20, 21
    alignment with head, 23, 26
    and weight bearing, 88
    compression fracture, 80-81, 86
    cord tethering, 82
    cord tractioning, 14-16, 22
    disc herniation, 80
Thoracolumbar fascia, 124, 136, 147
Thorax
    and lumbar spine, 160
    and subluxation of pubic symphysis, 185
    muscles of, 179
Three point weight bearing, 2, 117
Trabecula
    arachnoid, 5, 22
    of medullary bone, 120
Transverse abdominus muscle, 179
Transverse processes
    added stability and, 80
    as levers, 185
    of C1, 13
    rib articulations and, 77, 82
Trachea, 4
Tractioned
    cord
        and flexion, 16
        and inflammation, 81
        cervical, 57, 64
        thoracic, 14, 15, 22, 115
    uterus, 180
Trochanter, 180

U

Urogenital, 180

V

Vascular
    changes and alignment, 12, 13, 16, 21, 23, 24, 26
    condition of ventral horns, 20
    condition, improvement of, 81
    entrapped structures, 14, 19
    flow, motion and, 10
Vasoconstriction, 13
Vertebral canal, 8, 79
    and maintained curves, 45
    changing length and tethering, 18, 20, 57, 63, 70
    protrusions into, 35
    subluxation and shape of, 13, 17, 32, 54, 67, 79
Vertebral artery, 3
    cervical deformity and, 12, 23
    irritation of, 13
Vertebral column, 22
    absolute motion of, 6
    adhesions and, 20, 21
    and thecal motion, 7
    A-P, 2, 3, 19, 117
    loss of disc height, 75, 92
    motion and length change, 25
    motion and nutrient flow, 10, 23
    motion and tethering, 49
    muscle guarding of, 11, 22
    subluxation of, 13, 14, 15
Visceral
    and pelvic subluxation, 180
    nerve pathways, 81, 83
    problems, 83

W

Whiplash, 23
    vulnerability to, 16, 44

Z

Zygopophyseal joints, 10, 11, 12
    see also Facets